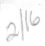

MANAGING
PROSTATE CANCER

MANAGING
PROSTATE CANCER

A Guide for Living Better

By Andrew J. Roth, MD

OXFORD
UNIVERSITY PRESS

OXFORD
UNIVERSITY PRESS

Oxford University Press is a department of the University of
Oxford. It furthers the University's objective of excellence in research,
scholarship, and education by publishing worldwide.

Oxford   New York
Auckland   Cape Town   Dar es Salaam   Hong Kong   Karachi
Kuala Lumpur   Madrid   Melbourne   Mexico City   Nairobi
New Delhi   Shanghai   Taipei   Toronto

With offices in
Argentina   Austria   Brazil   Chile   Czech Republic   France   Greece
Guatemala   Hungary   Italy   Japan   Poland   Portugal   Singapore
South Korea   Switzerland   Thailand   Turkey   Ukraine   Vietnam

Oxford is a registered trademark of Oxford University Press
in the UK and certain other countries.

Published in the United States of America by
Oxford University Press
198 Madison Avenue, New York, NY 10016

Library of Congress Cataloging-in-Publication Data
Roth, Andrew J.
Managing prostate cancer : a guide for living better / by Andrew J. Roth, MD.
pages cm
Includes bibliographical references and index.
ISBN 978-0-19-933692-0 (paperback)
1. Prostate—Cancer—United States.   2. Prostate—Cancer—Psychological aspects.
3. Men—Health and hygiene—United States.   4. Physician and patient.   I. Title.
RC280.P7R68 2016
616.99′463—dc23
2015016699

This material is not intended to be, and should not be considered, a substitute for medical or other
professional advice. Treatment for the conditions described in this material is highly dependent on
the individual circumstances. And, while this material is designed to offer accurate information with
respect to the subject matter covered and to be current as of the time it was written, research and
knowledge about medical and health issues is constantly evolving and dose schedules for medications
are being revised continually, with new side effects recognized and accounted for regularly. Readers
must therefore always check the product information and clinical procedures with the most up-to-date
published product information and data sheets provided by the manufacturers and the most recent
codes of conduct and safety regulation. The publisher and the authors make no representations or
warranties to readers, express or implied, as to the accuracy or completeness of this material. Without
limiting the foregoing, the publisher and the authors make no representations or warranties as to the
accuracy or efficacy of the drug dosages mentioned in the material. The authors and the publisher do
not accept, and expressly disclaim, any responsibility for any liability, loss or risk that may be claimed
or incurred as a consequence of the use and/or application of any of the contents of this material.

1 3 5 7 9 8 6 4 2
Printed in the United States of America
on acid-free paper

I lovingly dedicate this book

To my wife, Dr. Bunny Benenson. She is my precious life partner for all that is meaningful or mundane, making it all the more satisfactory. She helps me navigate the journey of twists and turns and ups and downs, with lighter falls and higher, brighter highs, not only in the writing of this book but as she has ever since we first met in our previous lives as community organizers. I am grateful to Bunny for enabling me to be a more rounded person and for enriching my ability to be a better physician, even a physician who publishes, sometimes at the expense of her own professional advancement, and for unquestioningly encouraging me to be a better, more caring, and loving parent.

And

To my children, Samara and Bram, whom I cherish and love, whose lives breathe life, sustenance, and hope into mine as they build their own renditions of healing the world.

CONTENTS

Acknowledgments | ix

Pregame: Overview and Introduction | 1

Part One: New Diagnosis and Early-Stage Disease

1. Why Me? Why Not Me? What Now?: And Why Is a Psychiatrist Writing a Book about Prostate Cancer? | 13

2. How Can You Make the Right Treatment Choice When There Is No Perfect Choice? | 29

3. Lifting the Weight of Waiting and Preparing for Treatment: Deciding Between Definitive Treatment and Watchful Waiting or Active Surveillance | 69

4. Prostate Cancer Anxiety, Depression, and Sleep Problems: Relax and Enter the DRAFT of the Emotional Judo Playbook | 95

5. Do I Really Need a Psychiatric Medication to Cope with Prostate Cancer? | 173

6. Keeping the Flames of Intimacy Alive | 203

7. Urinary, Bowel, and Energy Leaks: This Wasn't Supposed to Happen to Me | 233

8. Not for Patients Only: Spouses or Partners Can Manage Prostate Cancer Better Too | 255

Part Two: Later-Stage Disease and Recurrence of Disease

9. Coping with Recurrence of Cancer If the "Definitive" Treatment Doesn't Work: Going Hormonal | 273

10. Grieving for Loss of Trust, Physical Wholeness, and Sense of Immortality: Reinvesting in Your Future as a Wise Role Model | 295

Appendix | 331

Index | 337

ACKNOWLEDGMENTS

Time and time again, I witness growth arising out of tragedy. Many have told me about the "silver linings" of fuller, richer lives, as well as strength and purpose that appear from the distress that accompanies their cancer experiences.

I am indebted to my patients and their families who pursue the goal of living better with prostate cancer, even though there is neither a crystal ball to help them focus on an uncertain and frightening future nor any guarantees for optimal outcomes.

I am grateful for the excellent guides and teachers who have impacted my career and ultimately led to the writing of this book:

- My parents, Sherry Rotker Roth and Albert Roth, who modeled hope, faith, and courage as they lived with and then died from lung cancer.
- My parents-in-law, Dr. William Osler Benenson and Dr. Esther Benenson, who have exemplified healing and charitable hearts, inspiring me to become a physician.
- Dr. Henry Weisman, who resuscitated this grieving medical student and became a mentor and friend.
- Dr. Jimmie Holland, who highlighted the human side of cancer, who taught me to write professionally, who gave me feedback

on early proposals of this book and unfailing encouragement throughout my career.

- Dr. William Breitbart, who taught me about the importance of determination and persevering through endless drafts of research grants and manuscripts. He has imparted endless pearls of wisdom about complex clinical and training situations, as well as meaningful life goals.
- Dr. Howard Scher, who invited this junior psychiatrist into his prostate cancer oncology center in 1994 to address the emotional distress of his patients and their families. He taught me about prostate cancer and has supported my clinical and research work there ever since.
- It has been my privilege to work alongside the other superb clinicians, caring nurses, physicians, and researchers who work with Dr. Scher who helped me identify and learn how to manage the challenges of prostate cancer.
- Dr. Peter Scardino, a leader in surgical urological oncology and prognostics, who introduced me to the struggles men face with early-stage prostate cancer. His wife and coauthor Judith Kelman, founder of the Visible Ink writing program at Memorial Sloan Kettering Cancer Center (MSKCC) suggested ways to make this book more reader friendly.
- There were many friends, colleagues, and generous gifted souls who read versions of outlines, proposals, and manuscripts of this book, including James Eastham; Meyer Glaser; Mindy Greenstein; Pierre Lehu; Michael Morris; David Nanus; David Payne; William Pirl; Susan Slovin; Jeremy Winell; and Don Walker. I appreciate their thoughtful and encouraging comments on both content and form.
- I am grateful to Dr. Nathan Kravis, a valued colleague, supervisor, and therapist who has debrided inner scars from my past, helping to nurture seeds of vitality and clearer vision.
- Dr. Chris Nelson, who is a psychologist specializing in the care of older cancer patients and in male sexual problems, who has become a superb research and clinical teacher to me and to scores of psycho-oncology trainees and colleagues. He is also a valued friend and research and writing collaborator. His gifts of humor,

kindness, encouragement, and creativity are models and lifelines for me.

- Annie Kong, who is my physician office assistant, facilitates my ability to manage multiple clinical, educational, research, and academic writing responsibilities.
- Abby Gross at Oxford University Press (OUP), who asked to meet with me at an American Psycho Social Oncology Society conference in 2012 to see if I had any ideas for a book, and has nurtured this project, giving feedback on my proposal and reassurance in completing this manuscript.
- Special thanks also go to Molly Balikov from OUP, who seamlessly took the handoff when Abby went on family leave. They both helped me deliver this guide to the goal line.

I am blessed with family and friends who lovingly encouraged the completion of this book. Thanks to all of you and in particular:

- My brother-in-law, Peter Lynfield, who guided me with a sure and benevolent hand.
- My sister-in-law, Barbara Witke, who gave me an insider's view of how to bring a book idea to fruition.
- My cousin, Norman Grandstaff, who helped me focus and readjust ideas as needed. When he also became a prostate cancer patient, he not only gave me feedback on the accuracy of my suggestions, but also modeled coping with grace, clear-headedness, and courage.
- And lastly, my brother, Jack Roth, who was going to be the physician and writer in the family. He has taught me so much about healing and writing as we traversed the death of our parents, the birth of our own families, the span of our careers, and the completion of this book.

Thank you to all of my family, friends and colleagues who supported my writing efforts, with wishes that we go from strength to strength.

Pregame

Overview and Introduction

One crisp autumn day a few years ago, a 61-year-old successful businessman from the Midwest flew into New York for an unusual second opinion. He came into my office with a leather briefcase for a consultation. This was just weeks after his prostate cancer had been diagnosed. Mr. Jonah was well groomed, dressed in a neat suit and tie, and exuded energy and a sense of control as he took out a file of papers and sat in the chair across from me. He read the basic medical facts as if from a business profile: pre-cancer prostate-specific antigen (PSA) levels; date of cancer diagnosis; biopsy report; Gleason score; subsequent PSA levels; prostate cancer nomogram prediction of the probability of cancer remaining progression-free following definitive treatment of either prostatectomy or radiation therapy; family history; and other medical issues. He stopped himself and said, "I've been through these medical facts with two urologists, a radiation oncologist, and a medical oncologist. But you are my first psychiatric consultant. I want you to know some additional things about me and my life that are not in these papers." He began describing the loving relationships he has with his wife of 30 years and his two young adult children. He and his family were surprised and devastated by this cancer diagnosis. He was in good health otherwise, felt great physically and emotionally, enjoyed his career, and had vibrant dreams of a long and happy future. "I exercise 5 days a week at the gym,

I never smoked, and I don't drink much alcohol." There was no history of cancer in his family, and he was not ready to give up his career, lifestyle, or family.

A devastating reaction to a new prostate cancer diagnosis is not unusual, especially for men who otherwise have no major medical problems, who feel healthy, and who have no family history of prostate cancer. As Mr. Jonah would soon approach retirement from his beloved business career, his hopes and expectations of living a well-deserved retirement seemed shattered. But he was always a "go-to" kind of guy, so he naturally wanted to be proactive with the cancer. That meant having sufficient expert analysis of the medical aspects of his condition by the top professionals in the field at his fingertips, as well as understanding and addressing any relevant psychological components. Like a general going to war, he wanted to win this battle, and he was choosing his soldiers, weaponry, and allies wisely. He said to me on our first visit, "For a psychiatrist, you have seen a lot of men with prostate cancer. Please paint a picture of what I need to be concerned about or what I will likely be facing emotionally with this cancer. You know...the potential pitfalls and remedies so I can cope better with that distress if and when it arises." Mr. Jonah believed our consult would help him have the best attitude possible in his fight against prostate cancer. His request alerted me to the need for a book like this for other men with prostate cancer and for their families, who may have many of the same questions yet have no one to ask. For many years, I had been working with men with prostate cancer and their families at the request of Dr. Howard Scher, who runs the Genitourinary Medical Oncology Service at Memorial Sloan Kettering Cancer Center (MSKCC). He recognized the high levels of distress that men and their families had during visits to his practice, as well as in between visits, with anxious telephone calls to nurses and other staff members about PSA levels and physical symptoms. With the support of the Chair of Psychiatry at MSKCC, Dr. Jimmie Holland, he invited me to help these men, starting in 1994.

Prostate cancer may change lives dramatically. In the United States, over 200,000 men are diagnosed with prostate cancer every year, and it is estimated that about one of every six men will be diagnosed with this cancer during his lifetime. Improved medical, surgical, and radiological diagnostics and treatments for prostate cancer will help men live longer lives. More than two million men in the United States who have been diagnosed with prostate cancer are still alive today and are survivors of prostate cancer. But is just surviving enough? Prostate cancer impacts heterosexual men, gay men, married men, single men, as well as divorced and widowed men. Many have chronic physical and emotional effects of the cancer related to complications from their cancer treatment. Most men feel they should cope "just fine" with this cancer, just as they have with other challenges they've faced—but they don't. Our research group and others have found that about one-third of men with prostate cancer experience significant psychological distress, anxiety, or depression secondary to the cancer diagnosis, treatment decisions, unpredictable complications, or fear of recurrence of the cancer after treatment. This distress often goes undiagnosed and untreated. Other studies have shown that spouses or partners are even more distressed! Men and their spouses or partners are hungry for information about how to get the best medical outcome for their cancer—and they consume plenty of books and spend many hours online toward this end. This book focuses specifically on the emotional toll of this disease. It will help you, the reader, negotiate cancer-oriented information in the context of your unique life, and help you readjust your perspective as needed, especially if the ideal, hoped-for physical outcome is not achieved or not achievable.

Although prostate cancer risk varies in different groups—for example, men of African descent are more likely to have prostate cancer—all face the same concerns, such as controversial treatment decisions; coping with treatment complications; fear of recurrence; and overt threats to mortality. Most men, regardless of racial or cultural background, express unease with potential sexual side effects of their cancer treatment—they are concerned about erectile dysfunction and decreased sexual desire and satisfaction—as well as urinary and bowel concerns. When men get to my office it is common to hear them say, "It feels like one thing after another, doc."

Over 70% of men diagnosed with prostate cancer are over 65 years old. As baby boomers age, this number is expected to increase. Dr. Jimmie

Holland, the former Chair of Psychiatry at Memorial Sloan Kettering Cancer Center, has noted that it takes effort to confront and manage the double burden of aging and cancer. *Managing Prostate Cancer: A Guide for Living Better* will delve into the particular challenges that younger and older men and their families confront with prostate cancer. You or someone you love has prostate cancer, and that is why you are reading this book. Fear and anger about having prostate cancer and getting treated, and regrets regarding treatment because of ensuing complications, will be addressed in these pages.

Prostate cancer is usually thought to be a slow-growing tumor with a relatively good prognosis compared to that of other cancers. Many celebrities and public figures have talked openly about their prostate cancer and treatment, paving the way for other men to acknowledge their own experiences. This cancer has begun to come out of the closet, placed there because of its sexual nature and the general stigma of cancer itself.

Our research team has found that many men who rate themselves as distressed are not planning to see a psychiatrist unless specifically directed to by their physicians. They think to themselves, "Of course I'm distressed, I have cancer; depression is normal," not "I am in need of psychiatric treatment." So while looking for prostate cancer miracles, they suffer silently, fearing impending death with every PSA test. As a result of the work of our clinical and research team, many patients, oncologists, nurses, and social workers now better understand the link between the physical and emotional factors that patients and families experience with cancer treatment.

Managing Prostate Cancer: A Guide For Living Better lets men with prostate cancer know they are not alone or unusual, even though they may feel isolated when they experience ongoing frustration, distress, anger, and depression. The experiences of men and their families highlight the complexities of coping with a new diagnosis of prostate cancer, dealing with the trials of treatment decisions when there seem to be no definitively *right choices*, coping with complications of treatment and with recurrence of disease, and, lastly, coping with advanced cancer and end-stage disease. The stories and clinical illustrations come from my experience helping many men and family members cope with prostate cancer. These anecdotes are fictionalized in order to mask the identities of real patients. But because these patient accounts relate to matters that are common to most men with prostate cancer, those of you with this diagnosis may identify with many of these men, even though you feel your experience is unique.

This book will help you and your spouse or partner think through and better contend with the ping-pong effects of the medical and psychological frustrations of prostate cancer. You will be guided to develop a roadmap to cope with distress about your cancer and be provided with the tools to better survive prostate cancer crises. Some points will be stressed more than once, as is needed in actual psychotherapy, because "getting it" intellectually does not immediately change emotional reactivity. But unfortunately, a book cannot be interactive, like a live therapy session. It therefore cannot take into account what is happening with your specific medical issues in the present moment, just as information you gather on the Internet cannot. However, realistic advice is provided for improved navigation along your path of treatment decisions as well as results, based on the actual experiences of many patients and their families, as well as seeing mental health professionals.

Experiencing anxiety, depression, or demoralization or just feeling tired of fighting cancer can be frightening and leave you feeling disconnected from others. It is not unusual for psychological difficulties or concerns about the future to interfere with a man getting adequate, appropriate, and timely medical care for his cancer. Indeed, many referrals come to me from oncologists, urologists, oncology nurses, social workers, and psychologists when they recognize that a man or his family might need additional support.

What men with prostate cancer really want—the *guarantee* of a long, healthy life, with their prostate cancer definitively and safely behind them—is not available. There is no crystal ball that can forecast the certain, good outcome that every man hopes for—not even for those people who will ultimately get the result they want. The 5-year survival rate for prostate cancer diagnosed in local and regional stages is nearly 100%. But most men are not used to thinking in 5-year survival periods. Hopes and expectations are often dashed regardless of what the actual end result is, because uncertainty plagues the whole process, from diagnosis, to treatment, to ongoing monitoring with PSA tests after definitive treatments, which stimulate anxiety about possible recurrence of the cancer. Though psychological distress is not unique, it plays out personally for any given patient, based on his and his family's life histories.

So, in dealing with prostate cancer, if you come up short trying the usual coping mechanisms that have worked for other stressors in your life, this book will teach you how to recalibrate and try again to make it easier for you and your family to cope more successfully with your illness and treatment experiences. Signs of poor coping will be identified, and skills will be taught to more effectively move through one of the most challenging health crises faced by men, by using a technique I've named *Emotional Judo* (EJ). Even the question of when to seek emotional help will be addressed. Hopefully, you will be able to appreciate that every day of your life is precious and you will find more meaning and enjoyment even though you may be on a road you never wished to travel, and which seems to have little resemblance to the life or future you thought you had before your prostate cancer diagnosis.

Managing Prostate Cancer: A Guide For Living Better is divided into two parts comprising ten chapters. The first part (eight chapters) focuses on how to manage prostate cancer. It is for all men with prostate cancer, though the spotlight is on early-stage disease and primary treatment challenges. Men with early-stage disease may decide not to continue on to Part Two, as they may still have a chance for cure. But men with recurrent or advanced or metastatic disease will find the building blocks of managing their disease in both parts of the book and should read it from start to finish. Cancer management options and recommendations range from active surveillance with periodic PSA tests and biopsies to surgery or radiation therapy. Similar management skills are applicable to men finding out about biochemical recurrence. Sometimes the same patient will seek multiple opinions for one treatment decision, or he may require multiple treatments over time. Cure is a strong possibility for many, so the levels of expectations and the stakes are high, even without guarantees of perfect outcomes. The first three chapters of Part One present time-tested recommendations that can improve decision-making, help you get more value from doctors' office visits, and help you recognize and treat distress, anxiety, and depression. In Chapter 4 of this section I teach you the DRAFT with Emotional Judo technique, to identify and manage wayward emotions, self-defeating thoughts, and unproductive behaviors. Emotional Judo benefits men with all stages of prostate cancer.

Specific symptoms related to prostate cancer treatment decisions and coping after treatment can be very stressful. Chapter Sex, err, I mean Chapter 6, is devoted just to managing intimacy and sexual worries and complications posed by prostate cancer and its treatment. Chapter 7 focuses on managing the sometimes unmentionable urinary and bowel complications as well as the frequent complaints of low energy or fatigue. Although the entire book addresses reactions and concerns of both patients and family members, Chapter 8 is devoted specifically to helping spouses and partners, who may feel at a loss about how to help, what to say, what not to say, and how to care for themselves while they are being caregivers.

The second part of the book (the last two chapters) discusses issues related to cancer recurrence. Chapter 9 addresses the frustrations of finding out about and managing recurrence of the cancer and advanced disease. Chapter 10 engages readers in the grief and loss experienced when facing end-of-life issues. These chapters will help you transform fears of cancer progression and the subsequent dejection and demoralization of losing the hope of cure and of waiting to die into promotion of an attitude of living as rich and rewarding a life as possible. Part Two could even benefit men who *have* been cured, though some "do not want to even think about mortality if not forced to."

I am filled with considerable respect and regard for the men who struggle with this disease, as well as for their spouses, partners, and families, and the urology and medical oncology caregivers who have pushed the treatment of prostate cancer into a new paradigm since I began my work in this field over 20 years ago. Many men cope quite well with their illness. They accept things as they are, manage expectations realistically, deal with problems confidently as they arise, and do not feel burdened by prostate cancer or a need to talk about these issues.

I don't see those men very often. Oncologists in busy practices may not readily identify psychological distress in those who are struggling quietly, especially if there is no psychiatric consultant easily available. But family members know when there is distress. After all, most people, including physicians and nurses, believe "Well, I'd be depressed or nervous if I had cancer, so it is normal to be depressed." Prior to diagnosis many men have been accomplished and successful in their professional or work lives; expecting to cope with this illness on their own, with a similar skill set, is a reasonable response. Unfortunately, the expertise used in the job world, such as ingenuity, hard work, and forethought (thinking a few steps ahead to either prevent things from going wrong or to fix them soon thereafter), does not always help a patient in the world of cancer. In fact, these otherwise rational behaviors, with the anticipation of a clear cause-and-effect outcome, may be counterproductive in the health setting and lead to more stress. Feeling like you need to be the pilot of your own treatment is a frightening—and at times a foolhardy—endeavor. But with so many unknowns in cancer care, men feel they need to become experts themselves, hoping to elucidate easier or better choices.

It is important to state right up front that I do not believe there is any one "right" way or strategy to *cope* with prostate cancer, just as there is no one correct cancer treatment for all. It is beneficial to be aware of successful strategies you have used in the past to deal with other crises or challenges that had uncertain outcomes. If the strategies apply to your current situation, try them. If not, this book offers various approaches to cope with the many nuances that arise with prostate cancer. The techniques described can be useful for coping with other illnesses and life crises as well. If these suggestions resonate with previous behaviors, they may be easier for you to integrate and carry out now. If they do not, this is an opportunity to get outside your comfort zone. These recommendations are not dangerous; some will seem self-evident, yet you may not have thought of applying them to your cancer situation or realized how much trial, error, and persistence is required now. In fact, the more alien my proposals seem to your nature or past actions, the more perseverance and repetitive practice will be required to make them work for you.

As Sandy Koufax once said, "People who write about spring training not being necessary have never tried to throw a baseball."

Success is possible. If your distress remains very high or very intense, it may be helpful to seek the help of a mental health professional.

Many of the recommendations I make to patients to decrease distress and help them cope better are often countered with, "Doc, you make it sound so simple. Remember, this is CANCER." Some of these remedies do sound quite simple, and will sound like plain old common sense. But don't let simplicity get in the way of acting. When I am faced with trying to solve difficult problems, I remind myself of the KISS (**K**eep **I**t **S**imple **S**illy) method. I have tested many of these suggestions in my own experience as a patient. Although I did not have prostate cancer, I had to investigate and make treatment choices and deal with the ramifications of a benign brain tumor called an acoustic neuroma. There were similar threads of distress and uncertainty regarding decisions, as well as the acceptance and management of unwanted acute and chronic complications from my treatment. Though different, in many ways my ordeal mirrored what many of my patients with cancer struggle with. For better or for worse, I had a chance to test out and clarify many of the tools I have used to help men with prostate cancer and their families. Though simple to understand, I experienced how difficult these skills are to carry out. I briefly discuss parallel lessons learned throughout the book.

Developing new behaviors is burdensome because of the rigidity we develop in our habitual, customary actions, and because of the unrealistic expectations we maintain despite new realities. One patient wisely told me, "I've learned not to have expectations anymore...but I do like to have hopeful goals." Even when men are aware that their emotions or behaviors are unproductive and uncomfortable, they cannot easily adjust. That is where the simple ideas become difficult to execute. It takes a good deal of effort, trial and error, and a multitude of recurring attempts to develop new habits and sustain new patterns of thinking. Practice. Assess. More practice. Reassess. Continue to tweak and reassess. Learn from your mistakes and apply what you have learned. Practicing the same wrong moves over and over will always lead to the same busted play. Patients have asked me whether I can really "teach an old dog new tricks." Many of us think that as adults we are supposed to know this information already. Yet old strategies often do not apply sufficiently to cope well with a new formidable illness and changes in lifestyle. The guidance of a coach or teacher who knows what can be attained, point out mistakes, and show you how to correct and manage them, while being supportive along the way, can be priceless. This is a large part of a therapist's job. You can also use a healthy dose of patience. I will describe exercises to promote patience for practice. These exercises will also enhance your insight into the issues that distress you most.

The loss of various physical functions, or changes in those functions that are due to the cancer or treatment and that cannot be reversed or be resolved sufficiently to one's liking may repeatedly impact mood for many men, which in turn makes the medical dysfunction even worse. Dealing with these changes and grieving for these losses are vital to emotional and physical recovery.

Beware of anyone offering guarantees when it comes to your physical or emotional health—they rarely exist; "guarantees" set expectations so high that when they are not fulfilled, there is that much more disappointment. No pledges, no promises, no guarantees. But I do believe there is more contentment when goals, hopes, and aspirations are reasonable *and* flexible. Gratification is also more likely when you can persevere and accept a "new normal," rather than wishing things were "just the way they used to be" or should be drastically different than they really are now.

New Diagnosis and Early-Stage Disease

Chapter 1

Why Me? Why Not Me?
What Now?

And Why Is a Psychiatrist Writing a Book about Prostate Cancer?

If the world was perfect, it wouldn't be.

Yogi Berra

"YOU have cancer, prostate cancer."

The blood drains from your fingers and toes as your pulse rate goes up, trying to ready for the battle, not even sure what the battle is yet—while at the same time weighing your options, like getting the hell out of the doctor's office, and out of this new script life just wrote for you. Questions like "Are the tests even correct?"; "How can this be?"; "How can this be happening now? I'm supposed to retire in a year"; "Wasn't I a good person?"; "Wasn't I in reasonably good shape?"; "What good did stopping smoking 30 years ago do for me?"; and "Why me?" may repeatedly race through your mind.

Prostate cancer, or perhaps any life-threatening diagnosis, generates for most men and their families a host of conflicting feelings, ranging from a sense of disbelief, anxiety or fear, to sadness and anger. The questions can snowball:

"Will it kill me?"
"If it will kill me, when?"
"Did my dad have this?"
"Are my sons at risk; my grandsons?"
"Do we have a cancer gene?"
"Doesn't prostate cancer affect sex?"
"Did sex cause this cancer?"
"Will my wife or partner leave me if we can't have sex anymore?"
"How will my life change?"
"What does this mean for my retirement?"

Common Reactions to a New Prostate Cancer Diagnosis

"I need a second opinion."
"I need another second opinion to learn more about this and to figure out the right treatment choice."
"The biopsy was wrong."
"This is not happening to me."
"Why me?" (Yes, this does keep popping up for most men.)
"I will beat this thing."
"Maybe the PSA level will go down without treatment."
"This will really screw up my life and plans."
"This will kill me."
"Why me?"

The "Why me?" question often recurs in various forms over and over again during the days, weeks, and even months after a new diagnosis of cancer, and during most disease transitions over the course of cancer thereafter. Just about every person I have seen with cancer, including men with prostate cancer, has asked, "Why me? How could this happen or be happening to me? What did I (or my family) do to deserve this? How can God do this to me?" Disbelief is common in people newly diagnosed with cancer. Of course, a number of men have answered the question with another: "Well, why not me?"

After a cancer diagnosis threatens physical health, men are often the last to believe that they have psychological difficulties as well. If they begin to experience an unfamiliar emotion such as anxiety or depression, they are quickly concerned that they may lose their sanity after they have just lost the physical health that they have come to know and count on. Spouses or partners are usually the first to recognize the emotional distress in the newly diagnosed man. Adult children, and even younger grandchildren may also recognize it: "How come grandpa doesn't want to see us anymore?" It is not that grandpa is going crazy. But he may stop enjoying usually pleasurable activities. He may avoid social interactions. He may be more irritable or distracted than usual. He may be depressed. For the first few years I spent in the prostate cancer center at Memorial Sloan Kettering Cancer Center, the oncologist who invited me into the practice, Howard Scher, suggested I see the patients visiting for the first time to learn their medical and emotional issues. He knew their distress would be elevated. These men were either coping with new diagnoses or finding out whether the cancer that had been treated months or years before, which they thought had been cured, had now returned or progressed. Many did have high anxiety. I would visit these men in "real time," during their medical visits. In our busy hospital that meant seeing the patient in between visits by the nurse who was getting vital signs, an oncology physician fellow in training who would do a medical assessment and physical exam, and the oncology attending who performed a second, more focused assessment and exam. Sometimes my visits were divided over one or two of these "in and out" intervals, hardly the most conducive atmosphere for developing a traditional psychotherapeutic relationship. But that didn't seem to matter. My introduction and questions were fairly brief and basic:

> The last person you may have expected to see during your visit to an oncologist is a psychiatrist; I am part of this medical team because Dr. Scher has recognized that many men with prostate cancer and their

families are distressed and have difficulty coping, and we'd like to try to help.

The feedback the oncologists and nurses received from patients, and especially from spouses and partners, about my visits was fantastic. Even in broken intervals, I was able to acknowledge and validate the upset and frustration that patients, spouses, and partners had coping with the cancer. This holistic view of the situation was appreciated, and it was self-evident that all could benefit from support. Spouses and partners, who often feel as if they, too, have been diagnosed with the cancer, and feel the uninvited intrusion of cancer in their lives, ask, "Why me?" as well. They are often the first to ask, "Why us?" There is an appreciation that life will be different for them, their spouses, and their families. An important question that is not usually asked early on is, "How can WE cope with this?" Just the knowledge that help was available was sufficient to decrease stress to a more acceptable level.

The shock and disbelief that men with prostate cancer and their families have is similar to what most people with any newly diagnosed cancer experience. I've heard wise people comfort those who wonder why horrible tragedy could happen to them. They've said that when the question "Why me?" is asked and has no legitimate or acceptable answer, perhaps a helpful answer comes in the form of another, more therapeutic acknowledgment: "This really sucks, but what can I do now?—What can I do to cope well with whatever is handed me?" It can take weeks or months for most people to get to a point of accepting that cancer has intruded in and changed their lives, possibly forever. Prostate cancer does not have obvious notorious causes, such as lung cancers and smoking cigarettes (though there are certainly many people diagnosed with lung cancer who are not smokers, as well as smokers who never get lung cancer). Prostate cancer is not like head and neck tumors, where a history of heavy alcohol drinking and smoking tobacco combines to significantly raise the likelihood of getting one of these cancers. There have been findings that associate the development of prostate cancer with diets high in fat and red meat; however, these culprits are more like added ingredients to a soup, as they do not seem sufficient in and of themselves to cause the cancer to develop. The only clear, consistent ingredient is male gender and having a prostate. An important factor is often a family history of prior prostate cancer, especially in first-degree relatives, such as fathers or brothers. As noted in the Introduction, men of African descent are also more at risk of developing prostate cancer. And yet, even if we know we have a higher risk, when something catches us off guard and does not make sense in our lives, we still like to understand why it is happening now, and try to fit it into a rational context. If there is no past activity that we can easily and sufficiently, though not necessarily correctly, blame (like smoking or drinking), we then start looking for other possibilities. Common suspects for blame are related to the fact that the prostate gland is so important for men's sexual activity: "Was it because I had too much sex?, . . . too little sex? . . . sex with the wrong person or people? Is God punishing me for my moral lapses (either sexual or otherwise)?" Studies about prostate cancer do not show a consistent culprit, so men look for something else: "Did the cancer come because I have too much stress in my life? Is my job literally killing me? Is all the arguing I do with my wife killing me?" If we can find someone or something to blame, then the world keeps making sense and feels predictable, which is comforting, however misguided that may be in reality.

Many of my patients tell me they "have never been sick a day in their lives" before prostate cancer, and that is why they are having difficulty accepting the diagnosis and coping with this new health challenge. This contributes to high anxiety or low moods. And they are not alone. Studies estimate that about one-third of men with prostate cancer have significant distress, anxiety, or depression. Maybe they have never been sick with a life-threatening illness until now. Many don't recall how sick they were earlier in their lives, and many do not recall that they've been sick at all. Denial, unconscious forgetting, or conscious suppression of prior illness experiences can cloud one's memory. But we all have reactions to even a week's bout with the flu when we were "sick as a dog," or to a sprained knee or ankle after a jog on the treadmill, or to a jammed finger that may be debilitating or painful after a basketball game. We know these injuries will likely heal and we will move on. Men have told me that dealing with cardiac bypass surgery was much easier than dealing with cancer. The response is usually to forget about the episode when healed, perhaps because it is short-lived. Additionally, if they have seen parents, siblings, cousins, or friends suffer through serious illnesses, including cancer, they may wish never to be in the same circumstances. They use those past experiences of others to predict their future. But it is risky to generalize from another's disease to your own future. Even your own past encounters with illness do not guarantee future outcomes, as there may be uniqueness to every illness, to every occurrence of illness, and to a body's ability to fight an illness at different times.

Shock and disbelief as first reactions to a cancer diagnosis are universal. People wonder how their bodies could betray them by growing a tumor. Prostate cancer diagnoses occur in those who exercise regularly and maintain reasonably healthy lifestyles as well as among those who do not. This cancer is diagnosed in men who run marathons, who complete triathlons, and, paradoxically, who raise money for good causes like cancer research. Men who are otherwise healthy may erroneously feel insulated from the possibility that cancer or any life-threatening disease could get them, in their forties, fifties, sixties, or seventies.

It wasn't until I went through my own odyssey with illness that I really understood what previously I only saw from an empathic therapist's distance. When I first began writing this book, my qualifications were based on the years I had spent learning about the medical, surgical, and radiation therapies, as well as the psychological aspects, of prostate cancer. I could point to the many hours I counseled men and their families about how to cope better with all of its ramifications. Early on I wondered, however, as other therapists have in other contexts, "Can I really know what is going on in someone else's heart and mind if I haven't walked in his shoes? Could I really understand what it is like for a man to lose his erectile functioning or his urinary continence?" The answer was always a truthful "No, but . . ." I had a lot to learn. However, this did not get in the way of learning ways to help these men and their families cope better with the cancer—in fact, maybe it actually helped to have a little distance from it.

"Why Me?" Asked Dr. Roth

Nine years ago I was diagnosed with an acoustic neuroma, a rare benign tumor of the internal ear canal. That sounds quite treatable. It started with occasional ringing in my right ear, called tinnitus. After a month, the ringing was constant. It had one pitch, sometimes sounding like the static between two radio stations with varying volumes, none of which I had control over. At first it was more annoying than worrisome. My physician looked for causes in the medications I took but eventually ran into a diagnostic dead end. So I was referred to an ear, nose, and throat specialist who I expected would tell me the ringing was due to all the loud rock and roll music I listened to as a teenager. The Internet informed me that a common cause was a plain old virus. I didn't consciously notice another cause further down the list: "brain tumor." I hoped the doctor would be able to give me a medication to quiet down the static in my life, the auditory equivalent of what I as a psychiatrist do for others. He ordered an urgent hearing test, which showed significant hearing loss on my right side; I hadn't noticed how bad it was. He suggested an immediate magnetic resonance imaging (MRI) scan of my brain to rule out a tumor—an acoustic neuroma. It is rare—just 1 in 100,000. I was in great health. I had just completed the New York City marathon. I went into the MRI scan naïve, recalling so many patients I had treated to alleviate panic symptoms in these scanning machines. I came out a seasoned veteran. But in less than 24 hours my life changed. I had a brain tumor and now I had a treatment decision to make. Though benign, it is considered a brain tumor because it is so close to the brain—it can grow into the brainstem, causing death, even though it is designated as benign. It requires either neurosurgery or radiation for removal. One of my colleagues remarked, "benign tumor, potentially malignant treatment and course." I also had a watchful waiting or active surveillance option. It was difficult to feel the relief of "Thank God it's not cancer." I felt a need to do something and not let a tumor, benign or not, keep growing near my brain.

I clearly comprehended what I'd been counseling men about for years. I understood the seductive, captivating lure of the "Why me?" question, and so plainly felt the emotional sting and treacherousness of it; I was compelled to keep asking the question, expecting that there really could be a logical answer that would preserve the rational perspective of the foundation of my world. The more angry and powerless I felt without an adequate response, the more the question "Why me?" persisted, while looking for a sense of control to fix this problem. If I understood the "why" I could deal better with the "what." Yet I also recognized that there was no sufficient explanation; I had to grieve for the illusions I had: good lifestyles cannot prevent disastrous situations, and good luck cannot be counted on. "Why me?" was an elusive way of saying, "I just want things to be fine, the way they were before the illness." "Why me?" returned when complications that I did not think likely when discussed during consent processes actually arose after surgery.

The question "Why me?" peaks our interest when we are presented with dilemmas in which we sense an uneasy, complicated journey ahead where there may be unimagined and unimaginable adversities. Most of us tend to think that major life snags happen to others; that's a form of denial or suppression that may be necessary to move forward, day after day, without the distractions of potential traumas. Limiting major distractions about what may happen down the road is important after a cancer diagnosis in order to choose potentially life-saving treatment that can have potential complications. Being an aware consumer is essential, but accepting the possible and as yet unknown downsides is important as well. The rubber hits the road when you encounter actual side effects that were only hypothetical when you signed the treatment consent form, when a 100% successful outcome for you was still a possibility. What you expected to hear from your physician, "tumor removed, no complications," may no longer be a possibility.

Most people respond to new diagnoses and treatment with a plethora of unanswerable questions about the future, with disbelief, and, at times, with recurring uncomfortable emotions. These feelings are best managed when identified, acknowledged, explored, understood, expressed, and, hopefully, resolved. Learning the DRAFT with Emotional Judo techniques described in Chapter 4 will help to manage these reactions successfully.

Anger is a common reaction to a cancer diagnosis. Rage or resentment can go overboard and be misplaced, disorganized, unguided, diffused, or unbridled and, thus, potentially harmful. No particular emotion will change the facts. An argument or fight won't settle the matter. Yet appropriate anger is understandable and may clear the cobwebs to bring about temporary relief and clearer thinking. Men get angry with God, at their doctors, at stressful jobs, at their spouses, at their children, at other stressors in their lives, and sometimes at their fathers and ancestors for passing down the prostate cancer vulnerability. Acknowledging and addressing these perceived affronts might be therapeutic. However, without a clear protagonist, your anger may not naturally crescendo and decrescendo; it may boomerang inward, with unfair blaming of yourself in the form of depression or anxiety; it may also be directed hurtfully at close loved ones. "Getting it out" isn't always productive. Sometimes this can damage your ability to gather support from vital members of your team.

Some men think that they have been unfairly picked on, especially if they had good lifestyle behaviors—they did not smoke or drink; they exercised regularly and ate a reasonable diet low in fats and red meat; they had a reasonably satisfying sex life with a long-term partner; and they are decent, morally upstanding people. Men may feel this is a case of mistaken identity: "They got the wrong guy." This is scary. They may feel as if they do not have control over the most important aspects of their health. They have heard that proper diet and exercise will prevent heart disease or strokes. Indeed, healthy lifestyles may reduce the odds of some health disasters and even some cancers for many people, but that is not true for all diseases or for all people. Preventive health behaviors may have averted diagnosis at an earlier age or more advanced disease at diagnosis. It is impossible to know exactly where we stand in terms of genetic or biological vulnerabilities and other environmental protagonists.

My dad was 83 when he died of prostate cancer. I have checked my PSA test every 6 months since his diagnosis 10 years ago. It is not fair that

I am getting diagnosed with advanced prostate cancer at age 62. I was hoping to live until at least my seventies if not my eighties like my dad.

This scenario will be discussed more in Chapter 10 on grief. Most people have certain expectations about the future, at least regarding health, which may have nothing to do with reality. We all make assumptions based on family history and our own past health, but just as even the best horse race handicappers get fooled at times, a scenario like this can happen to us. As common as prostate cancer may be, with a majority of men developing some form of it if they live long enough, the types brought to attention in younger men often are more aggressive. Even if prostate cancer is *supposed to* happen to older men, it is rarely easily accepted. Increasing success in treating all medical diseases has set men up to live long enough to deal with the benefits and drawbacks of otherwise "normal" aging, like retirement and time for grandchildren and hobbies, as well as gait disturbances, poorer eyesight or hearing, weakness, and prostate (and other) cancer. Battling aging and cancer can make men feel as if they are fighting losing battles on multiple fronts, with their desire to enjoy their families and recreational hobbies now starkly threatened by mortality. The losses that pile up on men with prostate cancer include the loss of health (whether good or not so good, not so good looks better after having been diagnosed with prostate cancer) as they've known it, and the loss of a sense of security that "all is right with your world and with you," especially if they were able to tackle most problems when they arose or had the choice to ignore them. My grandmother used to say, "If you have your health, you have everything." The corollary to that is that with aging or diminished strength and energy that comes from cancer, you may feel more helpless. You may feel like you have little to live for. Losing any independence or autonomy can set in motion a snowballing fear of further losses. You may feel as if you have lost your sense of identity as an individual and as a man. You may fear the loss of the future as you imagined it, however cloudy or clear that image may have been before your cancer. Your presence at future special events like weddings, anniversaries, and birthday parties may be called into question. Maybe you just have an image of yourself, becoming gray (or bald), with stooped posture, sitting in a rocking chair by a fireplace with your grandchildren playing nearby. These images of the future are not concrete experiences that you can literally see and touch right now. However, they can be quite real in your mind. And their "certainty" is now in question.

For younger men there is a concern that, given normal life expectancies, they may have more time taken from their lives than from an older man. The previously mentioned 62-year-old man whose father died at 83 may grieve for his loss of health and hoped-for future more acutely than an older man with prostate cancer because he has to reset his "future frame" that much more. It is deceiving to assume that because his dad lived to a much older age before being diagnosed with prostate cancer that he, the son, should have the same trajectory. He has to deal with different variables than his dad's and accept his reality. As he started going into unfamiliar and, for him, uncharted territory, he had to deal with his anxiety. His sense of certainty was shattered. His dad hadn't had to worry about a life-threatening illness at a young age, before he completed a career, before he got to see his children grow up—all things the son expected for himself.

It is not uncommon for men with family histories of prostate cancer to be very careful about getting regular prostate specific antigen (PSA) tests. Some men want PSA tests scheduled even more frequently than the oncologist or urologist recommends. Some look to these tests with a degree of magical thinking: "If I take the test, I will not get the cancer." They are not really expecting a bad result; in fact, they may be looking for verification that everything is okay. If a cancer is detected, they are often quite shocked and angry. Rather than seeing that their steadfast persistence in getting these tests has served an important purpose—to detect a cancer at an earlier stage than might have otherwise been detected, so that they have a better chance at a better outcome—they are angry that they have to deal with the cancer at all. The wishful thinking was not so magical. Others await these tests with significant fear: "What if the PSA goes up? What if they find cancer?"

PSA tests have helped with earlier diagnosis of prostate cancer for many men. Unfortunately, PSA tests are far from perfect. These tests may not be sensitive enough to pick up some early-stage cancers (false-negative aspects of the tests)—somehow the cancer in these men avoids detection by the blood test. Sometimes these tests show false-positive results—higher readings that are not necessarily reflective of aggressive or dangerous cancers, yet lead to heightened worry and more tests and invasive biopsies that do not find cancer. Suffice it to say that these men feel further alienated from and betrayed by their bodies and genes. They feel misled by the sense of control they thought they had by obtaining regular blood tests. I will discuss the hypervigilance and worry some men have about their PSA tests, also called PSA anxiety, later in Chapter 4. This sense of doomed expectations leads to anger, anxiety, and depression; each of these emotions can be dealt with effectively.

Biopsies

Most men get very anxious while waiting for the results of their prostate biopsies. In fact, this may be among the most anxiety-ridden times people diagnosed with cancer go through. The result of the biopsy appears to hold the power of life or death—as if it were a death sentence. A positive (with cancer) biopsy means life has taken a major, unforeseen turn. Though death may ultimately come from this disease, it will not necessarily come from prostate cancer, and if it does, most likely it will not come anytime soon. Men lose sleep contemplating their future options, as nighttime is frequently the most fertile time for anxiety and worry to attack. There are fewer distractions (i.e., work, family, TV), and a man is left with his own thoughts and schemes of how to get out of this cancer mess. Endless thought-loops revolve around rethinking what he could have done or still could do differently: "I could have gone to the doctor sooner...eaten better...prayed to God more." Men may start to silently bargain or make deals with God about living a better life, if only the biopsy result is negative: "Maybe the biopsy will be negative; I'll pray harder. Tomorrow I'll start exercising and give up drinking alcohol." They may experience significant worry, depressed mood, poor sleep, poor appetite, and poor concentration and not be able to enjoy usually pleasant activities. Life can feel as if it is on hold until this cancer stuff gets figured out. The desire to go back to the way life was before the threat of cancer is a recurring theme throughout the course of illness. When the biopsy is positive, there is an impractical wish to make the cancer go away. Inadvertently, that "death sentence" men fear with a positive biopsy can come much sooner, as men start acting as if they were dying instead of living as full a life as possible until they die.

The prostate gland is about the size of a walnut. This fact about the prostate's rather small size was one of the few I remembered from my medical school classes about the prostate. "So what is all the fuss about something the size of a walnut?" I asked myself, back in 1994, when the chair of my department, Dr. Jimmie Holland, said there was an oncologist who wanted a psychiatrist to work in his prostate cancer program. Over the next few months, through the "real-time" prostate center experiences noted earlier, I learned much about the fuss. Men with prostate cancer are concerned with things that most people diagnosed with cancer are concerned about:

"I can die from this."
"My life will never be the same."
"I used to feel like I was healthy and now I am not."
"I don't want to die."
"I do not want to suffer and do not want to be a burden on my family.
    I don't want them to suffer. I don't want to suffer."
"When will I die?"

In addition, men with prostate cancer are worried about other illness-related problems. The prostate, when it is working well, has many functions, facilitating urinary and sexual function for men. When it is enlarged without any cancer (benign prostatic hypertrophy) it can cause urinary problems, usually with some degree of blockage, which leads to urinating frequently or with a weak stream. There are more frequent trips to the bathroom. A number of men have told me about their self-consciousness when in public bathrooms, such as on an airplane, because they feel they take so long to finish, and they know others are waiting for the door to open before the "fasten your seatbelt" sign goes on again. Anxiety can make a man take even longer to urinate.

Newly diagnosed men worry that an aggressive prostate cancer that is left untreated will eventually cause urinary problems as well as sexual problems. They learn that if the cancer spreads, it can go to bones, lungs, and liver, which can cause pain, trouble breathing, and debilitation. A man's self-definition; his sense of independence, sexual identity, and affectionate relationships; and his sense of the future he had planned on, as well as urinary and sexual functioning, may all feel threatened. Many of these functions may also be compromised by the surgery or radiation treatments aimed at curing the prostate cancer. These treatments have improved outcomes in the last 20 years; however, the risk of side effects is by no means down to zero—even with the best surgeons and the most advanced radiation technologies. It seems like there are new treatment modalities being developed all the time. However, as long as there is a significant amount of uncertainty, there remains a significant void for anxiety to fill. So questions like "Will I ever be able to have sex again?"; "Will I live the rest of my life wearing diapers?"; "Will my wife love me if I cannot have intercourse?"; "Will I die a painful death?" may intrude on quieter moments.

These potential life changes related to prostate cancer or treatments, that appear in the form of questions, are experienced realistically and emotionally as losses—physical losses, loss of hopes and expectations, and emotional losses. If you are like most men, even before your biopsy result comes back, you have already heard or read about the many treatment options for prostate cancer, including not having active treatment at all. Sometimes what is lost is temporary, and sometimes it is permanent. Sometimes the loss is complete, yet sometimes any loss feels like everything. Sometimes these losses are tangible, and sometimes they are just in men's imaginations, such as the future they expected that may now be in jeopardy. That you even have to think about possible treatment options for cancer is a loss of the less treacherous life you had been leading.

Acknowledging and grieving for these losses, the real and the feared, the probable and the possible, the partial or the complete, is normal and advantageous emotionally. It is also healthy. But it's not easy, and it's not necessarily intuitive, since most men tend to think about grieving only when someone has died. And death, for any particular man awaiting the results of his prostate biopsy, whether related to prostate cancer or some other cause, is likely a long way off. But these perceived losses impact actions, reactions, thoughts, and feelings going forward. Understanding this process helps men move forward with more awareness and more thoughtfulness, allowing for a more successful and fruitful life journey. Otherwise they are at risk of staying stuck in an imagined, depressing world of the future that could lead to a self-fulfilling prophecy, as they miss opportunities for fulfillment in the here-and-now. Their spouse or partner will also encounter grief about changes and losses with a unique and sometimes shared perspective and vantage point, because of the changes their loved one encounters. Understanding and dealing with these reactions will help everyone adapt and cope better, and help men move into the next phase of the cancer experience, making a treatment decision more clearly.

Chapter 2

How Can You Make the Right Treatment Choice When There Is No Perfect Choice?

Men and their partners tackle many medical bottlenecks when doing psychotherapy with me. They try to figure out their sense of the best cancer treatment decision for them. They come to a psychiatrist because there is usually no "one size fits all" choice agreed upon by the urologists, radiation oncologists, and medical oncologists who are consulted. In this chapter we discuss the importance of second opinions and how to go about getting them, while cautioning about the challenge of too many opinions. Treatment decisions are often difficult because there really is no clear "right" choice. These decisions often feel impossible to make because of the emotional and intellectual uncertainty surrounding the available options and outcomes. Sometimes this can lead to indecisive paralysis, and men get stuck between two extremes:

You miss 100% of the shots you don't take.

Wait for your pitch.

One of the first decisions men newly diagnosed with prostate cancer have to deal with is whether to get treated actively or not. If diagnosed early enough, many men can be cured, or live with prostate cancer for many years. In fact, many prostate cancers will remain dormant for many years, leading to the controversial question of whether these tumors should be routinely screened for with prostate-specific antigen (PSA) tests, or treated, in the first place. The goal in screening men with PSA tests is to diagnose the tumor at as early a stage and at as small a size as possible. To treat or not to treat a tumor is a complicated question. Deciding on which treatment to have is the beginning of a slippery slope of challenging decisions that contribute to worry. The PSA test is not perfect, and the current state of the art regarding the predictability of which tumors will be life-threatening is also not ideal when it comes down to one man and one family who have to make such an important decision.

One day soon there may be urine or other tests that use biomarkers to predict the likelihood of a positive biopsy and whether a worrisome biopsy will signal clinically significant cancer that needs to be treated sooner rather than later. But until then, men and their doctors have to decide whether getting a PSA test is a good idea, given their age, family history, and medical well-being, and what to do if the result is suspicious for cancer. This decision is all the more difficult without sufficient information to indicate whether a man could live with his cancer until he dies of something else, or if the prostate cancer will likely be the illness that kills him. The latter alternative might mean that he should accept the quality-of-life risks and get the tumor out before it starts spreading.

The decisional domino-like effect is one of the reasons there remains a controversy about screening the general population of healthy men for prostate cancer: a positive or suspicious PSA test needs to be followed up with repeated tests and a likely biopsy. Biopsies are procedures that come with risks and may cause discomfort. A biopsy that is indicative of prostate cancer needs to be considered for observation or treatment; treatment may negatively impact quality of life while not ensuring significant added value to quantity of life. From a population-based bird's eye view, general PSA screening does not add to longevity and adds to healthcare costs.

The next round of worry and fear related to decision-making begins after a positive biopsy. The biopsy result includes a description of the tissue sample and a Gleason score. The *Gleason score* is a sum of two numbers, representing patterns of cancer seriousness (each scored from 0 to 5). The total score (maximum is 10, the most aggressive type of tumor); is a reflection of how threatening the tumor might be; and helps the physician formulate the prognosis, along with other variables such as the PSA test, serial digital rectal exams, ultrasound tests, bone scans, positron emission tomography (PET) scans, and magnetic resonance imaging (MRI) scans. Dr. Peter Scardino and his research team, at Memorial Sloan Kettering Cancer Center, and others have developed statistical models that predict the likelihood of when a cancer might return after definitive treatment with either surgery, external beam radiation therapy, or seed implants. Sophisticated yet easy-to-use computerized nomograms are prediction tools that can help one understand which treatment options will result in the greatest benefit for men at various stages of prostate cancer. They are readily accessible online.

However, making a decision about which primary treatment to undergo, if any, is where the worry and aggravation really take off. By this time, men have tried wishing the cancer away, wishing for a negative biopsy, wishing for a magically corrected and normalized PSA test, and they are now feeling like they are facing either a life sentence of CANCER or, worse, cancer death row, rather than a medical diagnosis. I once saw a wonderful cartoon by Peter Mueller from *The Cartoon Bank* that summed up this wishful thinking many men go through. The cartoon shows an older gentleman on Santa's lap, saying, "I want a new prostate."

Any man who complains about urinary difficulties from an enlarged prostate or sexual difficulty from an older prostate or about prostate cancer might wish his life could go back to the way it was before the cancer or prostate problem began. As complicated as life may have seemed then, it now seems, in hindsight, like it was much simpler and clearer and safer. Before cancer, mortality could still be largely disregarded and one could be seduced by the "assurance" of living forever or at least until a ripe old age without a significant threat. For those men diagnosed with prostate cancer at an older age, this could be the first real indication of their mortality, even if they've faced other serious non-cancer illnesses previously. They now feel that dealing with prostate cancer is a much tougher challenge.

Which Treatment Choice Will Get Me Where I Want to Be?

It is easy to get a thousand prescriptions, but hard to get one single remedy.

Chinese Proverb

Men who are used to successfully making complicated and important decisions related to career, family, the law, finances, and other health care issues are suddenly stumped, because this life-and-death prostate cancer decision feels like it has an immediate impact on their ultimate mortality. It cannot just be seen as a deal that could go bad, a decision about a child's school problem, or even dealing with a summons for driving while under the influence of alcohol. There are no "mulligans" (do-overs) or an easy route to moving on to the next problem that arises and trying harder. People who have cardiac disease, congestive heart failure, or emphysema may have similar or even worse end-of-life quality of life than those with cancer; however, those illnesses and the aftermath of treatment decisions do not seem to be as frightening to most men. With the treatment controversy in prostate cancer, a treatment choice can feel like an impossible choice. When your cardiac arteries are clogged, you have a few options to open them up or to bypass them. Many men who come to me for help in coping with their prostate cancer tell me that cancer is a much more difficult challenge emotionally than the cardiac bypass surgery they had previously. If there were no complications from that treatment, it goes into the future as a "one and done, so let's move on."

Treatment Choices, More Choices, and the Fear of Buyer's Remorse

It is an equal failing to trust everybody and to trust nobody.

English Proverb

Trust yourself. You know more than you think you do.

Benjamin Spock, MD

Depending on the size and location of the tumor, a man may be a candidate for active treatment. Current treatment options are variations on surgery, including open radical prostatectomy or robotic-assisted laparoscopic prostatectomy; variations on radiation therapy, including external beam radiation therapy with or without radiation seed implants or enhancing hormonal treatment; cryosurgery (freezing the tumor); proton beam therapy (a form of radiation therapy that can deliver a very high dose of radiation to the cancer, minimizing damage to healthy tissues and organs near the cancer); or active surveillance, during which PSA levels are regularly monitored, without invasive treatment. Not surprisingly, different expert practitioners have different opinions regarding treatment, and sometimes a physician may have more than one opinion about the same patient. Men are not just looking for the right treatment choice but are also wanting to know that they are "fielding an expert team," from the urologist, radiation oncologist, medical oncologist, nurses, office clerks or secretaries, blood drawers, to the people who make sure the center or hospital is clean and safe.

Current Treatment Options for Primary Prostate Cancer

Surgery

Open radical prostatectomy
Robotic assisted laparoscopic prostatectomy

Radiation Therapy

External beam
　With or without radiation seed implants
　With or without enhancing hormonal therapy
Proton beam therapy
　High-dose radiation, trying to minimize damage to healthy
　　tissues and organs near the cancer

Cryosurgery

A technique for freezing and killing cancer cells

Active Surveillance

With PSA monitoring
With biopsy monitoring
No invasive treatment

Many men, fearful of making a wrong or bad treatment decision, find themselves on endless worry-loops, foreseeing worst-case outcomes for different options. The reasons used to decide on a particular treatment with a particular physician at a particular hospital are quite variable:

I like the doctor and he's an expert in the field with great statistics.
I think I can handle the side effects of Treatment A better than Treatment B.
I want radiation because I am scared of surgery.
I want surgery because the doctor gets to look inside and there is another
　opportunity for pathology re-examination, and then we really know
　what we are dealing with.
I feel more comfortable with surgery because the treatment is over and
　done within a short period of time.
I want radiation because my friend had radiation and he did very well.
I feel better with radiation because I won't have to have anesthesia, and
　the time it takes to recuperate from surgery will be about as long as
　the radiation will take anyway.

Men and their partners will think that if all turns out well, with few complications and a prolonged disease-free survival, hopefully dying many years later of a non-prostate cancer cause at a very old age, then they made the RIGHT CHOICE, as if that is how alternatives are defined: RIGHT or WRONG. But without a crystal ball, no one can predict future consequences and outcomes of any treatment decision. I suggest that even if there are complications that were not wanted or expected, or the cancer comes back in a few years, that a man and his partner look at themselves in the down-the-road, future mirror and honestly say, "I/we made the RIGHT CHOICE, even if I/we didn't get the result I/we wanted." The last thing a man needs when finding out about recurrence of disease or while coping with a frustrating complication is the extra burden of internally stimulated regret and self-bullying and blame, feeling as if he made a poor initial treatment decision.

Men are often paralyzed trying to make the RIGHT CHOICE—trying to make a decision that pits a better chance of cure or a longer life against the hope of fewer complications with erectile dysfunction (ED), urinary incontinence, or bowel dysfunction and therefore better quality of life. Some men feel they would even sacrifice years of life to maintain their erectile ability or to maintain urinary or bowel integrity, while others hold the longest life span as their desired goal. If any undesired outcome is realized, men feel remorse. This is illustrated in Figure 2.1. A treatment decision is eventually made at Time 1 between Choice A and Choice B. Assume he chooses A. At Time 2 (months or years later), if Option A leads to Outcome X and X is a cure with no side effects, feeling that A is a RIGHT CHOICE is a no-brainer. If there is a cure, but there are unfavorable side effects at Outcome X, many men may feel they made the wrong choice. They think, "If only I took Choice B, all would have been good." This is faulty thinking. They are looking back at Choice B from the same idealized, as yet unknowable-future vantage point they had at Time 1. It is assumed that Choice B (still with an unknowable result at Outcome Y) would have turned out better, just because it is not Choice A, which now has a known bad outcome. We can't go up both paths simultaneously, so we'll never really know if Choice B and Outcome Y would have been

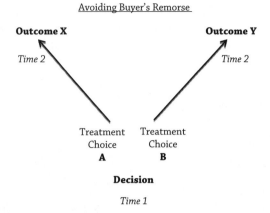

Figure 2.1. Avoiding buyer's remorse.

better than Choice A and Outcome X at Time 2. In fact, Choice B and Outcome Y could have been much worse than Choice A even at a future Time 3, with no cure and lots of side effects.

A few years ago, I evaluated two 40-something-year-old men newly diagnosed with prostate cancer over the course of a few weeks. The first had been married for 15 years, with two young children under age 10. He had a good relationship with his wife and placed a high priority on spending time with his children, though he was very busy as a manager for a local business. He felt it was unfair to have to make a decision between longevity and quality of life, and was angry that there were no assurances that either surgery or radiation therapy would yield his hoped-for outcome of a guaranteed cure. But he wanted the best shot at seeing his children grow up.

The second gentleman had lived with his male partner for the past 10 years. When the patient wasn't working, he spent most of his leisure time with his partner or with friends. Sexual intimacy was important to their relationship. This patient was willing to sacrifice some years of life for a "guarantee" that his sexual and urinary functioning would remain intact. No urologist or radiation oncologist could assuage either man's anxiety before making a treatment decision. They could not offer guarantees about cure, sexuality, or urinary function—just statistics.

These two patients chose different treatments, hoping their predictions would be correct—that surgery would give the first man an edge in longevity, and that radiation would give the second man an advantage for less impaired sexual and urinary functioning. There was no crystal ball that could predict a guaranteed outcome that would prevent buyer's remorse. Discussion of the pros and cons and the worries that went into each treatment option helped each of these men come to a decision so they could move forward with their individualized treatment plan. I would argue that regardless of the outcome in 3 months, 3 years, or three decades, they each made the RIGHT decision for themselves, given the thought, research, and consultation they put into the process. I also believe that these pretreatment discussions helped them accommodate whatever outcome they would face. In football, it is said that quarterbacks with shorter memories are more successful. That is true for tennis players and golfers as well. Spending too much time looking back at a bad play or a shot gone bad, or even a good one, might impair getting ready to take on the next challenge and see the opportunities to succeed at that one. Regret about unwished-for outcomes will not retrospectively help these men get what they want. But acknowledgment of the wish and expectation, as well as of the frustration, sadness, and anger aroused by a potentially disappointing outcome helps expedite emotional recovery so that people can move forward securely and safely more quickly.

Of course, neither urologists nor radiation oncologists nor medical oncologists can predict any particular outcome with certainty. They offer options based on statistics analyzed with an individual's particular medical characteristics in mind. Statistics are useful if you are not looking for guarantees or seeing outcomes as absolutes for your particular situation. You have likely heard that if there is a 1% chance of something going wrong (or right), and what goes wrong (or right) indeed happens to you, it is 100% for you. Unfortunately, we are likely light years away from a Star Trek healthcare system where diagnostics, prognostics, and treatments will come with iron-clad guarantees after the wave of a wand. Keep in mind that data about outcomes, in order to be helpful, must be applicable and generalizable in some way to your situation. So a 40% chance of a particular favorable outcome is a lot better than a 20% chance;

however, each number in itself has room for error; and even with the 40% prediction, there can still be a 60% chance of a different outcome. Population-based statistics about prognosis do not take into account some very important variables that are unique to you—your genetics, your current overall health, the medications that you take that may help or impede recuperation, your ability to recover from a treatment, your social supports, and your history of exercise, smoking or drinking, or lifestyle issues that can also impact recuperation and outcome. That is what you hope your doctor will do in recommending a treatment choice to you. Additionally, the outcome may not be a pure either-or endpoint; there may be gradations—such as some degree of urinary incontinence, or an erection that is strong enough for intercourse but without the same degree of presurgery rigidity or length. Maybe the cancer is not ultimately cured but stays relatively dormant for many years. Of course, many men view the world from an either-or/black-or-white perspective, especially regarding a bodily function prior to prostate cancer—it works or it doesn't work; thus any urinary incontinence or erectile problems may be experienced as complete dysfunction or failure—it doesn't work!

It would be ludicrous to ignore statistics altogether. They can give very important images of the lay of the land. As the author Nate Silver suggests in his book, *The Signal and the Noise*, it is useful to understand the difference between "the signal" (information that plays an important role in causal connections) and "the noise" (superfluous information that may be associated with effects, but often misleads in terms of definite causation) when trying to forecast outcomes. So it is helpful to accept the fluidity and inexactness of statistics as they may relate to your particular situation. Then you might derive practical benefit from the numbers and not be paralyzed, mesmerized, or demoralized by them. Statistics and nomograms can guide you to making more informed decisions while maintaining a realistic outlook and managing your prostate cancer as best as possible. But the numbers cannot tell the whole story, and therefore they cannot provide the crystal ball into the future that most men would like.

It is useful to ask yourself, "What scares me most about this treatment decision"? Is it a particular complication: "Will I be able to have a full erection again" or "Will I be able to control my urine?" Or, "What will sex be like if I have a weaker orgasm but I can't ejaculate? What will sex be like if I pee when I come?" Do you have a fear of dying earlier than anticipated or hoped for or of not accomplishing some major goal before death? Is there some other conscious or unconscious fear that accompanies your treatment decision, similar to a scene in a movie where an actor says one thing and a captioned commentary is seen at the bottom of the screen about what he or she is *really* thinking?

Concerns about surgery include getting anesthesia; prolonged recovery times; the need in the early postoperative recovery period for a urinary catheter; incontinence that can take months to improve; and ED that can take 6 months to 2 years to improve, perhaps never fully regaining presurgical rigidity.

Concerns about Surgery

Anesthesia
"Maybe I won't wake up."
"Maybe they won't give me enough and I'll wake up in the middle of surgery."
Prolonged recovery after the procedure (less with robotic procedures)
Need for postoperative urinary catheter
Urinary incontinence that can take months to improve and maybe not completely
Erectile dysfunction can take 6 months to 2 years to improve, perhaps not completely

---

Fears about radiation therapy include the need for daily treatments for many weeks, with the possibility of fatigue; urinary incontinence; and urinary bleeding and bowel problems either immediately or down the road. With radiation therapy there can be delayed ED years after the treatment has ended. One man described having to hold onto his urine early on during his radiation therapy as being "like torture."

Concerns about Radiation Therapy

Daily treatments for 2–3 months
Fatigue during treatments and for months afterward
Urinary incontinence
Urinary and bowel problems immediately or in the future
Good erections early on, but delayed problems years after treatment

Fears and anxieties can often be addressed quite directly. It can be helpful to speak with someone from the anesthesia team before the day of surgery about what happens during surgery today, in the new millennium. Doubts can be addressed for those who have not had anesthesia previously, or for someone who is afraid of "being put to sleep forever or not being able to wake up," or for the man who had ether as anesthesia when he was a boy 60 years ago for an appendectomy and had an uncomfortable experience. Anesthetic agents and techniques continue to change and improve decade by decade.

If you've had the good fortune of never having had surgery or any major medical problem previously, and you've never had to deal with hospitals, it may be helpful to speak to another patient who has already gone through the surgery or radiation regimen that is planned for you. Finding out what another's experience was like may address incorrect yet widespread assumptions that our fearful, adrenalized brains imagine will happen to us. Though it would be foolhardy to generalize from one patient's experience to what lies in store for you, this conversation might clarify issues, give some guidance, validate your experience that this is scary stuff for most men, but not lethal. It may also dispel some untrue myths or beliefs.

Talk to the Experts about Your Concerns

Urologists
Radiation oncologists
Anesthetists
Patients who had the procedures you are thinking about choosing

Many men have found that creating a pros and cons list of each treatment option is helpful to get a different and, hopefully, better view of the decision landscape. One patient told me, "Some men think better in a linear fashion; I think better in a circular fashion. By visualizing things from a different perspective, I understand better." You can include the known statistics of each item in this list, but also note how important each element is to you, your family, your life, and your lifestyle, now and in the future. I've formulated a sample pros and cons list to give you an idea of how it is done (Table 2.1). You can rate those items to signify how important those pros or cons are to you.

TABLE 2.1 SAMPLE PROS AND CONS LIST FOR TREATMENTS AND COMPLICATIONS

Surgery		Radiation	
Pro	**Con**	**Pro**	**Con**
Second pathology report	Urinary catheter (not sure I can handle that)	Fewer urinary problems (important to me)	Possible bladder problems
Hands/eyes-on view of tumor and possible tumor extension (sounds good to me)	Increased risk of immediate ED (can last 2 years)	Daily staff support (I think I might need a lot of support)	Delayed ED (can be years later) Likelihood of adjuvant hormonal therapy
?Longer track record; 10-year life expectancy for good prognosis	Urinary problems (not sure I could stand using diapers)	10-year life expectancy for good prognosis	Possible bowel problems (diarrhea, bleeding) (I don't think I could handle those)
The tumor is out	Anesthesia		9 weeks of treatment (how will I work?)
Short-term hassle	Wound healing		Fatigue (I hate feeling tired)

So my bottom line message is this: Beware of statistics but be aware of them. As Mark Twain once said, "Facts are stubborn, but statistics are more pliable." Even predictive nomograms that take into account multiple variables such as PSA levels and biopsy information such as Gleason score cannot show you a three-dimensional version of your life. Patients can feel shattered when told by one urologist that they are not good candidates for a radical prostatectomy, and then have hopes, suspicions, and apprehensions raised when told by another urologist that they are good surgical candidates. There is a sense of devastation if you find out your illness is either too advanced or not in a good location for a treatment option you were hoping to use. It may be even harder to hear that you are not a good candidate for a particular treatment because you are not in good enough shape or not young enough. This can be another dashed hope or expectation.

Another statistical dilemma is trying to figure out if a surgeon's statistical outcomes or results are a measure of the surgical skill of the surgeon, or a measure of how complicated the patients are, or both. Complex cases may lead to higher levels of ED or urinary incontinence. Men with prostate cancer often juggle consideration of many unequal variables and multiple tradeoffs: better or worse longevity with one option or physician or cancer center vs. better or worse quality of life with another treatment option, physician, or cancer center; one complication more likely with one treatment or practitioner may be felt to be more tolerable than another more predictable complication with a second treatment or physician.

Some men with prostate cancer are told that they are not good risks for nerve-sparing surgery, for a variety of health reasons. These men feel let down and already behind the eight ball, as if they are now going for the next best treatment, feeling rejected and scared. But without a crystal ball, questions without clear answers will linger:

"How can I know for sure what the best treatment option is for me?"
"Will I be able to deal with the discomfort of not knowing for sure?"
"Will I hit a home run, or strike out?"
"How am I supposed to understand the doctor's statistics for me?"

Before the Doctor Visit

If there is a reliable family member or friend who can accompany you to the visit, ask them to do so. Two heads are often better than one, especially when I consider how many people tell me that their brains "turn off" once the doctor starts talking, and sometimes as soon as they entered the exam room—just from anxiety about what they think the doctor will say or hope he or she will not say. A family member or good friend will help you better absorb and digest all that the doctor has to say. Review with a family member or friend before arriving at the doctor's office what questions you might have or want answered before you leave the doctor's office. If you have many questions, ask your physician if he or she wants the list in advance so enough time can be scheduled for your visit. Write the questions down beforehand to save anxiety later on. Handheld electronic equipment like a Blackberry, Android, or iPhone or a similar device can be useful for this purpose. This will allow your visit to be more productive, and your questions will be more comprehensive and thoughtful. It will help if you or your companion takes notes on the doctor's answers. After the visit, compare notes and understanding of what was said.

Prepare for the Office Visit

Choose someone to accompany you to the office visit.

Prepare a list of questions the day before the visit.

Allow extra time for travel.

Plan for a longer than expected time for your visit.

Bring a notebook or electronic tablet and take notes during the discussion with the physician.

Debrief with your companion after the visit.

Don't schedule pressing engagements for immediately following the appointment.

If you have a difficult night sleeping before the doctor visit, and don't usually have strong coffee, the day you visit the doctor might not be the morning to start. Caffeine can jump-start anxiety; it can also stimulate a strong need to urinate frequently. The same is true for alcohol. Using alcohol to calm you or to fall asleep the night before a doctor's visit may be counterproductive. Alcohol can get in the way of having the clear head you will want for discussing issues that can affect the rest of your life. Alcohol also will make you need to urinate more frequently. If you feel anxiety or distress, acknowledge it rather than attempting to hide it. You can use the DRAFT with Emotional Judo techniques described in Chapter 4 to relieve some or all of your anxiety; trying to ignore anxiety leads men to feel overwhelmed by it. If you do feel overwhelmed, let your doctor know so you can get assistance.

The Waiting Room Wait

Some men go into a urologist's or oncologist's waiting room feeling like cattle waiting for slaughter. However, you can take some control here. It is no secret why these areas are called "waiting rooms." In fact, entry rooms of most medical practices should probably be called "really long waiting rooms," and not because of their size. Once you complete your wait outside the examination room, you can then look forward to even more waiting inside the exam room. And if you are being cared for at an academic center, you will likely see a nurse and then a resident or fellow trainee before you get to see the attending physician you made the appointment to see in the first place. I strongly believe that these academic environments provide a model for assuring excellent quality of care through a system of checks and balances with multiple reviews and more than one set of eyes. But patients used to the one-doctor routine get frustrated. Visits usually take longer than expected. Periodically, patients or family members already look and feel tired, frustrated, and sometimes angry in the waiting room, and they haven't gotten any news, good or bad, yet. Inadvertently, what was already an upsetting situation (a new cancer diagnosis) has been made into a more inconvenient and life-interfering scenario.

Give the doctor visit your full attention, and anticipate all aspects of the visit. Even though you may wait longer in the waiting room before your visit, allow extra time (for you and those who come with you) to get there. Many couples complain about the other person wanting to be too early or having worries about being too late. It is difficult to correctly anticipate traffic delays, public transportation snafus, or parking problems. Remember, your partner is not the enemy. Be ready for compromise. When you make the appointment, ask what the time range might be for how long your visit might take. Do not schedule a business luncheon or pressing engagement for immediately after the expected end of the doctor's appointment. This will make the entire visit more stressful than it needs to be if your doctor is running late, and you will obsess about whether you will get out in time to make your next engagement. You might start fuming as the minutes tick away. We might all treat doctor visits a little differently if waiting rooms were called "activity rooms." Bring "busying" activities with you. These may include business projects; laptop computers; a Blackberry, an Android or iPhone, or similar handheld device for e-mail or texting (talking on cell phones is discouraged in open waiting rooms because of the noise and discomfort for others); or a device loaded with music, books, audiotapes, or downloads and games. Magazines, puzzles, or paperwork come in handy as well. Pack a few snacks (this is a good place to catch up on your green tea supplements if brought in a thermos) that you like. Bring a few types of diversions so that if you are disturbed by the environment or bored by one activity, you can find another that may work better. Do not spend time online (assuming wireless service is available) searching prostate cancer–related information. It will likely heighten your waiting room angst. If you want to read about or research non-cancer issues, fine. You are not studying for a test and will not benefit by becoming a prostate cancer expert now. That is what your doctors are for.

Waiting in a doctor's office is a great opportunity to meditate. If you are not familiar with a meditation technique, look into the one I describe in Chapter 4. It is okay to skip ahead and start learning and practicing that now if you'd like.

If you find yourself waiting for more than 30 minutes, ask the office clerk if you have time to take a short walk around the building you are in or outside if the weather is nice. Give the clerk your cell phone number in case you are called for your appointment. Depending on the time of day, you might even have a chance for lunch or a snack or some window shopping outside. Some hospitals have taken a tip from the restaurant world and give out flashing beepers that alert you when you can go into the exam room.

Passing the Time in the Waiting Room and Waiting in the Exam Room

Bring busying activities: books, games, music (with ear buds/ headphones), distracting work projects.
Meditate.
Bring snacks.
Ask to take a walk and be called on your cell phone when it's your turn to go into the exam room.

Stop Keeping Up (and Down) with the Joneses: Don't Get Caught in a Thought Trap

There are hazards, like golf course sand traps, that can get you feeling down or nervous. You are likely not the only one waiting to see your doctor. And if you are in a clinic situation, there may be many men with prostate cancer or people with other cancers waiting to see their doctors. It is almost impossible not to notice who else is waiting. But it is important to remember that most of us are generally poor interpreters of what someone else's situation is just by looking at them. But this is what men do all the time. It is not productive and it can be very anxiety provoking. It is easy to compare yourself to men who look healthier than you and wonder if you will have their good luck. You may make negative self-comparisons with others who look stronger and healthier ("the grass is greener syndrome") and wonder, "How come my luck was not as good?" It is even more unsettling to see someone who looks more ill than you and wonder if that is the road you will be heading down, and when. To be forewarned is to be forearmed. Men don't always realize they've been making comparisons with other patients that have nothing to do with their reality until they notice themselves fidgeting more and stewing about their visit. On the one hand, it is hard not to notice others. On the other hand, you are not obliged to keep looking and daydreaming about "what if...."

When you see other men in a brief cross-section of time who look sicker than you and you wonder, "How much longer 'til I get as bad as them?" you are indeed assuming that the other man is sicker and more debilitated than you and that his condition is permanent. Keep in mind that comparing from your own situation to another's, or vice versa, is risky because there is a very large margin for error. Men with prostate cancer may have different cell types and different stages of disease at any point in time as well as at the time of diagnosis, and they may have had different treatments and different regimens of the same treatment. Medical care always needs to be individualized. This is why Internet hunting can be so frustrating. Men tolerate the same treatments differently and have diverse complications. Every man comes to his prostate cancer experience with a different genetic and physiological makeup, having had unique life experiences and losses, as well as having developed his own coping patterns for dealing with those experiences. Each has distinctive support systems and health problems. Men have unique needs for the amount and type of information that will help them make the best treatment and life decisions for them. The need for control or the ability to give up control in making a treatment choice varies from man to man. Many factors are shared among men with prostate cancer; however, there are many variables that make people distinct that must be accounted for, not only by the patient's physician but also by the patient himself and his family. For instance, when Mayor Rudolph Giuliani was diagnosed with prostate cancer, the New York news sources reported that he decided to have brachytherapy, a type of radiation therapy that entails short-term placement of radioactive seeds into the prostate to kill the cancer cells. Men who had already chosen prostatectomy (even years before brachytherapy had become more refined and acceptable) were questioning their past choice, and newly diagnosed men who were recommended to have other treatments (i.e., external beam radiation therapy or prostatectomy) demanded to know why they were not getting "the Mayor's" brachytherapy. They were fearful of not getting the best treatment. If you start to freak out because you think you made, or will make, the wrong treatment choice, remember some of the thought traps you might be stepping into: buyer's remorse and making the RIGHT CHOICE. Uncertainty can pull you in the wrong direction.

In Chapter 4, you will learn to use the DRAFT with Emotional Judo techniques to handle these stressful periods. You will learn strategies to deal with feelings of regret or fear that you made a wrong decision because it differed from someone else's. You will learn how to

1. **D**etect the anxiety or fear
2. **R**ecognize where the anxiety is coming from
3. **A**cknowledge the rational and irrational aspects of your thoughts: "I am worried that I did not (or will not) make the correct treatment choice; I am worried because I want to live a long and healthy life and now I am scared that hope is compromised; I am worried because my friend's erections did not get better after surgery and that might happen to me"
4. **F**lip to the more rational, glass half-full aspects of your life and health circumstances, often beginning with the word *however*: "However, I sought expert opinions and asked around and I read a lot of material. I am feeling pretty healthy otherwise. I've made excellent decisions in the past. I have to believe that my treatment was/will be the best choice for me when I made/make it" and
5. **T**ransform the somber, anxious feelings or thoughts through distraction into something more life-enhancing right now: "Let me pull out my crossword puzzle while I'm waiting," or "Let me take a walk with my partner or call my daughter."

As noted earlier, information from other patients and the Internet can be very useful. Others can help you understand some general parameters or responses, as well as to see that one can get through the treatment, overcome complications, and be able, after the tincture of time for physical and emotional recuperation, to speak about it in an encouraging way. However, it is important not to take any information too literally and to *try not to generalize* from any one situation to your own.

> While waiting to see the radiologist for a second opinion for primary treatment, I saw this man who told me he and all his friends had radiation therapy, and they all did very well with no urinary problems and no sexual problems. "Everyone should have it," he said, and I felt the cards were stacked against surgery.

If you asked this man who had the radiation how many of his friends he was discussing, he might have said two or even three. Had we spoken to his friends we may have found out that their pre-cancer health and sex lives were different from that of gentleman who was waiting for the second opinion, or we may have found out that their prognoses were significantly different, or perhaps that you cannot always count on what men tell their friends about their sex lives or urinary function. Just as statistics can be confusing and inadvertently deceptive for a man who wants to know where he will stand in the future as a unique entity, it is problematic to generalize from the experience of one or a few men and believe that is how you will wind up. Have you ever purchased an item you were disappointed with that a friend raved about? Or have you listened to a highly recommended *"could-not-miss* song," or read a *"great* novel," or seen a *"fantastic* movie" and felt let down? It doesn't mean one shouldn't listen to others' experiences and recommendations about their choices and perhaps try some out; however, the listening about health issues must be done with a discerning ear—this is information that you will assess in the context of your body and lifestyle, but will not be a blanket guarantee of a particular outcome. "My friend recommended a doctor very highly. I didn't like her—she didn't spend enough time answering my questions." This sounds like common sense. It is. It is important to keep these concerns in mind to avoid this all-too-common thought trap of overgeneralizing.

During the Doctor Visit

When you have face-to-face time with the nurse and physician, remember to pull out your list of questions or points you want to discuss. Write down the facts, the answers to your questions, and other things you are told by your consultant. Being prepared may help alleviate some symptoms of *white coat syndrome*, a term usually referring to the increase in blood pressure many of us have as we go into a physician's office, just because we are nervous about what will ensue, the results of tests, the potential diagnoses of severe illnesses that may require onerous treatment.

> Q: Can a doctor get white coat syndrome?
> A: Yes, when he becomes a patient.
>
> I, too, had "white coat" syndrome or "doctor's office" anxiety. I hadn't yet lost complete hearing in one ear, yet I didn't "hear" a lot of what the doctor said because I was nervous—about understanding what was being said; about having good questions to ask; about fearing I would forget what was said. It's true. Even psychiatrists can be anxious when they are patients. But I did not want my anxiety to sabotage the best outcome I could get. So when I visited doctors about my neuroma, I had all of my symptoms, questions, and concerns written down in my Blackberry, to make sure I didn't forget any of them. I was less anxious because of my list. It felt weird going through all of the questions, especially as I knew doctors had full waiting rooms, but it was necessary for my care. I assumed that the other patients would get adequate attention for all of their questions as well.

Not everyone is naturally assertive, but try to cover as many bases as possible. If you do not understand what the staff is telling you, especially medical jargon or statistics, politely ask them to stop and clarify! Ask for an explanation, so you know that you understand. Once you start to feel lost, it can be difficult to get back on track. If you still feel like a question has not been answered, try to rephrase it. It may be that there is not a good answer to your question, or that what the doctor is saying is not what you want to hear. Try to clear up as much as possible. It is a good practice to repeat, and preferably rephrase, your physician's or nurse's answers back to them in your own words. That way you and they know that you understand. Some patients like to record the conversation so they can listen to it at home and not have to worry about catching everything that is said in the office. A possible downside to this is you may be more passive during the discussion and you still may not understand what was said when you listen to the recording later at home—resolving questions or statements in real time is important. Listening to the recording later can be very time-consuming. Alert your doctor to your desire to record the visit. He or she may have sufficient information written down already that you can review when you leave. But as with most optional strategies, try it if you think it might help. If it works, continue it. The flip side of not being assertive enough is being too aggressive or challenging in your discussion with the physician. You may inadvertently risk not developing an alliance with the person you may be counting on to give you life-saving treatment.

There has been much research and teaching about how to improve communication between patients and physicians. Doctors, in general, and oncologists in particular, now learn specific communication techniques in medical school and all the way through their training to aid understanding and improve rapport with patients. Researchers have highlighted the importance of clarifying medical situations and treatment recommendations. You are looking for an understanding dialogue and clarifications with your oncology team that will facilitate optimal treatment and care for you. Don't be shy about making that list of questions before you go to see your doctor. Then, do not be too intimidated to ask your questions.

Possible Questions to Ask Your Oncology Team

If I don't have symptoms, how do you know this cancer is bad?

Why should I do anything if I have no symptoms now?

Is active surveillance a reasonable treatment choice for me? Why? Why not?

With active surveillance, how often and for how long do I have to have follow-up PSA tests and biopsies?

Are there potential consequences of not doing active surveillance?

How long will recuperation take after surgery?

How long will recuperation take after radiation therapy?

What's the likelihood of recurrence? How and when will we know?

Are there any other treatments that might work?

What changes should I make to my diet? Alcohol use? Tobacco? Exercise?

What are the consequences of not doing the suggested treatment?

What can you do to decrease the side effects of adjuvant hormonal therapy?

What does this cancer and my treatment mean for my son(s); grandson(s)?

Specialist Questions

Urology

How many prostatectomies do you do in a year?

Do you do the nerve-sparing technique?

Do you only do open prostatectomies, or robotic surgery as well?

How many of each do you do per year?

What are your particular statistics regarding erectile dysfunction or urinary continence with open prostatectomy, with robotic surgery?

What is the range of time it takes until erectile strength is sufficient for penetration?

How many men can get erections as firm as their pre-surgery baseline?

Why would you choose a particular procedure for me?

What are the likely down sides of each procedure for me?

How do you see the pros and cons of surgery vs. radiation therapy for me?

Radiation Oncology

Would you recommend external beam radiation, brachytherapy, or a combination? Why would you choose a particular one or combination for my situation?

Why do you recommend both types sequentially?

What about CyberKnife™ or proton beam therapy for me? I hear about them on the radio.

Are those therapies very different from regular radiation therapy?

How many of your patients get urinary or bowel complications? How severe are they?

Are those complications treatable? How well?

What is the range of recuperation until full energy returns?

What are the risks regarding erections with radiation therapy?

What are the likely down sides of each procedure for me in particular, apart from the general statistics?

Do you suggest adjuvant hormone treatment? Why or why not?

How long do I need to take the hormones, before and after the radiation therapy?

What are the long-term consequences of those hormones for me?

How do you see the pros and cons of radiation therapy vs. surgery for me?

Although it is important to choose a surgeon who has done many of these procedures, it is equally important to make sure the person does it well. As best as you can, try to find out if the surgeon takes all comers or at least enough men who are similar to you in age, health status, and stage of disease, and what the track record for complications is.

It can feel embarrassing to discuss bodily functions like ED and urinary and bowel function—even with a doctor. It is also difficult to con-
vert statistics into what might actually happen to you. But it's important
to have these discussions. Consider practicing or rehearsing at home if
you think it might help.

It is reasonable to ask all of the doctors any or all of the following:

"If there are any complications from the treatment, how do you deal with
     and manage them?"
"Do I get to speak to you, a nurse practitioner, or a trainee if there are
     problems after I get home?"
"Are there specialists you recommend for erectile or urinary problems if
     recovery is stalled?"
"Is there anything you recommend to prevent these complications?"
"How long do the problems last?"
"Are there any exercises or diet changes that I should be starting now?"

In an existential dance with the physician, men often fumble around
the question of time frames. The most obvious yet most unanswerable
question is "How long do I have to live?" Other questions include the
following:

"When do I get out of the hospital?"
"When will my treatment be over?"
"When will the catheter come out?"
"When will I be continent of urine again?"
"When will I be able to have sex again?"
"How often will you monitor my PSA?"
"If this treatment fails, what will we do next?"

All of these are reasonable questions; however, not all of them will have
accurately predictable answers when you ask. And not all of them have
to be asked, even though they pop into your head periodically. Ask yourself how the information will help you cope better and live a better life.
Pinning your doctor down to specific dates and times may not be helpful,
as this does not take into account the unpredictable and dynamic nature

of healing and biology. If you are curious, or feel you need to know information because of planning for the future, ask the doctor for a time range, and make sure you hear the latter date in that range, which will take account of the complications that may occur. And try not to watch the clock.

If you don't want to know certain information, it's good to let your doctor know that as well. Some men do not want to hear time frames, knowing there is a wide range of accuracy of predictions. Others will hear predicted time frames as literal deadlines, which may not facilitate a better lived life.

Let your doctor know what you do want to know:

"I want to know if the treatment is not working, but I don't want to know every detail about where the cancer is progressing to."
"I'm a visual guy—if you can show me and explain what's going on in my scans, I will better understand what's going on in my body and how we are going to treat my disease."

Most people do not like thinking about advanced directives when they are relatively healthy. So why bring up an end-of-life topic in the section of this book written for men with early stage prostate cancer who may still be cured? Decisions about advanced directives are best made at exactly this time. It is no different than considering writing a last will and testament when you do not expect to die, but you know it is important to prepare for the unthinkable when you have all your faculties and can have clear discussions with your family and oncology team. Assigning a healthcare proxy is important, as is explaining your choices to significant others, especially if your wishes are not to follow your accepted next-of-kin lineage (i.e., spouse, parents, adult child, sibling, etc.).

One healthy 68-year-old man said, "If something goes wrong with my surgery, I don't think my wife would be able to sign a Do Not Resuscitate form for me at the proper time. I made my wishes very clear to my brother, who will honor my wishes. It was not an easy discussion with my wife; however, she understood. Hopefully, it won't need to be put into place."

Many men seek multiple second opinions from urological surgeons, radiation oncologists, and medical prostate oncologists. Unfortunately, there are legitimate biases and disagreements among these medical practitioners about the best treatment for any particular man with a particular stage and type of disease. Many urologists lean toward prostatectomy, while radiation oncologists may more often endorse radiation (external beam, brachytherapy, or seed implants). Patients are often looking for a clue that makes them more than a statistic. They are looking for an advantage, as one looks for a magical tip or sign before placing a bet on a horse race. For instance, ears are primed for the urologist who says, "If you were my father (or brother) I would tell you that you should definitely do XYZ treatment as opposed to ABC." A radiation oncologist who says, "If I were in your shoes, I would have the surgery," or, conversely, a urologist who says, "I'd suggest you go with radiation," could cause a patient to think: "Someone who would actually cross professional lines must really believe that this is the correct and best decision for me." But beware, some practitioners who "cross lines" may be telling you more about their inexperience, lack of knowledge, or discomfort with the complexity of a procedure, rather than the best choice for you. After seeing urologists and radiation oncologists, some patients look to medical oncologists as the tiebreakers, who have nothing to gain or lose by what treatment one initially chooses.

Active Surveillance or Watchful Waiting

The non-active treatment route has been known by at least three terms: *watchful waiting, expectant monitoring*, or *active surveillance*. Watchful waiting and expectant monitoring are essentially two names for the same process. They are recommended for older men who have significant medical illnesses and less than 10-year life expectancy at the time of prostate cancer diagnosis. There is less aggressive follow-up than for younger men getting active surveillance. The fear of potential quality-of-life deficits from active treatment is weighed against the hope of a longer life span. It is this very controversy that has fueled the debate on the benefits of population PSA screening noted earlier. In multiple large-scale population studies, the unpredictable trade-off of longer life span did not seem to outweigh the cost (financially and in terms of quality of life) of active treatment (either surgery or radiation) once a cancer is found. Once found, it must be followed and perhaps treated. With active surveillance, men receive frequent PSA tests and recurrent biopsies to observe for any changes in disease status or prognosis that will signal a need for active treatment. Anxiety can build before each PSA test and can take time to resolve even when good news is received. One of the larger risks of active surveillance, or non-active treatment, is that a man does not take it seriously because his situation does not warrant treatment. Physicians are concerned about men who are not compliant with strict follow-up and ongoing monitoring and one day find that the cancer has progressed to advanced stages, and a chance for cure is no longer possible.

Helpful Hints for the Two Sides of a Couple

Patient

Does anyone like a back-seat driver? It is difficult to say where a partner fits into the treatment decision process. On the one hand, it is your body that has the cancer and YOUR life that is threatened, right? On the other hand, your spouse or life partner will have to live with this cancer too—with the treatment decision and any complications that ensue, as well as the prognostic outcome—often as a caregiver in the immediate treatment period and perhaps for years to come. Yes, it's about THEIR life, too. Thoughts of possible life alone are common, even if this is early-stage disease. If there are sexual or other long-term side effects, your spouse or partner will deal with those as well. Your partner is the confidant of the lover who may be angry, sad, or complaining about the unwanted changes or outcome. Given how these decisions affect a family, it is useful to discuss the advantages and disadvantages of treatment options as a couple, as they may impact both of you. At this point, most

partners say they'd rather have their loved one alive for as long as possible and sacrifice sex if needed. Many men can't believe that, as they see
sex as a crucial part of their identity as men and as a couple, even if they
are not having intercourse very often anymore. The fear of taking away
erections and sex feels like life will only be filled by an unexciting, embarrassing void. Honestly discussing this potential loss is vital. Appreciating
the physical and emotional links that sexual intercourse has provided,
yet discussing how essential physical closeness and intimacy have been
and can remain, allows for a more realistic and acceptable picture. You
are not heading into a vacuum but toward a transition to a different kind
of loving that may have unforeseen benefits.

Some men see urinary incontinence as an even more important problem than sexual functioning that might influence their treatment decision; others see it as a secondary, cumbersome problem. It is difficult to
imagine what urinary incontinence will be like and how it might influence your day-to-day life. An honest discussion with your partner can be
enlightening. Some partners deal with urinary incontinence as they age
as well. But the abrupt complication from prostate cancer treatment may
have significant meaning to a man, making it difficult to accept a partner
saying, "Well I got used to it and so could you."

Partners

Avoid telling your husband or partner, "Don't worry honey, everything
will be fine." Unless there is a legitimate crystal ball that you've been
hiding in the drawer for just this occasion, you are likely to be met with
anger and bewilderment the more scared your partner is: "How the hell
do you know?" It's a little like saying, "Don't think about a pink elephant
for the next 2 minutes." This gives our brains an inadvertent dare and
holds the power of suggestion.

If you can, let your husband or partner know you are there
for him and will help with decisions if he wants, and that you
will do what you can to try to make this work out well. Ask him,
"How can I help?" though very often he will not know the answer.
Validate the unfairness of this. Offer to sit with him to determine

what needs to get done and whom to call, to develop a pre-visit list of questions, to develop his pros and cons lists (described earlier in this chapter), or to do some research. If he is paralyzed by fear, proposing that you do some legwork may be welcomed. Otherwise, you may come across as pushy and demanding, even though you are trying to be helpful. Many men feel as if their diagnosis has taken away their sense of being in control of their destiny, so any opportunities for reclaiming that control are usually appreciated, unless they are too paralyzed by fear. With too much anxiety, distinctions among options are not recognized. Splitting the tasks can help both of you feel as if you are in this together. Too often men inadvertently do not appreciate how a spouse is also affected by the diagnosis and the powerlessness that she or he also feels against a formidable opponent. As a partner you can offer to set up doctor appointments; do online research to try to distinguish the wheat from the chaff of suggested treatments; offer to accompany your partner or husband on physician visits; offer to set up social visits, and to respect when he does not feel like socializing; ask who is okay to talk to about your (pleural) new crisis so that you can get support when he can't offer it. This last question allows your husband or partner to have some control over who knows about this crisis in your lives.

Men and Partners

Addressing these matters together can assure each of you that you are not in this alone. Caring communication about needs or desires or dislikes is extremely important. But remember, no one is perfect. Nerves that feel frayed during this sensitive period can lead to misconstrued intentions and bickering with attacks whose wake seems never to disappear and that gets refueled with subsequent arguments. The helplessness and vulnerability that lie just below the surface are easily scratched and offended. Though we will discuss dealing with couple conflict in Chapter 8, a helpful saying we use in psychotherapy is, "Strike when the iron is cold." Let tempers cool before you discuss the issue again. Pushing on a sore spot is a distraction that your home team does not need now.

My wife was a priceless ally for me when I was deciding on treatment for my acoustic neuroma. She did what couples that come to see me for consultation do. She was mostly helpful, but sometimes not; most of the time it worked for me and us, sometimes it did not. She helped find second opinions and set up appointments, but also heard when I thought we had seen enough doctors. She accompanied me on office visits when she could. We argued at times, usually when I got frustrated at not having my own crystal ball. I am grateful she did not hold a grudge. We also hugged a lot.

This is not a bad time to review the lives you have had together: Recall when you dated, made a commitment to each other, your careers, the joys and angst raising children, important decisions you made together in the past, and other significant health issues that you, or others close to you, have dealt with. It is not a "life flashing before my eyes" moment portending death. It is reaffirming your strengths and acknowledging weaknesses, highlights and hassles, prideful commemorations, embarrassing or remorseful memories, as well as your ability to ride with the waves and punches of your life together. This can be an important signal to each other that in the face of this mortal warning and perilous time, you each continue to have a partner.

Many couples socialize with other couples but do not often socialize just with each other as the familiarity of years creeps into a long-term relationship. One way to defuse the distress about the future is to rediscover "the date." Fight the urge of resistance and inertia and go out to the movies, dinner, a concert, or for a walk in the park together. Reinforce the essence of your bond, the vows you may have made to each other years before—in sickness and in health, for better or for worse, 'til death do you part—as well as your hopes and recommitment for the future, since many of us do not fully acknowledge "sickness," "worse," or "death" when committing.

Single Men

It may be difficult to find a confidant to talk over these issues with if you are not in a committed relationship. Think about your usual social network for support. Good friends can be extremely helpful both for listening to the treatment options you face and to accompany you on medical visits. Other family members, such as siblings, cousins, nieces, or nephews, have been very helpful to my single patients. Some men who have good relationships with their primary care doctors will use them as sounding boards for decision-making dilemmas to see what makes sense to them. Discussing these issues with a therapist can also be beneficial.

Magical Thinking and Leaving No Stone Unturned

Many of the men I counsel have spent numerous hours, days, and months in libraries and bookstores, on the Internet and on chat sites exploring the ins and outs of prostate cancer treatments and complications trying to find as much information as they can to give them some edge to come up with the RIGHT TREATMENT CHOICE—to get a hoped-for, sure-fire outcome for their cancer treatment. They are looking for the option that has a strong likelihood of cure, a warranty of no recurrence, and no untoward or lasting side effects or complications (especially sexual dysfunction or urinary or bowel problems). Their search is geared toward gaining better control of the situation and decreasing their anxiety. Decision-making tools discussed earlier, like predictive nomograms that take into account various medical variables, as well as anecdotal information, are helpful to identify useful diagnostic, and treatment variables and their impact on outcome, but they do not offer the assurance or personal individual guarantee that most men want. Unfortunately, distress rises with the recognition that an ironclad guarantee for any man does not exist.

You can feel bewitched by the coincidence of prostate cancer–related ads that pop up on your computer. It may have more to do with software surveillance cookies than with coincidence or synchronicity.

When I heard a commercial come on the radio for radiation therapy for prostate cancer, I paid extra attention. I had never heard the commercial before, and I felt like this meant something special for me.

Many men spend a lot of time on the Internet looking for information that will "talk to them." They don't want to leave any stone unturned in finding the right answer for their treatment. They read blogs from patients and look at websites from highly respected as well as not so highly respected places, not really being sure what is credible and perhaps, more importantly, what will make a difference for them. We all need to recognize why we are pulled toward or pushed away from certain doctors, hospitals, or treatments: "The urologist I saw grew up in the same neighborhood in Chicago that I did, and he went to the same medical school as my friend Lou. He must be good." Or: "The radiation oncologist had a cancellation right before I called so I can get an appointment this week instead of the usual 3 weeks. This must be a good sign."

When I had to decide about my own treatment choice, I recognized the fantasy I had for some magical, wizard healer to come out of the woodwork, like a genie out of a bottle, and tell me, "For the best outcome with the least likelihood of complications you should go to Dr. So and So and have the QRX treatment and everything will be all right. Dr. House, where are you?" I was looking for the crystal ball, though I knew it did not exist. I often thought, "I don't know how to make the right decision. I just want to know that everything will turn out fine." I feared losing my hearing. What would that be like for a psychiatrist? I feared having a facial droop. My mind was beginning the process of grieving for the loss of my health as I had known it. No one was dying here, but I was losing a lot, even if my hearing stayed stable and there was no facial droop from the surgery. I was losing tangible and intangible parts of my life. I was mourning the loss of being able to take my health for granted; I had had 49 years of waking up day after day, assuming I would be more or less as healthy as I was the day before. The questions mounted: "What would it be like to go from stereo to monaural if I lose my hearing? Will I be able to play the guitar and sing on key? Will the ocean sound the same in just one ear? What will I do if I have a permanent frown from a facial droop? Shit! I am not a blank-slate therapist."

Most of my prostate cancer patients take urinary continence and getting erections for granted before their cancer diagnoses and treatment; fearing the loss of natural bodily functions is part of the package. When supportive friends or family say, "I can imagine what that would be like," internal responses may be, "No, you can't." If they say, "I can't imagine what that would be like," you may ponder how unfair it is that this is happening to you and get pissed off. Your anger may bubble over, making it more difficult to get support.

With many medical opinions in hand, even with some not being covered by insurance plans, and many hours of research, men become fairly competent lay experts on prostate cancer—yet they still may feel confused about which treatment is best for them. They may want some omen or apparition to lead them to the best treatment outcome. It is hard not to overthink this problem. Men often have to be given permission and adamant advice to stop seeking more information; the RIGHT TREATMENT CHOICE is not just another mouse click away. It is usually not hiding in another wakeful nighttime hour in a darkened bedroom. At some point, you will make a choice based on a combination of your research, your gut feeling, faith, and which physicians and sources of information make the most sense to you. Your choice will be the RIGHT TREATMENT CHOICE! Yet being RIGHT will have little to do with actual outcome. Your choice will make sense, even if it feels clouded by fear and anger; without a true crystal ball, there is no way to predict the future. If a good prediction were out there, then all of the physicians you consulted with would have been in agreement about that "one good choice." Since there is no way to predict the future, you can only take your best shot with whatever information you have at the time.

Some trustworthy cancer information sources include the American Cancer Society; the National Cancer Institute—PDQ; and the Prostate Cancer Foundation. There are many others; however, even these cannot point you to the "correct" way. Unfortunately, there is too much information out there, much that is credible and much that is not. When you consider that most of that information is not targeted to you as a unique individual, it is easy to see how you can easily become overwhelmed and frustrated. There are plenty of books with excellent information about prostate cancer, but they, too, will come up short in terms of accurate predictions for you.

> I heard my own voice giving me the same advice I give to my patients when I, too, could not find the clairvoyance to choose the "ideal" treatment. I realized this when my internist supportively suggested yet another second opinion when I mentioned my difficulty deciding between surgery and radiation. I thought about it and eventually said, "No thanks. I'm done searching." Information-overload became overwhelming and a little paralyzing for me, too. A pro/con list helped me gather all of the important data points onto the table, see them in different variations, and not fear that I'd lose them if I didn't continue to review them over and over again in my mind.

Reacting to a New Diagnosis and Starting to Get Your Sea Legs

Many men with prostate cancer have a variety of emotional reactions to a new diagnosis, as do people with other types of cancer. They may have some degree of denial or disbelief initially; some may have depressed or anxious moods, anger, difficulty concentrating, or problems with sleep or appetite. They may not feel like socializing anymore and question, "Who should I tell, and who not? Can I keep a straight face and say 'everything is fine' when a friend asks, 'how are you?' Why does he have to ask?" More often than not, men do not have a major psychiatric disorder at the time of prostate cancer diagnosis, though the anxious and depressive feelings they do have can be intense at times, feel alien, and interfere with daily activities at home or at work. Men who have never felt these emotions as strongly as they do now can be quite upset about them and wonder, "If in addition to losing my physical health as I've known it, have I also lost my mind and emotional health as well?" Men ask me in a hope-seeking manner, "Are these emotions NORMAL? Am I crazy doc?" I usually answer that I've been doing this work for more than 20 years and the more I do it, the less I know what "normal" is. Distress decreases when hearing from a medical professional that these emotions are commonplace and understandable. I really can certify that these emotions do not make these men "CRAZY." These transient emotions resolve to a large degree after a few weeks as men are given time to adjust and adapt. Distress continues for some men until they begin or complete their primary treatment or recuperate from their treatment. Uncomfortable emotional reactions may recur at other crisis points, such as before PSA tests, or if a man finds out that his PSA is rising and that his treatment did not work as hoped for, or if there are more or different complications than anticipated.

Over time, most men will develop their "sea legs" for coping with these crises and their aftermath. The image of sea legs gives men a useful illustration or goal to head toward. It implies an acceptance that the familiar comfort of the world as one knew it before cancer has changed, and that the turbulence of the crisis may continue to simmer for some time. While the sea may never find a solid calmness, you will be able to stand and roll with the waves without feeling seasick or falling on your face or overboard, even though you may not feel as rock solid as you did before. In fact, though you didn't ask for this insight, the perspective you gain from adapting to this crisis may help you with other crises in the future or even let you help others with similar dilemmas, even though it may seem too early to think about paying it forward. The sea legs image also incorporates the tincture of time that helps you process and accept your new normal and move forward.

When these uncomfortable emotions last more than a few weeks at a significant enough intensity to interfere with your daily life or getting your cancer treatment, you may have developed a depressive or anxiety disorder that is *not* normal and which should be addressed and treated by a mental health practitioner. Chapters 4 and 5 will discuss these clinical entities in more depth.

Many spouses think, "He's in denial; he goes to work like nothing is happening, though his surgery is coming up next week. He's not flustered at all." A better descriptor than "denial" of this phenomenon might be "suppression," a healthier defense mechanism that is under more conscious control. These men compartmentalize well—they go to their doctor's appointments, make treatment decisions, eventually take their treatment or medications, and are able to pursue their daily work and home lives apparently without skipping a beat. When at work, they mostly think about work. When with family, they mostly think about family. Denial would be better represented by a patient thinking he does not need to set up or keep doctor appointments, or by someone who consistently does not follow through with medication suggestions or important lifestyle changes.

The night is usually the time our brains reserve for worry and anxiety, when there are fewer distractions and ample time to wrap problem-solving powers around an insurmountable challenge. Many men can become trapped in wishful or "if only" thinking:

"If only my PSA test did not rise."
"If only my biopsy was negative."
"If only the Gleason score was a 6 instead of a 9. Maybe the lab made an error" (though labs may be just as likely to make errors in the patient's prognostic favor as against a good prognostic outcome).
"Why didn't the insurance company let me get a biopsy sooner?"
"Why didn't I go back sooner for another PSA test?"
"If only the PSA goes to zero on the next test."

Sometimes a man may be repressing the information. He knows there is a cancer in him. He may forget to set up timely medical appointments, or forget to properly prepare for procedures, but his mind is very aware of the threat. This is a less healthy defense mechanism than suppression. Just because a man does not want to make a suboptimal decision does not mean that he is in denial. He is more likely feeling overwhelmed by anxiety about the potential consequences of his decision. Behaving as if there were no cancer to grapple with—there are no second opinions, no further PSA tests, and no plans made for treatment; or if a decision is made for treatment, appointments are missed—might indicate denial. When asked, these men may argue that they were never told or have any knowledge about the importance of follow-up: "I never heard."

Is He in Denial, Repression, or Just Suppressing His Concerns?

Denial	Repression	Suppression
Does not believe there is a cancer; makes no attempts at further workup or treatment	Knows there is cancer but *forgets* to do proper follow-up. He seems not to understand the severity of the situation.	Knows there is cancer, does proper follow-up, but can focus on other activities even though he is concerned about the cancer and/or treatment
He may present in the future with advanced cancer.	Treatment may be delayed or delivered suboptimally because of decreased compliance.	A good coping mechanism for the patient, but it may be difficult for family and friends

Chapter 3

Lifting the Weight of Waiting and Preparing for Treatment

Deciding Between Definitive Treatment and Watchful Waiting or Active Surveillance

Ninety percent of this . . . is half mental.

Yogi Berra

So you have made your treatment decision. If you've chosen an active treatment like radiation or surgery, you've scheduled a date for the start-up radiation simulation and will start radiation soon thereafter, or a date to be admitted for surgery. You likely have at least a few days if not weeks to wait for these relatively elective procedures and to complete preparatory tasks. For those of you who were eligible for and chose active surveillance or watchful waiting, your "treatment" has already begun. Just as anxiety can rise while waiting for biopsy results, it can rise again while waiting for surgery or radiation or your next PSA test. Waiting, whether in a waiting room or at home, can be psychological torture if that is all you are doing. Time on your hands is worry on your mind. Your mood, anxiety, and thoughts can be all over the place once a decision is made. Trying to maintain "busy-as-usual" is a nice idea. But you may have to be more proactive about how to spend your pretreatment time or while undergoing active surveillance. Idle worrying about treatment and its aftermath is not always productive and can interfere with concentration or enjoyment of other activities. You could wind up feeling like you are sitting out a jail sentence, allowing the cancer to have additional consequences on your life.

During the first days or weeks after diagnosis, some men look stoic, trying to let everyone (including themselves) know that they can handle this ordeal; they want to project a sense of calm so that, hopefully, others close to them will be calm as well. But this period may be like waiting to get back on the playing field during a rain delay or the equivalent of the military quip, "Hurry up and wait." Men often have a "numbed" mood or move into a type of automatic pilot once the treatment decision is made, just wanting to get the treatment started and over with, yet still wishing they were not in these shoes—this leads to feeling high anxiety.

> You know, doc, no one in my family ever had cancer. I've played tennis twice a week all year long for 40 years and have been in great shape since college. I never smoked and rarely drink. Since my diagnosis, I don't feel like exercising at all. I feel betrayed by my body and I wonder, "What's the point of trying to stay healthy?"

This period of waiting before treatment begins is like a Petri dish designed to breed anxiety. Worry and concern have free reign, asking and trying to answer many of the unpredictable and thus unanswerable questions. So if a man is asked, "What is there to worry about?" if he is truthful, he might answer, "Everything and anything!"

Common Treatment-Related Concerns and Questions

How will the treatment go?
What will the doctors find when they look inside?
What complications do I really not want to experience?
Which complications will actually occur?
How will I live with the complications that I do get?
What would it be like to wear diapers?
How long will the complications last?
If complications are permanent, can I cope with them?
What if the treatment doesn't work and the cancer comes back?

There are no definitive answers to these questions—certainly not before you have treatment. Yet your mind may spend a lot of time trying to answer them, often with all kinds of responses. Sometimes the focus is on best-case scenarios, but too often the focus centers on worst-case outcomes. That your brain goes *there* is understandable. You want a good life in the future. You worry you will not get it because of this cancer. Maybe you are trying to prepare for the worst and hope for the best. When you find yourself spending an inordinate amount of time worrying about the worse-case scenarios in the future and not participating in life now, you are then unintentionally stealing your good life from "now."

If you are going to have surgery, it is useful to ask your doctor or nurse beforehand about time frames—ranges of how long potentially upsetting events might last—if you haven't asked or received this information already.

Questions to Ask the Urologist about Surgery

How long might the urinary catheter be in place?

How long will it take for an erection to return? The far end, not just the best case.

How long will it take until I get my energy back?

How long will it take until I stop using urinary pads?

Are there any activities that will make urinary leaking worse? For how long?

I heard that Kegel exercises are important. Can you teach me how to do them properly?

How often should I do the Kegel exercises?

Ask your treatment team if you can speak with other patients who have already undergone the treatment you will get. They have dealt with the complications you might be at risk for. Ask these men how they dealt with indwelling catheters or how they dealt with the initial phases of urinary incontinence after the catheter was removed. Ask them how they dealt with uncertainty and, now that they're through, what advice would they give you. Ask them how they dealt with their frustration, worry, and anger about all this:

> I can't imagine having a tube up my penis for 10 days. It seems like it would be really painful. How bad was it?

I've never spoken to a man who enjoyed having a urinary catheter in place. But knowing that it is there for a reason, that it will come out, and that other men survive it can make the unthinkable more bearable.

Feeling like you are putting the cart before the horse is what anxiety does, as people try to visualize and sculpt better outcomes down the road. Sometimes it helps to get more information. Though some information-gathering about possibilities can be a good distraction, too much can distract you from your current life and lead to increased worry and distress and to a less satisfactory life. Have you ever seen a shortstop boot a ground ball because he looked at his first baseman in anticipation of his throw before he had the ball in his glove? Or a football pass receiver who drops a pass because he took his eye off the ball, looking at a defender up the field? Once you've made your treatment decision, it's good to remember the phrases "Keep your eye on the ball" and "See the ball, hit the ball." Focusing more on the present is one of the first steps toward helping you turn down the volume on your worry and perhaps change the station to something less worrisome, and maybe even to something pleasant. The theory of this practice, or cognitive behavioral therapy, suggests recognizing any irrational aspects of your thoughts about specific or even unclear concerns that lead to anxious or depressive emotions and then trying to lasso and rationally revise them.

Many of the thoughts you have about prostate cancer are understandable and even rational, whether they are accurate predicators or pictures of your future or not. However, you know your thoughts have run amuck when anxiety derails you from moving forward and you find yourself neglecting opportunities to nurture your life today. Men may stop socializing with friends. They spend less time doing pleasurable activities, reserving more and more time for computer searches about prostate cancer. Potential worst-case outcomes are often given as much or more attention and weight than more probable and more acceptable outcomes. As noted elsewhere, some men find it helpful to have a "Prepare for the worst, hope for the best" attitude. I think this attitude is fine if it does not become a psychological self-fulfilling prophecy. Preparing for a worst-case scenario in the future does not mean giving up now. Anticipatory grief for those potential losses (the worst) may be inevitable. Living as fully and meaningfully as possible, should those losses actually occur, may become your objective or mission. Exaggerations, generalizations, and catastrophic thinking may hold sway over a brain that is used to feeling more in control of your thoughts, behaviors, and emotions. Most of us believe that we have command over the things we do and the outcomes we reach in life. An accurate retroscope may show that we have much more impact on what we do than on the outcomes we reach. It is difficult to manipulate all the many variables that go into how naturally occurring events in our lives, like cancer, eventually turn out.

The Big Three Worries: Sex, Urinary Incontinence, and Bowel Problems

Urologists and radiation oncologists are aware of and concerned about the sexual consequences of prostate cancer. Today, most are comfortable addressing these issues with patients and their partners or spouses before and after treatment. This is often the most fearful complication men face. Some dread the loss of their sexual identity if they can't get hard enough to have intercourse. Others who masturbate frequently for pleasure or for relief of stress or anxiety are distressed about the potential loss of this emotion-controller; their heightened distress about losing this habit matches how effective this regular behavior was in relieving tension and giving pleasure, however temporary the benefit. Some men feel addicted to sex or masturbation, similar to other compulsive behaviors like smoking or drinking, and cannot see living without it.

Doctors may recommend use of one of the erectile-stimulating medications (i.e., tadalafil, sildenafil, vardenafil) even before radiation starts and to continue using it after radiation or surgery, much like a vitamin for sexual vitality. In the past, men would wait to see if there was an ongoing problem and then try the medicine. By that time it may already be too late. The goal is to keep the penile muscles and vasculature active and with good blood flow until all tissue and nerves have healed sufficiently for erections to return. The goal is to avoid the "If you don't use it, you'll lose it" syndrome. If your doctor hasn't mentioned this precautionary program to you, ask about it. Reading books by John Mulhall, a urologist at Memorial Sloan Kettering Cancer Center who specializes in erectile dysfunction after prostate cancer, can be helpful. Sexual functioning *after* prostate cancer treatment will be discussed more fully in Chapter 6.

Before treatment, men also worry about how they will deal with urinary incontinence. Many predict they will skip social engagements because they fear leakage and odors, and they feel it is too much of a burden and shame to carry pads or diapers around to absorb leaks. Most men who are able to get beyond this initial fear and concern find that they have fairly normal social lives, though there may be some inconvenience associated with having to anticipate and plan for accidents. This is another opportune time to ask another man who's dealt with this issue about his experience: "Are there any special techniques you figured out to cope better with this until the urination improves?" Asking about what brand and types of diapers or pads other men recommend and why can help you realize that, as you're wondering whether this will happen to you, you are not alone, and this is survivable. You are capable of preparing for this complication even as you hope it will never happen. Coping with urinary problems *after* treatment is discussed more fully in Chapter 7.

Before radiation therapy, men worry if they will develop bowel problems: "How could I deal with that? No way am I gonna shit in my pants!" As with urinary accidents, bowel accidents are frightening and feel regressive and infantilizing. Sometimes, speaking with another patient who has dealt with this may relieve the anxiety that screams, "I cannot live if that happens to me." Managing bowel problems *after* radiation therapy, should they occur, is also discussed in Chapter 7.

Exercise

It's not unusual after a cancer diagnosis to feel as if your body and, at times, your genes or ancestry have let you down or betrayed you. Cancer is a wake-up call for many. We are mortal beings. Good health before cancer may have allowed you to hide behind the common human tendency to ignore that you will die one day; but cancer reminds all of us that we are mortal. Improving our lifestyles may help us live longer and healthier with whatever illnesses are set in motion by our genes and environment. This can be a timely moment to optimize your quality of life; alternatively, you can let the aging process take its toll with a business-as-usual attitude. Positive lifestyle tweaking can be just as important for your emotional well-being as your physical health.

As you wait for surgery or radiation therapy, it may be unrealistic to maintain the same exercise regimen you had previously. And if you are like most men, there is a good possibility you do not have any regular training regimen right now.

Though some men are "scared into health," there is no reason to expect that you will be able to get into the best shape you've ever been in, let alone good enough for a triathlon or marathon, now that a cancer diagnosis is in your life and treatment is in the offing. However, it is important to appreciate that being in *better* condition or *better* shape before you start your cancer treatment will give you a *better* chance of an easier and faster recovery, whether you are heading for surgery or radiation therapy. You do not need to be in elite physical condition, but you will reap both psychological and physical rewards. Apart from the benefit of distraction from your worries, you will optimize body functions that can make physically challenging interventions (i.e., long stretches of lying flat for radiation simulation; anesthesia for surgery; or fatigue that can set in from either radiation or a surgical procedure) easier to tolerate and, hopefully, more successful. You may get back on your feet faster. It's not too late to get in *better* shape!

"All things in moderation" is a useful mantra here. Try some activating pursuits even if your motivation and interest are low. One of the first things I tell my patients is "Get moving"—even it means taking a10- to 15-minute walk daily.

Some men try to suddenly get into shape for upcoming treatment even though they have not been in good physical shape for years. They dust off the old stationary bike or treadmill in the bedroom or basement that's been useful as a clothes hanger but not as an exercise machine. At least it is a place to start. But they have to be careful not to do too much in too brief a period of time without proper guidance, risking injury. Some get another gym membership that will hopefully not go to waste like the ones before, because there is now a very tangible motivator.

On the contrary, other men, already in good shape before their diagnosis, paradoxically decide after their diagnosis to give up good exercise habits. They become demoralized. The strain of many doctors' appointments, tests, and procedures and of researching the best treatment options makes them feel they don't have the time or energy to stay in shape the way they did even months ago:

> I did a triathlon months before my diagnosis, but I became too busy, angry, and overwhelmed with doctor visits and treatment decisions to focus on maintaining a vigorous exercise regimen.

Unfortunately, they decide that "too little" or "less" is worthless, so they do nothing. Or, like the previously mentioned tennis player, they feel that if being physically fit could not prevent prostate cancer in the first place, there's little point in staying in good condition—why bother working hard to stay in shape any longer? They become couch potatoes.

Many men don't get pleasure from their exercise routines, so cancer seems like a good excuse to back off. Men who loved playing 36 holes of golf on a weekend decide that it is too much of a hassle to play, so they don't play at all. Some don't like talking about their cancer and fear that a close foursome on the golf course or a doubles tennis game will threaten to bring up the cancer discussion. Some loved running or enjoyed going to the gym. Now they are consumed with anticipation of urinary leaks in public even before surgery.

Others are aggravated about new aches and pains that may mean their cancer is already spreading before they've even had treatment. They become overly cautious. Many find themselves glued to their computers, looking at prostate cancer symptoms, blogs, and statistics, as if they were stock market quotes. When I hear about these behaviors I am reminded of a couple of phrases I used to hear when I was younger: "Two wrongs don't make a right" and "Don't throw out the baby with the bath water." There's no way to do a comparison study of your past to see how much worse off you would be if you hadn't exercised or eaten better before your cancer diagnosis. It is possible that being in better shape prevented other diseases that could have compromised the better life you did have before cancer. Other illnesses could have made getting through prostate cancer even more trying. Smarter, healthier living, and being in better shape now could make getting through prostate cancer treatment less challenging. But without that retroscope, you'll never know.

Yet, this is the time to either stay in shape or to start an easy exercise routine (even starting to take short walks if you don't work out at all)— before treatment starts. "Something is better than nothing!" is a formula I suggest as a battle cry for healthier living habits that will help you get through whatever lies ahead physically and psychologically a little more safely. If you have been non-active physically, think about doing a little bit more than you had been doing. You don't have to become a gym rat spending hours pumping iron and running endlessly on treadmills. "Something is better than nothing!"—this is true whether facing a prostatectomy or radiation therapy, and is also true if active surveillance or watchful waiting is your treatment choice. If you have been more active previously and find too many time or energy constraints now, maintaining a "good enough" attitude and staying in reasonable, or *better*, physical shape may be an excellent compromise.

An important approach to managing prostate cancer is to manage expectations. If expectations are too high, you will become frustrated when circumstances are far from optimal. Recalculating and managing expectations appropriately will help you feel better and think more attentively.

For those men who are not used to doing much exercise, or who are not used to keeping to diets, again: "Something is better than nothing." Rather than waiting to see if you feel like exercising tomorrow, choose a time, a type of exercise, and a place. Make it happen. Exercise and healthy diets do not necessarily prevent cancer or prevent it from coming back, but being in better shape can help you cope with treatment and keep your other vital organs in better shape.

> Physical exercise was a welcome distraction from the worry of my upcoming surgery, even if short-lived. Whenever I thought about the tumor and possible complications, I was able to shift away from those worries to the exercise.

Your cancer can be an important health marker for your partner or spouse, too—and maybe for your entire family. Why not exercise together? Fitness experts say that one of the best ways to get motivated to exercise is to commit to doing it with someone else. Try taking a walk together in the morning or early evening. Or get a family membership at a local gym, but plan to go together. If your spouse already has an established exercise routine that seems inappropriate or unrealistic for you, you might be able to find a friend near home or a work colleague who could also use a 30-minute walk at lunchtime.

Patients at our hospital recently helped start an exercise group for men, called PEX, that pays attention to the unique needs of male patients and survivors to rebuild muscle strength, improve balance, and increase endurance. PEX involves a fun and challenging workout that improves their health, physically and mentally.

If your partner is not interested in or is resistant to exercising, your suggestion of exercising together, even with recognition of the mutual benefits for physical, emotional, and couple's health, may come across as coercion. That can lead to tension, frustration, and anger. Make the offer. Let it rest. Then make the offer again a little differently—remember that this will be good for your partner as well as for you. If there is still no uptake, let it rest again. When there is tension, and increased potential for arguments, remember the recommendation to "strike when the iron is cold." This nonconventional technique will be discussed more in the chapter on couples communication (Chapter 8). Arguments about disagreements are not fruitful when one or both parties are tired, frustrated, or angry. Wait for a cool-down period. Let it rest. Then try again a little differently.

Diet

The benefits of attitude adjustments carry over to diet as well. Men who have eaten a healthy diet in the past also say, "What was the point of eating well, since I wound up getting cancer anyway?" There have been reports about certain foods and nutrients being healthier for those with prostate cancer (i.e., fruits, vegetables, whole grains, limited red meat, high soy protein, green tea, and low, yet healthy fat). Some men who have been on relatively unhealthy diets for many years decide to go wholly organic and natural regarding food and become extremely diet-conscious. This works for many. Unfortunately, some of these men lose pleasure in eating and feel like they've now sacrificed something else to cancer, while others enjoy the shift, experimenting with new recipes and feeling like they are doing something to help their bodies feel better.

A prostate-healthy diet is also cardiac, blood sugar, and whole-body healthy as well. If you are scared of dying of prostate cancer, why not see this as an opportunity to stay healthier overall, even though there are no guarantees about how much it will help with prostate cancer?

Other Lifestyle Choices

If you are a smoker, start thinking about cutting down or quitting altogether, even though tobacco is not a major cause of prostate cancer. You will ultimately feel better. There are medications and smoking cessation programs that are specific and effective to help people quit smoking.

Smokers sometimes defensively point out to me that many smokers don't get lung cancer or any cancer, and many non-smokers get lung cancer. They provide me with anecdotal experiences rather than the statistical evidence about the consequences of tobacco on our vital organs. Though nicotine may give a temporary, short-lived physical or psychological lift, there are safer alternatives and, if needed, safer medications to feel good. Some men will go to the other extreme, feeling remorseful and angry about their tobacco use. One patient told me, "This isn't the time to quit smoking—I'm too nervous. Every time I've tried to stop before, I put on weight, and that is not healthy. But I can feel my breathing is more difficult today than 2 years ago. Do I want to get cured of prostate cancer just to find out I have emphysema?" Clearly, there is ambivalence. Smoking may be one of the most difficult habits to break. Support and encouragement for making a healthier choice soon can still benefit your future. Quick and dirty works for some, while slow and steady is the answer for others. A sign hanging in our smoking cessation program, "If at first you don't succeed, quit, quit again," has been reassuring for many men. Even starting to think about stopping is an important first step toward eventually quitting.

Alcohol is not known to be prostate-toxic; however, it can compromise overall nutritional health as well as challenge liver, brain, and other organ functioning. Yet it is also another tough addiction to kick. Heavy drinkers often have problems after surgery when they no longer have access to alcohol. Determining who is a "heavy drinker" is subjective; labeling is often in the eyes of the beholder. Men who have even two to four alcoholic drinks every day risk withdrawal symptoms if they stop drinking abruptly the day before or the day of surgery. Potential withdrawal symptoms include tremors, confusion, hallucinations, anxiety, restlessness, sweating, pacing, high blood pressure, high pulse rates, and seizures. Withdrawal from alcohol can be life-threatening; it can complicate what might otherwise be a straightforward surgery to remove your prostate, especially when it comes on abruptly, as it usually does postoperatively. If your medical team is informed about regular alcohol use, sedative medications can be prescribed and slowly decreased in a scheduled fashion to prevent serious withdrawal from alcohol after sudden cessation. Shorter hospitalizations, assuming all goes according to plan, will prevent many cases of withdrawal, as men get home sooner and can resume their drinking habits. Alcoholics Anonymous is still one of the most successful programs to help people stop drinking and stay sober over the long haul, but its use should be considered and initiated weeks before surgery. It also provides a beneficial worldview that helps people deal with other life trials, like cancer.

It may seem impossible at a time of crisis, such as with a new cancer diagnosis or the start of treatment, to cut back on tobacco or alcohol use, which are often used as emotional crutches to relax, de-stress, or unwind. It is not easy to give up that outlet when you are fighting cancer, facing perhaps the biggest confrontation of your life. That is why support from a counselor or a therapist can be a vital assist.

Improving Lifestyle

Manage expectations and don't try to do too much too soon.

Something is better than nothing: do some exercise; tweak some of your diet.

Plan to make exercise and diet improvements. Don't wait until you feel like it.

If you are taking care of your cancer, why not the rest of you?

It's a great time to cut back on or stop using tobacco, alcohol, and other substances.

Who to Tell?

Men often find themselves in a predicament, not knowing who to tell and what to say about their cancer—to family members, friends, and colleagues. Women dealing with a new cancer diagnosis do not have as much difficulty with this. Men often feel that too much discussion trivializes what they are going through, overwhelms them, and is likely not very helpful because it won't give them the answers they are looking for: "Talking doesn't fix anything!" However, too few discussions can arouse internal ruminating, which then increases anxiety, sadness, and, for many, feelings of powerlessness that make some men feel they will explode. They get into reflexive thought patterns bemoaning their "bad luck" and sometimes guiltily or angrily wondering why others don't have to deal with this problem: "I was the youngest of my friends to get cancer...it's not fair."

Many men find social activities uncomfortable and even distasteful while waiting for treatment. Will they be happily diverted from their preoccupying cancer thoughts or reminded of them? Will they feel uneasy about whether they feel pressure to talk about their cancer condition in front of just anyone, whether or not they are the closest of friends or family members?

Discussions Men Dread, or "Not Music to My Ears"

"How are you feeling?"

Once someone knows you have cancer, are going through treatment, or have recovered from treatment, they feel it is socially correct to ask, "How are you feeling?" whenever they see you. Sometimes a question is just a question. But for a man with cancer, the question may feel like so much more. It may set in motion an anticipatory, "I hate when people keep asking how I'm feeling," before going out to meet friends or family. This question stimulates too many internal responses about circumstances many men would like to forget for a while: "Some people don't really care how I feel, but they feel the need to ask; even if they do care, I don't always want to tell, but I don't want to be rude."

In therapy, men and I discuss alternative ways to take more control over the situation or to try to make sure that it doesn't keep repeating. It is acceptable to say:

> I know you're asking because you care about me, but a funny thing happens when people ask me how I'm feeling. It brings my mind back

to the cancer and I go down my checklist of what is not right with me now, or what I am concerned about down the road—so a supportive question inadvertently makes me feel worse and more tense, though I know that is not anyone's intention. So I want to let you know what you can do that I'd really appreciate and that will really help me. Whenever you see me, skip "How are you feeling?" or even "How are you?" and just go straight to something like "It's nice to see you" or "A great day for a drive" or "How about those Yankees, Mets, Jets, Giants, or Rangers (or local team/sport/politician of your choice)" or "How are the kids?" I will let you know if there's something about my health that I want to talk about. I am very comforted to know you'll be able to talk about it with me when I'm ready and if I need to; but you'll really help me if we stay away from the cancer talk for a while. Then I can relax.

Because "How are you?" is such a socially common phrase, it is not easy for people to stop asking in one of its many variations, like "How ya doin'?" So you may need to give reminders.

"Don't Worry, Everything Will Be Fine"

When you do let people know your healthcare concerns, they can become fearful themselves or feel powerless to help. They try to say something comforting that doesn't always help: "Don't worry, I'm sure everything will be just fine." Men commonly think in response, "How do you know? You have no clue. Where's your crystal ball?" This silent reaction is often felt quite forcefully. Just as with the "How are you?" question, it is fine to guide the person who means well toward what is beneficial for you:

I know we both want everything to go well for me, but when people tell me not to worry, It's hard to shut down or substitute my thoughts even for a few minutes. When people try to assure me not to worry, I start to believe there really is something to worry about, because my angst comes from the uncertainty of the future. The next time I tell you what I'm concerned or anxious about, validate or *confirm what I am saying. Tell me something like "I hear what you are worried about—I might be too." Or "I guess not being able to know what will happen is scary." Or "I hope that next PSA test comes back better; what can I do to help?" Or "Would you like me to go to a doctor's appointment with you? Debrief afterwards? Feel free to give me a call afterwards, good or bad news. We can take a walk, go to a movie, or play some poker."*

Your friend or relative may not act on these suggestions, but at least you have tried to maintain some control over where the conversation goes and therefore where your thoughts may go. You'll feel less like a victim. In a polite way, you get to tell someone what will help you and, maybe most importantly, you don't have to be fearful about being inadvertently ambushed without having a response you are comfortable with. Validating someone's understandable anxiety or other uncomfortable emotional responses in tough situations helps to relieve the anguish. Then the conversation does not have to get to the point of the anxious person trying to be convincing about how bad things *really* are or what they're really worried about. On the other hand, it is not helpful when a potential ally goes to the opposite gloomy extreme: "Of course you should be worried. Cancer can kill you. Remember that celebrity who died of prostate cancer." Or they want to tell you about their uncle's difficult and demoralizing experience with cancer.

Spouses and partners often have different communication needs and styles from those of the man with cancer. Because they don't want to pressure their partners to talk, or if they know that secrecy is desired, they feel trapped with information and emotions that they cannot share. A conspiracy of silence in the couple can lead to arguments about many issues, including the cancer. A partial conspiracy of silence—"It's OK to tell Mary, but not that blabbermouth Bob," or "It's OK to tell your brother but not my sister," is asking a lot of people who may not be used to keeping information confidential. Sometimes keeping accurate track of confidants and stories can be challenging. It's an essential discussion for a couple to have and to be clear about being on the same page. Some men have told me that confiding in friends was a chance to "find out who my friends really were. Some friends were right there with me throughout my ordeal, and others surprisingly disappeared." Even some business associates or colleagues who have gone through prostate cancer treatment previously may be good to speak with and get support from, if confidentiality in your job is not paramount. Men find that some relationships become strengthened not out of pity, which they fear or detest, but out of genuine connection and caring.

Good communicators and good listeners don't grow on trees (as my parents used to say about money or anything else that was valuable). They are gems to be appreciated. Men with prostate cancer can find these gems in some physicians, some nurses, some friends or family members, some colleagues, therapists, and even some strangers at cancer support groups or in clinic waiting rooms. But none come with a seal of approval that you can identify beforehand. It is most frustrating when people you expect to be most helpful or supportive turn out not to be. Some can be duds, and some hurtful. But it may be worth taking the risk more than once to find that gem, because feeling understood and supported when you feel confused and frustrated can be priceless.

Some men feel shame and anger about having a sexual organ tumor; this can feel embarrassing and depressing. Men shy away from commiserating and discussing these issues with others and lose ways of finding support. Envy and anger toward healthier men and couples keep potential supports at a distance. In fact, the sexual overtones of prostate cancer and its treatments often cause ambivalence about discussing cancer-related issues, even with healthcare providers. Men with prostate cancer fret about what other men think of them, now that they may not be able to "get it up" like they used to. Men are not used to talking about sexual problems when cancer is not in the picture; when it is, the situation can be even worse. Some men wonder, realistically or not, if their wives or partners will stop loving them or if their partners will leave them if sexual intercourse or sexual activity is not a part or as much of a part of their relationship as it was previously.

Dreaded Discussions or Communication "Red Flags"	
Problematic/Red Flag Statements or Topics	**Suggestions of How to Deal with Red Flags**
How are you?	Skip that question and start with a non-health-related chat.
Don't worry, everything will be fine.	Ask for your concerns to be validated, not dismissed.
Who to tell/not tell: family, friends, and colleagues	Discuss and be clear with your spouse/ partner.
Sexuality and other delicate topics	Nurture the gems in your life with whom you feel comfortable talking about delicate issues. Use a journal for therapeutic writing and angst relief.
Discussing "hot" topics when upset	Strike when the iron is cold. Cool down before discussing "hot" topics.

Some men find that writing down thoughts, fears, and concerns in a journal releases the pressure of their distress when they do not get relief talking with others. Some call this therapeutic writing; if you put it down on paper you don't have to keep track of it as often or so intensely in your mind. Sometimes you gain more clarity about or distance from a situation that seems otherwise murky, by jotting it down on paper (or on your computer).

As noted earlier, it is useful to keep yourself (your mind and body) occupied while waiting to begin radiation or have your surgery. Sometimes formal meditation brings solace. You may feel too distracted and unable to focus on usual pleasurable activities, but the attempt is worth it. Find activities to do, or get together with friends to relieve tension. It is useful to prepare your own *quick list* of activity options before you'll need them. You can then pull out the list when you start to get antsy or nervous. Being in the midst of angst without a plan is like being up a creek without a paddle. With a list, you don't have to feel on the spot while you are freaking out to come up with brilliant, entertaining, or interesting ideas. Your *quick list* might include easy-to-accomplish "go-to" activities that do not require much preparation, equipment, or even thought: put on some music; go for a walk (alone, or with your spouse or partner or a friend) outside, around your block, or up and down your apartment house corridor; drive to a mall and walk around there if the weather is bad; call up a friend or relative to chat or get together; go to the movies; do some exercise; play a game of solitaire or another game on your computer or with your partner; do a puzzle; read a book; listen to a book-on-tape/CD; go to a concert or out to dinner; attend a sporting event; or take a bath or shower. Watching a show or movie on television can be good distractions for some men; however, for others these activities are too passive—men find themselves not really paying attention to or enjoying the show—they might even tune out the show and tune back into their own persistent worries. Return to old hobbies or find new ones, such as playing an instrument, building things, or doing artwork or photography. When a man is bored or not active enough, he can become irritable and frustrated—this is usually counterproductive for both him and his family.

Try to Relax

Being in the midst of high anxiety is not the ideal time to learn a relaxation exercise or meditation. However, it does not hurt to try. Just don't expect a quick fix. It is better to start sometime, ideally when your anxiety is not peaking. If trying to learn how to relax makes you feel more anxious and aggravated, stop. Find a CD, or a teacher or therapist who can work with you in a supportive environment until you learn the basics. Then practice, and practice some more until you get it into your muscle memory. See Chapter 4 for a relaxation or meditation exercise you can learn and practice.

"Quick List" Activities

Increase distraction and pleasure, decrease worry.
Listen to music.
Exercise—start low and go slowly, but go.
Walk your dog.
Call a friend.
Play a card game, any game.
Read a book.
Listen to a book on tape/CD
Surf the Internet for non-cancer-related sites.
Take a shower or bath.
Watch TV.
Watch a movie.
Listen to the radio.
Go for a drive.
Go to a park.
Go window-shopping or an indoor mall.
Play an instrument.
Build things.
Do art work.
Make photographs.

Faith

Religious observance and spirituality may not be a common topic in a book authored by a psychiatrist. However, depending on its place in a man's life—currently and in the past—it may be a very important tool for coping better with prostate cancer. Faith, spirituality, and religious observance can span the spectrum from atheism with no belief in a "higher power," to those with a strong sense of a humanistic or natural-istic connection, to those who hold fast to traditional religious faith and rituals in the face of calm or crisis. In between these extremes are many who grew up with some training, education, or observance yet lost it or have seen it dwindle over the years. Those who are angry at God for causing their suffering with cancer may now be detoured from a connection that once was, and potentially could be, an important provider of support and emotional or spiritual sustenance. Many of the more religiously observant patients I see believe that God is in control of everything that happens in the world, and we humans do not have to understand, and maybe cannot understand, the reasoning behind the good or bad that happens in our lives, including cancer. This belief helps them more easily accept their fate, whether outwardly good or difficult, including a prostate cancer diagnosis. This is faith. These patients pray when they are scared and, in doing so, find strength and comfort.

Even without formal religious observance, meaningful prayer can be an important activity that helps men cope better with medical treatment. Many men have told me that a prayer in an MRI scan (even a prayer repeated over and over again) helped relieve anxiety and got them through the scan. In fact, some studies have shown that those with cancer who self-identify as having strong faith, have more satisfaction in their lives than do others with similar levels of pain, fatigue, or depression who have less faith. But these people are not the majority of men I see. So, does this mean that all other men with prostate cancer should find religion? No. But this does raise an important question: Where does religion or spirituality fit when severe illness is present, or when someone is confronted with mortality? This is easier to figure out if religion or spirituality has been a part of your life previously, or you still have some inclination toward faith, organized religion, or spiritual activities. If you've lost faith during your life, finding comfort in religion now that you have cancer can be more complicated. This is especially true if these beliefs were given up recently because of anger at God for "bringing on" this cancer.

I am always searching for ways to help people cope better with their medical struggles and often with their lives in general. If they can cope better with their cancer, I believe they will lead better lives. One way to do that is to take note of the good that has been in your life on a consistent basis—you do not have to be religious to do that. Recognition and appreciation of the natural miracles of life can be used as a strength-training or anxiety-reducing tool. Gratefulness for what has gone well and continues to go well in your life, including the wonder of existence itself, can help balance stressors and disappointments. These perspectives can quickly start filling a glass that seemed half-empty (or even empty) to one that is at least half-full. Same stuff, different vantage point. Religious or spiritual beliefs do not have to be the basis of this exercise. But they may help someone comprehend and act on this point more easily and thereby overcome this predicament more easily.

But even the committed faithful can run into problems of faith. I was once asked to see a religiously observant man with newly diagnosed prostate cancer. He was refusing surgery and radiation therapy despite multiple opinions unanimously recommending active treatment. Every urologist and radiation oncologist he saw felt he needed an active treatment. Neither watchful waiting nor active surveillance was a good option for him. But his faith in God was unquestioning and he made the statement: "God gave me this cancer and God will take it away if I pray hard enough. I do not need any formal human cancer treatment." He was angry with his family and his doctors for not accepting his decision to forego a definitive treatment. He had a difficult time seeing how to get beyond his anger and the blinders it created. We discussed the parable about the very faithful man who was living in a rural community. There was a horrible storm and the rain would not let up for days. The man's house flooded and he needed to climb onto the roof in order not to drown. A helpful neighbor passed by in a rowboat and said, "I've got room for you. Come on board and let's get out of here." The pious man, looking at the fierce wind and rain, replied, "Thank you, but I am praying to God and I know He will save me." Another person came along in a speedboat offering a ride to safety, as the water was so high that the man's head bobbed on top of the water. The man, seeing the boat shake from side to side in the water, said, "Thank you, but I am praying to God and waiting for Him to save me. I know he will. I have faith," and he refused the ride. A little later, as the man was treading water and was having a difficult time staying afloat, a helicopter came along and the pilot told him to grab the rope ladder that he dropped down to him. There was no sign of the rain or winds letting up, and it looked like the man would drown if he did not climb up immediately. The man looked at the rope and again proclaimed, "Thank you, but I am praying to God and I know He will save me." The man drowned and woke up in heaven. He looked angrily at God and said, "How could you do this to me? I was so devout and faithful. I kept praying for you to save me and you didn't. How could you let me down?" And God replied, "You fool. Who do you think sent the people in the rowboat, the speedboat, and even the helicopter?" My patient eventually went for surgery, recognizing within his framework of beliefs that there was a place for his faith in his choice for treatment, and maybe God had created a surgeon who could treat his illness.

To date, there is no consistent scientific confirmation to show that having faith or even a positive outlook affects the biological course of cancer in a significant and direct manner. Perhaps faith or attitudes lead to better lifestyle choices and behaviors that may prevent a cancer, lead to earlier diagnosis, or improve someone's ability to tolerate a treatment regimen. Prayer may decrease anxiety and enable more optimal treatment tolerance. If prayer or religion is or has been a meaningful part of one's life in the past, this may be a good time to revisit or retrieve it.

Many patients have their faith shaken with a new cancer diagnosis. They may have attended church, a mosque, or a synagogue regularly and have been good citizens in caring for others or donating to good causes that help the poor or sick. Now they are stricken with an illness that may portend extreme suffering and death. "How can God do this to me?"—this is a religious twist to the "Why me?" question. Many people want to feel as if the world we live in is rational most of the time; they look for answers that will make the unthinkable and unbelievable, the unacceptable, the unexpected, and the irrational tolerable and bearable. Some believe that any suffering they go through today will ease their passage into heaven when they die. Belief in these answers, if they come, helps us plan for today, tomorrow, and the distant future. It is difficult for many to accept the existential angst of not knowing or understanding God's ways or plan, as God may be so infinitely beyond human understanding. This may be especially true if one's belief means accepting that God is an accomplice in the suffering of often-innocent people. In the "see it to believe it" world we live in, faith may fall short of satisfactory answers.

Supporting expression, and examining the emotions behind these questions, is part of the psychological healing that men and their families need. Sometimes people of faith express their emotions to God, with or without a clergy intermediary, with or without a therapist, and feel as if the communication link with God is crystal clear. They feel rejuvenated and less isolated. Sometimes the best support I can give to someone is to help him figure out which is the most appropriate rowboat, speedboat, or helicopter for him, and how to get in it, whether he believes it is heaven sent or not.

Readjusting Your Coping-Scope

> Why can't we just rewind life to 2 months before the diagnosis and turn on a different show or channel?
>
> Can't we just rewrite this script?

As you get closer to your treatment, you may again be haunted with concerns about whether you are making the right choice. Frankly, this sense of mystery will likely resurface many times when you most or least expect it. There will likely be frequent backward glances, wondering if the treatment choice you made was the best one. Remind yourself again that given the disagreements among excellent clinicians, there is no preordained *absolutely perfect* treatment choice that will yield definitive desired results for any man. There may even be more than one good choice for you—that's why data don't support only one. This doubt may go on even after treatment as the buyer's remorse discussed in Chapter 2, when a man looks back months or years after treatment (or after a decision for active surveillance) with regret if something does not go the way he wanted—either because of long-term complications that compromise quality of life or because the cancer has returned or progressed out of control or, worse, both happened. Remind yourself about the psychological trap of potential regrets. They are understandable and common in the short run. But if they continue to gnaw at you, these misgivings can steal pleasure and meaning from your life now, perhaps more than the less-than-optimal results you might have in the future, which you could ultimately adapt and adjust to. Regrets may also make you doubt future decisions. Ultimately, there is no accurate way to know how any path of an early decision tree will turn out in reality—the route finder we have on GPS navigation systems is not available. So come back to now, find your *quick list*, give yourself a break, and get distracted.

Chapter 4

Prostate Cancer
Anxiety, Depression,
and Sleep Problems

Relax and Enter the DRAFT of
the Emotional Judo Playbook

"My back hurts…the cancer must be back…I'm gonna die."

Sometimes a sore back is just a sore back. This patient who believes
that his painful back suggests that he is losing his battle with cancer
is living daily with the expectation of a downward spiral into death.
He awaits the catastrophe. Insomnia, anxiety, and depression arise in
healthy people, but they can occur more frequently in the medically ill.
The incidence is highest in those with life-threatening illnesses such
as cancer. These understandable reactions to stressful, upsetting circumstances can also be caused by medications used to manage medical
problems. For instance, steroids, which treat inflammation or nausea,
and opiates, which treat pain, can both cause mood changes, including
depression, mania, and irritability. Electrolyte or hormonal abnormalities, pain, fatigue, or nausea can send your mind into dark or unpredictable directions. I occasionally see patients who really do suffer "one

problem right after the other," leading to fears of a downward spiral into a "predictable" abyss. The worry-wheel can start spinning after only a couple of things do not go as planned or hoped for, leaving the person feeling depressed or anxious about being on one of those rare, rocky, catastrophic roads.

This chapter discusses how and why worry and distress arise in the world of prostate cancer treatment, and how to deal with these uncomfortable emotions. Emotionally charged "thoughts traps" lie ahead, unless a man has no complications or side effects from his treatment. Men have plenty of concerns, even with a relatively uncomplicated outcome. A short list of these worried thoughts includes the following:

"How will I handle anesthesia since I won't be in control?"
"Won't a urinary catheter hurt?"
"Does radiation hurt?"
"Will I have pain afterward? For how long?"
"When will my erections return? Will they ever return?"
"How long will the urinary problems last?"
"I freaked out in the last MRI scan. Do I need MRI scans after treatment?"
"How will I deal with the uncertainty of my prognosis?"
"Am I naïve or in denial if I think everything will turn out fine?"

To worry is human; to get stuck in thought traps can be a landmine. These worries can occur 24/7, during daylight hours as potential distractions from work and family, and at night, often interfering with sleep. Once prostate cancer treatment commences or concludes, pretreatment worries often have their post-treatment sequels.

Whether you've had an open prostatectomy, robotic or laparoscopic surgery, or radiation therapy, you should expect to endure some recuperation period after treatment. But it is also time to begin living the rest of your life. Cards and gifts arrive from family, friends, and colleagues. Visitors stop by. Internet tools like CaringBridge offer free, personalized websites to help patients and spouses or partners keep interested others informed about medical updates. Some of my patients have even set up their own Internet blogs to efficiently let others know about their medical experiences and journey through illness. Spouses, partners, family members, and friends often keep a close watch after you come home. Hopefully, they make sure you rest sufficiently as you start to get moving again. Partners and other caregivers are expected to function as in-home, though untrained, nurses' aides. Now that's a tall order that may frustrate you and her or him. Sometimes significant others push too much and too hard, and it may be useful to negotiate parameters. Recognizing and appreciating the amount of work and support extended by partners is wise and recommended; they, too, may be exhausted after just a few days of your recuperation as they try to maintain their other responsibilities such as outside jobs. Remember, they are not used to being caregivers for someone who is not used to needing care. Spouses with young families who deal with prostate cancer need to make sure that children are well taken care of and supported emotionally as well.

Partners may be the ones you let your guard down with—sharing your deepest fears and, unfortunately, also your irritable moods. Your spouse or partner is likely to hear your worries about when and if complications from treatment, whether expected or not, will improve; yet she or he may not feel comfortable sharing her or his own fears and concerns about your recovery with you so as not to increase your burden.

Your closest supporters will also perceive your fears about whether complications that linger will ever get better. Those close to you are likely to know that you are wondering if and when your energy and mood will get back to your old baseline and how long that will take, whether you talk about it or not. They'll also be concerned about whether you'll be able to define an acceptable "new normal" baseline or standard for your life regarding sexual, urinary, or energy issues, or even general preoccupation with medical problems, depending on what complications you have to confront after treatment.

You will learn how to recognize distress, anxiety, and sleep difficulties and get information about non-medication formulas for improvement. Chapter 5 will address more severe anxiety and depressive syndromes and pharmacological techniques for managing them.

Distress

It is not easy to tell the difference between anxiety and depressive symptoms. In fact, they often go hand in hand. Different people may understand anxiety and depression differently at different times. We have found that men in particular do not easily admit to feeling anxious or identify that emotion as anxiety. They often do not recognize feeling depressed, either. This may be culturally and biologically based—some men say, "Tell me what you mean by depressed (or anxious), because I have never felt that before." The terms *depression* and *anxiety* can feel derogatory, as signs of weakness or non-masculinity, so they are invisible, denied, ignored, minimized, or interpreted as some other entity. When men do say they are anxious or depressed, I ask them what *they* mean by these terms, as there are wide ranges of emotions that may be experienced.

Symptoms that are not severe enough to be labeled as an official psychiatric disorder can still be troublesome and interfere with your ability to get treatment for your cancer as well as enjoy and get on with your life afterward. These emotions can interfere with sleep, energy levels, the ability to enjoy activities, and the ability to focus and concentrate on daily chores or projects. Many men and their families try to figure out whether the degree of emotional angst being experienced or expressed is "normal" or not, and, in fact, men often ask me, "So doc, isn't that normal?" I've been telling men for years that trying to distinguish between normal and abnormal may be a misleading venture. I'm not sure that there is a norm. Though labels may provide a sense of stability, they are often not beneficial because symptoms can change from day to day. What you're feeling is common and understandable. Let's figure out how to help you feel better.

When someone confronts mortality because of a cancer diagnosis, regardless of whether or not they will be cured, they may have significant yet "normal" anxiety or depressive symptoms. If those emotional reactions are ongoing and interfere with treatment decision-making, work or home life, sleep, or focus, they can be addressed to soften, lower, or remove altogether the barriers to getting on with one's life.

In many cancer centers around the world, nurses and oncologists now use the word *distress* to describe many of the concerns patients have about cancer. Our research group at Memorial Sloan Kettering Cancer Center measured how upset men with prostate cancer were about their cancer. These men were more amenable to the word *distress* than to *anxiety* or *depression*. Jimmie Holland, Alice Kornblith, Laure Batel-Copel, Elizabeth Peabody, Howard Scher, and I reported on the use of a simple 0–10 visual analog scale that looks like a thermometer, that was called the *Distress Thermometer* (Figure 4.1).

Men could easily self-score how distressed they were, with 0 being "no distress" and 10 "extreme distress." We felt that the thermometer could "medicalize" the issue for men. We hoped that medicalizing the process, as well as using the word *distress* instead of *depression* or *anxiety* would decrease any embarrassing psychological stigma attached to describing an uncomfortable emotion. Men were eager to fill out the thermometer. Not surprisingly, we found considerable distress among the men in our center. But those found to be distressed did not readily want additional help or support. The National Comprehensive Cancer Center Network (NCCN) has defined medical distress as "an unpleasant emotional experience of a psychological, social and/or spiritual nature which extends on a continuum from normal feelings of vulnerability, sadness and fears to disabling problems such as depression, anxiety, panic, social isolation and spiritual crisis." The Distress Thermometer has been adopted and

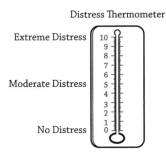

Figure 4.1. Distress Thermometer. From Roth, A. J., Kornblith, A. B., Batel-Copel, L., Peabody, E., Scher, H. I. and Holland, J. C. (1998), Rapid screening for psychologic distress in men with prostate carcinoma. *Cancer*, 82: 1904 -1908. Reprinted with permission of John Wiley and Sons.

adapted by the NCCN and the American Cancer Society as an important screening tool for emotional distress for patients with cancer.

You can use a scale of 0–10 to rate your distress from time to time as you go through various exercises in this book or just to see where your distress is at any time of day. It's like a mood ring, just more accurate.

Anxiety

Anxious feelings can be minor, with a heightened awareness about actual or suspected dangerous or threatening situations. The full avalanche of anxiety is reminiscent of the primitive "fight or flight" reactions of our ancestors. But not every perceived danger is a lion in the jungle ready to pounce and devour us, where our options are to throw the spear accurately, being ready for the battle, or to get the hell out of there fast. Our brains and hormonal alarm centers have evolutionarily hard-wired us for these responses, though today they may be inappropriate or mismatched for less imminently threatening situations. Although these reactions are meant to be protective, they can also be internally destructive. Numerous areas of the brain, including the sympathetic and parasympathetic nervous systems, the amygdala, and midbrain periaqueductal gray regions, as well as the serotonergic and norepinephrine neurotransmitter systems, are involved in these alarm processes that can result in anxiety and panic, depending on our biological and genetic susceptibilities. Our emotional experiences with past traumatic or stressful events, including how we handled them and how they were resolved, likely also play a role in how we enter the stress of a cancer experience. All of these factors may explain why a cancer diagnosis is viewed as a trauma for some and as a major life stressor to others. Remember that our study on the prevalence of anxiety in men with prostate cancer showed that about one-third of men had significant anxiety. That means that about two-thirds do not report significant anxiety or depression.

Just as a sailor watches the luff and stall of their boat's sails to assess the strength and direction of an otherwise invisible wind and then uses that wind information to guide the boat more efficiently, so, too, can men be better served by recognizing and acknowledging the different aspects of anxiety—the many variables, instigators, and intensity of distress in different settings—rather than just letting that angst knock them off course by ignoring it or collapsing from it. That is what men hope their experienced physicians will do when treating the obscure winds of cancer. Sometimes, as mentioned earlier, the gentle breezes of anxiety can be quite useful as an alerting mechanism for preparedness. Emotional preparation may be beneficial for an upcoming test such as an MRI scan or a bone scan, or for receiving the results of a recent scan, a biopsy, or a PSA test; however, it may also be a good warning for the need to focus on a wider range of issues. I often tell patients that if I had experienced no anxiety in medical school, I might have flunked out. No pressure, no study, no pass. But if I had had too much anxiety, I might have felt intellectually paralyzed, incapable of reading, understanding, or retaining information—again, increasing my likelihood of failing. Optimal levels of concern and vigilance to properly meet the needs of a specific situation can lead to improved function and living. For instance, the man fretting about an upcoming PSA test who worries about missing his grandchildren's life milestones if he dies of prostate cancer may find that spending time with his grandchildren or speaking with them on the phone is the ideal distracting antidote to his concerns, rather than avoiding them because he is worried about a test.

Psychotherapy may not be needed for mild forms of worry and anxiety, unless these symptoms begin to impact the satisfaction and integration a man feels in his life, or unless a man wants a supportive bridge to get through this life-changing experience. Some men are not used to identifying these feelings as anxiety because in other non-life-threatening scenarios they might instinctively transpose the worry into some type of productive action. But when it feels like they are spinning those wheels into worry, they may benefit from a therapist pointing out the ups and downs and intricacies of being on a different playing field now—that is, the world of being a patient with cancer, rather than a construction worker finishing a complicated job while facing a deadline, a plumber finding the source of a flooded basement, a business executive making risky financial decisions, or a husband making a decision about family issues.

Complicated medical issues like cancer, and how your body responds to treatment, are different from your usual life stressors. When people don't respond to illnesses or treatments in the hoped-for manner based on the stats, we sometimes say that "human bodies don't always read the textbooks." Thus a man who tries to figure out the "correct" formula to predict the optimal medical outcome may be on a misguided mission. When there are unexpectedly good outcomes, most are glad that "the body didn't read the textbook." With therapy, you can sense and cope better with those situations over which you do not have as much control as you would like. You can discover the circumstances where you feel more vulnerable because predictive factors are not iron-clad for treatment decisions, and you can cope better and make the RIGHT CHOICE for you. Hopefully, you'll be able to spend less time trying to forecast your medical and life results and more time building meaningful and memorable life experiences. You can better understand and manage the areas in this medical arena so you can bring into play a sense of appropriate control. You can also learn how to deal with the frustration of situations that don't go the way you want and seem out of your control or your doctor's control. You can handle these situations even if you see them as caused by fate, the will of God, or the fortune or ill fortune of human luck. The emotional playing field can be acknowledged, acted on, and perhaps even mastered so you can improve compliance, comfort, and success. Once understood, the emotions that arise become less upsetting and frightening and can start to work to your advantage.

Prostate cancer and overwhelming anxiety can represent a real threat at your front door. When our ancestors in the jungle ran into threats, like a lion, they had to be ready with a spear to fight (and kill) the threatening animal or be fleet-footed and prepared to take flight quickly. This phenomenon as it relates to prostate cancer is described by psychologist Suzanne Chambers in her book, *Facing The Tiger: A Guide for Men with Prostate Cancer and the People Who Love Them*. Fight or flight is a survival instinct. Most of us do not run into lions or tigers today, but that physiological defensive mechanism remains intact and on alert for dangerous or threatening situations. So your internal wiring may substitute another stimulus (i.e., an upcoming PSA test or a MRI scan) for the tiger. Certainly a rising PSA test or a worsening bone scan is worrisome and upsetting. Adrenalizing responses that get your heart and blood pumping activate you in an attempt to help you figure out the best strategy to handle a dangerous situation. However, an overly intense response may have you fighting or fleeing unnecessarily in unhelpful ways, such as to the Internet, which also may "paralyze" you, leaving you like a "deer in the headlights" with panic symptoms that either make you feel horrible physically and emotionally or impair your ability to deal with the threat. You might not get your next PSA test or have difficulty staying in an MRI scan. Your ultimate goal of promoting your health will be thwarted or compromised. Few people have nerves of steel. But managing emotions is possible and could be an advantage in managing prostate cancer.

Signs of high distress, anxiety, and panic include jitteriness, restlessness, ruminating about the past or worrying about the future, pacing, agitation, irritability, insomnia, decreased concentration, "butterflies" or a knot in the pit of your stomach, diarrhea, poor or excessive appetite, hopelessness or helplessness, social withdrawal, *palpitations, *shortness of breath, *sweating, *facial flushing, *tremors, or *a sense of impending doom (symptoms with an asterisk are indications of panic attacks). These adrenaline-stimulated, flight-or-fight signs of anxiety are often mistaken for heart attacks, strokes, or other worrisome medical conditions, which can lead to multiple visits to the emergency room.

PSA Watching and Anxiety

If you keep scoreboard-watching, you can't focus on what you need to do on the field.

How do distress and anxiety encroach on a man's world of prostate cancer? After prostate cancer treatment, men are at risk for PSA watching and PSA anxiety. If a man had surgery, he looks for the PSA level to disappear, which indicates that the cancer is gone and the surgery was successful. If the PSA reaches a nonmeasurable amount, he then fears a rise in this blood test level, a sign that the cancer has likely returned. This anxiety can be so pervasive at so many points along a prostate cancer trajectory that it steals much of the joy of living that prostate cancer survival otherwise affords.

Signs of Distress, Anxiety or Panic

Jitteriness
Restlessness
Ruminating or worrying (about the past or the future)
Pacing
Agitation
Irritability
Insomnia
Decreased concentration
Upset stomach/diarrhea
Poor or excessive appetite
Hopelessness/helpless
Social withdrawal
*Palpitations
*Shortness of breath
*Sweating
*Choking sensation in your throat
*Facial flushing
*Tremors
*Sense of impending doom
*"Butterflies", a knot in the pit of your stomach; diarrhea

---

*Symptoms of panic attacks.

I can't stand this anymore! For 2 or 3 weeks before each PSA test I get very upset and restless. I have trouble sleeping, I'm irritable and I just don't think straight. My concentration is shot. My wife says I'm a terror to live with. All I keep thinking about is my combat experience in Vietnam—when I was in a ditch with bullets flying over my head and I was never sure whether a bullet would get me. It seems random, but you know someone will get hit. I keep wondering when or if I will get hit by the PSA bullet.

Our research found what oncologists had been describing to each other for many years—that many men get very upset about changes in their PSA levels. Sometimes the changes would be clinically inconsequential and the high anxiety and worry seemed out of proportion to medical realities. We call this *PSA anxiety*. Concern over PSA tests has also been described as "PSA-dynia" and "PSA-itis." Men get worried about a particular PSA test and whether the PSA level will go up. And if it does go up, they wonder, "How high will it climb?" Patients often do not view PSA levels as the early warning system it is meant to be—a trigger that allows a physician and patient to formulate a plan to be aware of and treat the cancer sooner if it returns or progresses; in the past, before PSA tests, this could not be done until much further down the road. It was like closing the barn doors after the cow has escaped. The hope that you won't ever have to be concerned about prostate cancer again is shattered with a post-surgical elevation in PSA. Many a patient has told me, "Well doc, if it were your life post-surgical, you might be feeling the same thing."

PSA anxiety might be aroused even more easily in men who have undergone radiation therapy. Their PSA levels do not always go to zero after treatment. They find their own bottom baseline, or *nadir*, which is their equivalent of zero. Over time, potential increases will be measured against that baseline; however, there's nothing as reassuring as a zero.

I cannot say how much I'd worry about my own PSA level if I had prostate cancer, given the life threat that these men fear. But I am uneasy for a couple of days until my own PSA screening results come back.

There are unfortunate consequences when men obsess about their PSA tests and are distracted from living their lives more fully *today*. They demonize each test by equating it with disaster, as the knowledge of their own mortality is reawakened. Men who get extra PSA tests to make sure they have the "correct" number are often looking to see that the PSA has not gone up—they want reassurance that everything is fine, not an early warning in case there may be danger. They understandably want the good news, not the bad. Men bring elaborate charts of their PSA test results to the urologist or oncologist's office, sometimes in multicolored logarithmic formats, to best highlight the clinical response to their different prostate cancer treatments. This process may be calming and a good channel for cancer worry for some men. The patient may feel it is informative for his oncologist. However, too many men spend too much time obsessing about their PSA tests and results. They spend hours and sometimes days calculating and analyzing how each test compares with changes in the past and with possible predictions of the future. This process, just like the multiple hours spent on the Internet reading blogs about others' responses to different prostate cancer treatments or looking for new treatments, may take the idea of an informed consumer too far. These men become preoccupied about a projected, potential catastrophic timeline interpretation of their PSA tests as if they will die soon, rather than living meaningfully now.

Urologists and oncologists have tried to get patients to focus on the significance of trends of PSA levels, rather than on any one result. Our research found that PSA anxiety is correlated not with a singular PSA result but with the trend of recent test results. Those men who had a pattern of fluctuating results over their last three PSA tests—that is, either (a) a pattern of three rising levels, (b) a pattern of up-down-up, (c) a pattern of down-up-down, or (d) paradoxically, three falling PSA levels—had significantly higher anxiety in a study designed to measure prostate cancer–related anxiety. The men who had stable PSA scores had less anxiety—stability likely heralds a sense of routine predictability and calm; change triggers anxiety. People tend toward stability and certainty, just as individual atoms settle into the most stable state possible.

Physicians, nurses, and patients have all asked me why a trend of falling PSA tests would be more highly correlated with anxiety. This does not make intuitive sense if lower is better. The relatively high levels of anxiety among men with falling PSA levels may indicate that patients who are still in the active phases of treatment are concerned that their improvement will continue. Perhaps they are so focused on the future that they invert Newton's laws of gravity: What goes down one day may go up on another—and maybe soon. There may be a time-insulating element involved in this phenomenon. If the PSA were to trend and stay down for a long enough period of time, these worried men might eventually adjust, just as those with stable PSA levels. This has not been studied sufficiently enough to know for sure.

Are You Depressed?

New diagnoses of cancer can make most people feel sad, down, depressed, or demoralized. Differences in intensity and duration of mood changes may indicate whether these emotions are likely to resolve on their own or if professional help is needed. In a person without medical illness, a treatable depression is diagnosed when a depressed mood has been present for at least 2 weeks, most days and most of the day, and the depressed person cannot enjoy usual pleasurable activities. They may have changes in sleep patterns, appetite, concentration, and energy levels, also called neurovegetative symptoms, caused by physiological or biochemical changes in the brain.

People with cancer may feel less hope about the future than they did before their diagnosis. That may be appropriate, at least for now. When these symptoms are linked physiologically to the cancer or its treatment, similar to the neurovegetative symptoms noted earlier, their helpfulness in terms of identifying a depression is somewhat decreased. The more significant clues of a severe depression include feelings of worthlessness or helplessness; severe, nagging guilt about being punished for something you did or did not do in your life (not mere regrets for things we feel we should or should not have done, which occurs to most of us); ongoing despair; a sense of hopelessness about the ability to find any meaning, joy, or purpose in life; and constant thoughts of death or dying or the wish to die or take your life. An inability to do or enjoy usual pleasurable activities because of symptoms such as pain or fatigue is frustrating and may be depressing—but it does not always add up to a clinically significant depression. A useful question that helps me distinguish these is, "If you could take a magic pill to give you energy or take away your pain, what would you like to do?" If the answer is "I don't care; it doesn't matter," this is likely a significant depression that is lacking future orientation or hopefulness. If the answer is, "Of course, I'd like to get out and garden or see my children or grandchildren," this may look like a bad depression to those around you; however, it is more likely related to your medical symptoms and can resolve if that connection is clarified and if those physical symptoms are addressed more vigorously.

When depressive symptoms are constant (most of the day for most days), and the intensity is moderate to severe (i.e., the symptoms interfere with your ability to carry on with daily life activities and enjoy them, even in the context of cancer), it makes sense to get professional help. Psychotherapy can help. Some will try an antidepressant under the guidance of a physician who will regularly monitor for the benefits and watch for and attend to possible side effects. Antidepressants in cancer patients work best on those biochemical changes associated with persistent depressed mood, thoughts of dying, worthlessness, and hopelessness that may or may not coincide with neurovegetative symptoms. Many individuals will seek the help of psychotherapy and an antidepressant.

Many people with cancer have thought, "Maybe I or my family would be better off if I were to die," or "If it gets bad enough in the future [usually with very personal criteria for what 'bad enough' means, such as too much pain, not being able to care for oneself, or being a vegetable like the uncle who had dementia], I would kill myself." These are serious thoughts, but are futuristic reflections that are common in cancer patients who agonize over one day losing a sense of control or putting up with the compelling distress in their lives. These occasional musings bring temporary relief to the present with a sense of control of the future: "I won't have to take it if I don't want to" (i.e., the uncertainty, the prognosis, the losses, and the changes). Your physician and family should take these thoughts seriously. If there are fears of future helplessness, they can provide reassurance by committing to relieving any suffering as best as possible.

Current thoughts and plans of suicide are more concerning and may indicate significant depression. If you have a major depression and a concrete plan about how to commit suicide with any intention to do so, your doctor and support people should act on that immediately to ensure your safety, and treat the depression that is causing this overly bleak view of life. Rarely, as noted earlier, severe depression can be caused by medications used to treat the cancer (i.e., steroids, hormones, pain medications). These depressive symptoms can be resolved by changing the dose of the offending medication, by changing the medication altogether, or, when those options are not possible, treating with an antidepressant. The despair and suicidal "rationale" that look inevitable during a significant depression dissolve after it is treated, and life looks very different.

How Do I Know When to Get Professional Help for Depression?

For those with fatigue or other physical symptoms (like pain or nausea) that interfere with usually pleasurable activities, ask yourself: "If I could take a magic pill to give me energy or take away my pain, what would I like to do?"

If the answer is "I don't care; it doesn't matter," it is time to get professional mental health help. If it does matter, it is important to ask your doctor for help with those uncomfortable symptoms.

Duration of symptoms: >2 weeks
Intensity of symptoms: moderate to severe most days, most of the day

Common Symptoms of Depression

Depressed mood
Loss of interest (not related to physical symptoms of pain, fatigue, nausea)

Inconsistent Symptoms of Depression in People with Cancer

Weight loss or gain may be related to the cancer
Insomnia/hypersomnia
Psychomotor agitation/retardation
Fatigue
Feelings of worthlessness/guilt*
Persistent thoughts of death/suicide*

Common Symptoms of Depression in the Elderly

Stomach aches
General aches and pains
Diffuse somatic complaints
Malaise/weight loss
Persistent and intense hopelessness about the future*
Late-night insomnia
Mood variation
Anxiety/agitation

---

* Occasional thoughts of hopelessness about the future or questions about feeling worth-while, or even wondering if it would be better to not be alive anymore, when adjusting to new levels of health are common when dealing with cancer. Persistent thoughts of hope-lessness, wanting to die, or suicide are hallmarks of depressive episodes and should be addressed by a mental health professional.

Once You Identify Distress, Anxiety, or Depression What Do You Do about It?

We can't solve problems by using the same kind of thinking we used when we created them.

Albert Einstein

All of the therapeutic techniques described in this section will be help-ful before, during, and after you complete your cancer treatment. Days or weeks before and during return visits to the urologist or oncologist, or to get a PSA test or PSA result, or to get an MRI or bone scan, you may be fraught with worry. The coping techniques discussed here include methods to avoid thought traps that prolong worry rather than resolve it. We accomplish this by tweaking and correcting or recalculating recurrent, exaggerated, generalized, irrational, and troubling thoughts and thought processes; by using behavioral activation; with problem-solving strategies; and with relaxation procedures that diminish daytime anxiety and nighttime insomnia. If the information I provide does not help sufficiently with your distress, get professional help. Psychotherapy and possibly medications for anxiety or depression can bring relief that then allows you to get back on track with your life as you manage prostate cancer.

Get DRAFTed with Emotional Judo

The approach I use to help men with prostate cancer manage stress is called *Emotional Judo (EJ)*. It is an integrated mingling of various schools of psychotherapy including insight-oriented therapy, cognitive behavioral therapy (CBT), acceptance and commitment therapy (ACT), problem-solving therapy, and mindfulness meditation. This method visibly maps out how to cope with distress that arises with prostate cancer experiences. I like the visual image of a big, bad opponent (the cancer, anxiety, distress, etc.) that is menacing me being flipped, as in a judo flip. Since your fight or flight adrenal mechanism may be in high gear, you can try to run away, but the opponent will still be there waiting for you later; or you can try to hit back, but risk getting clobbered. Instead, with the right moves, you can use the opponent's strength to your advantage and cut it down to size. Then you can move on with your life. These techniques can be used at home, at work, while taking a walk outside, as well as in a medical office waiting area, or in the hospital.

Many types of psychotherapy are available to well-trained general mental health practitioners to manage emotional difficulties related to prostate cancer. However, mental healthcare professionals not familiar with cancer settings may not be aware of the intricacies involved in diagnosing and treating the distress that is specific to these men and their medical problems. The trick is matching the patient and/or family member, as well as the cancer conditions and physical and social circumstances, with the therapy type. Mismatches and frustration happen frequently because one size doesn't fit all. Insight-oriented psychotherapy relies on increased understanding and expression of current feelings, motivations, beliefs, fears, and desires, and on the connection with past emotional conflicts. Although this therapy derives from psychoanalysis and Sigmund Freud, it has evolved into many variations of intensity, style, emphasis, and length of treatment. This therapy helps people consider their reactions to their cancer in the context of the broad continuum and complexity of their entire lives, including other illness experiences, losses, and reactions to death. Many at this crucial crisis in their lives appreciate this primarily nondirective, exploratory method.

Others hypothesize: "My life was fine before this cancer. A silent therapist who explores unconscious childhood slights won't help me in my cancer crisis now. I want someone who is more active in my treatment." For instance, a more reflective therapeutic approach might be less appreciated than an active cognitive-behaviorally oriented treatment that teaches relaxation techniques or attempts to recalibrate suboptimal, unhelpful automatic thoughts and behavioral patterns that don't fit the current situation for someone caught in the inertia of a recuperation period from radiation therapy when his energy is diminished, or someone who fears getting into an MRI machine. The eminent psychologist Aaron Beck initially conceptualized the theory and practice of CBT, which is based on the premise that our thoughts, behaviors, and emotions interact and influence each other. Where the thoughts, emotions, and behaviors derive from is less important than in insight-oriented therapy; recognizing the irrational nature of the thoughts, emotions, or behaviors is key to solving problems and fruitful change. Thoughts influence emotions, which can influence behaviors, which can influence thoughts or emotions in all directions and many permutations, like a web. There are many excellent books on how to use cognitive behavioral techniques to deal with various life stressors and uncomfortable emotions. A number of my patients have found *Feeling Good: The New Mood Therapy*, by David Burns, to be very helpful. Those interested in a formal CBT approach that focuses on localized prostate cancer in particular may look at a book coauthored by Frank Penedo: *Cognitive-Behavioral Stress Management for Prostate Cancer Recovery Workbook (Treatments That Work)*. This book discusses cognitive behavioral stress management (CBSM) and relaxation training for those who have difficulty readjusting to life after surgery as a result of treatment-related side effects. It provides stress management skills, including improving awareness of automatic but unhelpful thoughts, and practicing more rational and less anxiety-provoking coping strategies. The book teaches progressive muscle relaxation, imagery, and meditation. Relevant issues for men who have had prostate cancer, such as sexuality and communication, are also addressed. There is a corresponding workbook, with exercises, monitoring forms, and homework assignments.

My colleague Chris Nelson has adapted acceptance and commitment therapy (ACT), a therapy initially developed by Steven Hayes, for men with prostate cancer. This therapy helps people accept what is out of their personal control and commit to action that improves and enriches their lives. It is derived from CBT principles and uses mindfulness meditation techniques to help people notice and accept what is happening, rather than wishing things were different. Dr. Nelson's ACT adaptation specifically helps men get over the hurdle of erectile dysfunction, using penile injections, if needed, after prostate cancer treatment.

Often, diverse therapeutic approaches integrated thoughtfully by the same therapist can help patients find comfort and healing by specifically targeting what's needed at the time and for the specific situation.

A useful skill to learn for using any of these therapies is how to relax. It will facilitate many of the suggestions that follow if you are too tense to carry them out. Mindfulness meditation is a popular form of meditation that helps reduce stress and tension. Mindfulness-based stress reduction (MBSR) stems from Eastern meditations and yoga traditions as formulated and popularized by Dr. Jon Kabat-Zinn in his book, *Full Catastrophe Living: Using the Wisdom of Your Body and Mind to Face Stress, Pain and Illness*. MBSR is effective in providing relief to people with medical illness and physical symptoms such as pain and nausea. Dr. Kabat-Zinn has written many books and has made many recordings for learning and practicing mindfulness. I have read or listened to many of them, and I try to practice it regularly. Think of this exercise as part of emotional aerobics (E-Robics). Listening to his CDs is a good way to learn this type of meditation and will strengthen your brain *muscle* to better handle stress.

Thoughts, behaviors, and emotions play on each other in multidirectional or cyclical modes. When I am down emotionally, I feel like doing less physically. When I do less, I think I am not productive and feel more useless. Once the seeds of these emotions, behaviors, and thoughts germinate, sequelae of the original thoughts, events, or emotions propagate like weeds that overtake a garden—this becomes a classic self-fulfilling prophesy. These thoughts, emotions, and behaviors may be irrational, over-exaggerated, and not pertinent to the current set of circumstances, though they seem believable and appropriate as you feel more down or nervous, continuing the spiral. Described as "automatic" or patterned and habitual, over years of reinforcement in different situations and circumstances, the thoughts, emotions, and behaviors develop a life of their own so that they feel quite natural, routine, and almost predestined for us: "This is just the way I am; I always feel depressed; nothing goes my way." These false perceptions are like bad habits that seem normal or justified just because they are familiar. These patterns can be quite seductive yet potentially self-sabotaging emotionally when it comes to cancer issues:

> If I just put more time into figuring out the best treatment, or what I will do if my PSA goes up, I will be better prepared and will discover the correct solution.
> If only my PSA didn't go up again. Why didn't that treatment work better for me? I must be jinxed.

There are a limited number of replays that are useful before making a call. But your brain doesn't always realize this—neither your intellectual brain, which tries to see your way clear to cure by using your usual problem-solving powers, nor your emotional brain, which may feel the anxiety-provoking recoil of inappropriate shadows of imminent dying.

You can try to "short-circuit" these patterned thoughts and behaviors, consciously shifting your focus to activities that either have meaning, purpose, or enjoyment for your life in the here and now. This practice will enhance your present and future, and hopefully your family's present and future as well. It will keep you from getting stuck in the past or the far-off future so you do not miss the here and now. There are specific algorithms in formal CBT that help people reassess irrational thoughts and learn to reformulate ones that are more fitting to the person, time, and situation. For some people, it is difficult to work on the current thoughts and emotions without understanding the impact of conflictual relationships and life experiences from the past—that is amenable to insight-oriented therapy. The Emotional Judo method takes into account features from all of the previously mentioned approaches. Later in the chapter I will delineate a step-by-step description of the DRAFT with EJ technique, but first it is important to start with a primer in meditation. If your thoughts or emotions are spiraling in distressing ways, it is good to have a few options to diffuse the angst.

Relaxation or breathing exercises and meditation are useful devices under your control for bringing on calm when you are freaking out. I'm not looking to make a yogi out of anyone. I just want to help you take a little bit of the edge off so you can carry out the other recommendations with more clarity and calm. Some patients tell me this practice reminds them of the transcendental meditation (TM) they did many years ago that they loved so much, but which they packed away with their youth. They hadn't thought of using it in this crisis. Dust it off, if it feels more familiar and do-able! Otherwise, try the following exercises.

First, Let's Take a Break to Meditate or Relax—Warm Up

Relaxation or meditation is a useful skill to learn. If you didn't skip to this section earlier in the book to learn how to better tolerate doctor's office visits, now is a great time to start. Becoming more aware of your thoughts and emotions and what you are doing while you are doing it can help you change what you think, feel, and do. Your ability to catch impulsive, often self-sabotaging reactions will improve, and you will be more able to deflect them and stay clearer and calmer and feel improve, more in control. You may find that you are more alert and better able to deal with the ordeals of prostate cancer.

Sit Up (or Lie Down) and Relax

Relaxation techniques have been shown to decrease anxiety, improve responses to stressful situations, improve alertness and concentration, and decrease physical discomfort such as pain and nausea. Learning relaxation exercises and practicing them routinely when your anxiety is less intense will make the techniques that much more accessible and successful when you have more distress. Taking a conscious breath is like taking a "chill pill," as one of my colleagues described it. Relaxation or mindfulness breathing facilitates using any of the thought, emotional, or behavioral boosting skills of Emotional Judo that follow. Before you start, measure your distress on a scale of 0–10, where 10 is the worst distress you've ever felt. When you finish the relaxation exercise, measure your distress again. In fact, you can measure your distress daily or multiple times per day. It may give you a weighted handle on how well you are feeling emotionally. If you're not sure how to proceed or whether you even want to proceed, breathe.

Relaxation exercises help men "consciously relax." I know this sounds convoluted, perplexing, and paradoxical. Isn't relaxing supposed to be effortless? Relaxation exercises are closely related and very similar to meditation, visualization, guided imagery, self-hypnosis, and other de-stressing methods. Just as there are many roads that lead to Rome, there are "different strokes for different folks" when it comes to meditation and relaxation. Men tell me they were aware of doing meditative breathing when they practiced yoga as well as more rigorous martial arts. Some remember when their wives were going through Lamaze breathing training before they gave birth. Any of these approaches will facilitate a heightened sense of concentration or focus while decreasing distress. Practiced efforts over time will allow you to feel more relaxed as you turn down the volume of the emotional and physical noises of distress and tension that cancer ushers in.

There are many good books to read, as well as tapes or CDs to listen to that can teach you how to relax or meditate and many great classes available locally and online (see the Appendix for some suggested resources). Though I have not done an exhaustive study of these some methods, I imagine that most are excellent variations on a theme and can get you to a similar place—becoming calmer and thoughtful when you are anxious or upset. Herbert Benson found in *The Relaxation Response* that even focusing on or repeating a word or phrase for 10 minutes at a time, once per day, helped decrease anxiety levels considerably. Mindfulness meditation or MBSR directs you to bring continued attention and awareness to your breath, which, like an anchor, is always present. Rather than focusing on a mantra, word, or phrase, you bring continued refocusing on your breath, the anchor that is always present. When you lose focus, or you find your mind drifting, which will likely happen often over short periods of time, resuming awareness of your breath guides you back to the wakeful present.

Reading about relaxation or breathing exercises is not enough. Then they are just good, helpful ideas. Putting the ideas into use in a personalized fashion is called for in order to bring relief and get you back on track with your life—in this case, with more control over your cancer-related anxiety or distress.

Imagine that your doctor has written a prescription for you to practice this technique once a day, for 20 minutes at a time. Most patients are more likely to comply with a prescription for a medicine than with "just good advice." If you need to start with a lower daily dose, even 5–10 minutes a day, that's fine. Just start!

Prescription for Relaxation Therapy

Rx:	Relaxation exercise
Sig:	One session daily (10–30 minutes) plus brief calming breaths as needed throughout the day
Dispense #:	Unlimited per month (no insurance approval needed)

The exercise that I will describe here is like a sampler or demo model. It includes a few variations, like a tasting menu, that will give you a flavor of the meditation or relaxation exercises that I practice with my patients, containing sections on mindfulness, using a mantra, and using passive muscle relaxation. Find more detailed descriptions and guidance on tapes or CDs, or in books solely on this subject from your local bookstore, library, or online. If there is a variation or option you like and think you might use, go with it. The following example is designed to show you what relaxation or meditation can be like.

I will describe three common relaxation techniques, in three parts, so you can see which, if any appeals, to you. The first part of this exercise suggests focusing on your breath, an enduring signal that is always present. When you notice that your attention is not on your breath, its constant presence in the background of your awareness stands like a guiding buoy to redirect you back to your breath, or like an anchor to grip on to when your thoughts have gone astray. This is the bedrock of mindfulness meditation. Re-attending to your breath and continually becoming aware of your breath, which persists whether you are aware of it or not, draws your thoughts back from wherever they have drifted to. Your breath, in its constancy, is with you whether you are in an MRI scanner, in a doctor's waiting room, lying awake in bed while everyone else is sleeping, or feeling back pain while sitting at your desk.

Try not to get into the trap of expecting or waiting for something to happen, such as sublime relaxation or ecstatic happiness or to be worry-free or thought-free. The more you try to force your thoughts on one route, the more they may go on just the opposite course. Just let them go with gentle redirection, back to awareness of your breath.

The second section of this relaxation example uses a repeated word, phrase, or mantra technique to help maintain your focus. Mantras originated with Eastern religions and often have a spiritual connotation. In this exercise, like the breath in mindfulness, the words or mantras essentially serve as mind place-keepers. When your thoughts wander, which they do naturally, it is good to have the target to come back to. These techniques are not brain-clearing devices. They are exercises that use a physical (the breath) or mental (the word, phrase, or mantra) device over and over again, to modify or detour the angst of worries, thoughts, recurring regrets, or uncertain expectations. They might be described as emotional or thought circuit breakers. You then have a chance to halt or diminish the seductive, yet menacing nature of snowballing distress.

The third segment is a passive muscle relaxation exercise designed to ease tension in any tight or achy muscles or joints from your toes to your head. You will visualize different sections of your body and see and feel the tension that may be in them releasing and leaving from that part of your anatomy.

You may read the following script to yourself or record it on your smartphone or a computer and then play it back and listen, so you don't distract your attention by reading. You can also have someone read the exercise to you the first few times you try it, or make a recording of his or her voice. Depending on which feels more comfortable, you may sit or lie down for this practice. However, while lying down, some men are more prone (no pun intended) to falling asleep, so they prefer sitting up in a comfortable chair. If it's nighttime and you are having trouble falling asleep, see a variation on these techniques in the sleep section later in this chapter to quiet your mind and eventually bring on sleep.

See which of the three methods you prefer—following your breath, using a word, phrase, or mantra, or passive muscle relaxation. Does one speak to you more than the others? Experiment with each to see which you like more and which, over time, is more helpful. Some men will make a unique combination that works for them. When I teach this to patients, spouses, partners, or adult children in my office, I narrate all of them. For the second method of repeating phrases or mantras, I include choices: Calm; Relax; Peace; Serene; Ohm. If none of these rings true or feels right, make up your own.

Prepare

Sit on a chair (or lie down if that is more comfortable) and arrange your arms and legs so you feel at ease. Place your hands on your knees or lap and your feet on the ground (if you are sitting and they reach the floor). You may lie on a couch or mattress; recognize that you may be more likely to fall asleep this way—the idea of this exercise is to heighten your awareness so that your brain is pulled in far fewer directions of worry or agonizing thoughts so you can relax more. Coach yourself to stay awake. It helps to have a gentle-sounding timer or alarm nearby that will go off in a set amount of time (10, 15, 20, 25, 30 minutes or longer) or have someone who will gently tell you when the time is up, so you do not have to continually watch the clock mentally or worry that you will fall asleep. You can find timers on your smartphone or computer. There are even meditation apps that you can download. Close your eyes if you feel comfortable with that. If not, pick a spot somewhere in front of you to focus on. I usually prefer the eyes-closed method as it removes visual distractions, even if it is more likely to bring on sleep (although that's why I usually don't lie down). Mindfulness and heightened attention can even be practiced while walking or doing some other activity, like waiting in your doctor's office, driving a car, riding in an elevator, or waiting at a crosswalk for the traffic light to change. *But don't close your eyes!* You can induce a sense of calm and alertness by focusing on your breath, the word or phrase you've chosen, or breathing a relaxed feeling into a tense, uncomfortable, or achy part of your body.

The Relaxation Exercises

Part One: Observe Your Breath

Notice your breath. Your breath is your anchor or buoy for this exercise. It is always with you. It signals where to come back to when you are distracted by your thoughts or emotions and find yourself no longer focused on your breath. Your breath is here now while sitting in your chair or lying on a mattress. Become aware of it. Take a few, slow, long, easy breaths. Breathe in through your nostrils and out through your mouth. You can continue like this or breathe in and out just through your nostrils or mouth. Comfort is an important aspect of this process, especially if you are not feeling well physically. You do not need to breathe too deep, too shallow, or too anything. After those first long breaths, just breathe as you would normally. Notice the breath. Be aware of your breath. As you focus on the inhalation, notice that your stomach or abdomen rises or expands a little. It contracts or falls as you exhale. This is often called "belly breathing" and helps your lungs expand more and get a fuller supply of oxygen. Just because you notice your abdomen expanding does not mean you have to exaggerate it at all or "make it happen." It will happen naturally. Just notice the breath as it is. Notice what the breath feels like—is it fast or slow, moist or dry, loud or soft, cool or warm? Is it different when you breathe in compared to when you breathe out? Observe the breath entering your nostrils or mouth when you inhale, and then exiting your nostrils or mouth when you exhale. Decide which is easier for you for you to focus on. If you have breathing difficulties or congestion, breathe any way that feels comfortable. Or you may want to focus on another part of your body that is not concerning and visualize that part of your body breathing.

If focusing on your breath is not working for you, skip down to the next section and use the word/phrase/mantra repetition as your stationary beacon. You may find that your attention begins to wander after a few seconds or minutes. This is natural and happens to everyone. After all, our minds are accustomed to thinking thoughts and feeling feelings. There may be everyday problems to solve. Concerns about health, upcoming PSA tests, finances, or loved ones may come to mind. Mundane musings such as "What am I going to do for dinner?" or "Did I shut the light off in the kitchen before I sat down to meditate?" may also appear. We are often seduced by our thoughts, emotions, plans, and concerns, and try to follow them to a logical conclusion that seems just around the corner yet never seems to come. That's often how the "worry snowball" grows. However, whenever you find yourself not focusing on your breath, bring your attention and awareness back to the breath, again and again. Don't get upset with yourself when you find you have wandered. Follow your breath all the way in, and then follow it all the way out. Follow it all the way in, and follow it as you let it out. Take note of where your mind wanders to if it does wander, and what you are thinking about or feeling. However, don't linger there. RETURN TO THE BREATH. Even if it feels like you are doing this many times within a few short minutes, RETURN TO THE BREATH. If your eyes open, simply close them again. Follow the breath.

Be aware of this moment. And then the next moment. And then this one. Continue to focus on your breath.

Part Two: Follow a Word, Phrase, or Mantra

You may find it easier to maintain your attention by repeating a word, a phrase, or mantra. The word or phrase can be *relax, calm, peace, peace be with me, serenity*, or any word or phrase that feels comfortable to you. It can be a sound like *ohmmmmm*. A word or phrase with religious or spiritual significance such as *ahhhhhmen* or *shalommmmm* from Hebrew, or *saaalaaam* from Arabic may feel right to you. When the words are elongated you might feel a vibratory effect of the sound within your body. Just notice the vibrations. If your mind wanders, gently bring your awareness back to the word or phrase or mantra. There is no goal to achieve, no need for a perfect performance. You are not looking to "get to" or attain relaxation. It will come with more time and practice. All you want to do now is focus on the word or phrase, and be aware of this present moment, and then the next one. If you find that the suggested words do not work for you, choose another that feels more suitable.

You can combine the first two parts and breathe a relaxed feeling in, and then breathe out anxiety; breathe in calm, breathe out tension; breathe in peace, breathe out distress.

Part Three: Relax Your Body from Your Feet to Your Head

Now let's transition into the passive muscle relaxation part of the exercise. You will concentrate on relaxing various muscle groups from your feet to your head. Some people prefer to purposely and actively tense all muscles before starting this exercise or before each muscle group (this is called *active muscle relaxation*). With your eyes closed, picture your feet. Become aware of how your feet feel. Are they achy or uncomfortable? As you breathe in, repeat your calming, relaxing word, phrase, or mantra; breathe a relaxing, calm, peaceful, or serene feeling all the way down into your feet; then with your exhalation, see yourself breathe whatever tension, tightness, or distress is present in your feet out through your mouth or nostrils. Breathe in the calm...breathe out the achiness. Breathe in the peace...breathe out the tension. Do this a few times, and then move upward in your imagination. Breathe in a calm feeling to each major body area...breathe out the tension or tightness. Focus on your ankles for a few breaths: breathe in a calm, relaxing feeling into your ankles, and breathe out whatever tension or distress that may be there...do this a few times. See them relax. Now become aware of your shins and calves. Breathe in a calm, peaceful feeling into your shins and calves and breathe out whatever tension or achiness that may be there...do this a few times. Focus on your knees for a few breaths: breathe in a calm, serene feeling into your knees and breathe out whatever tension or tightness may be there...do this a few times. Focus on your thighs. Breathe in a calm, relaxing feeling into your thighs and breathe out whatever tension or distress may be there...do this a few more times slowly. Now focus on your pelvis. Breathe in a calm, relaxing feeling into your pelvis and breathe out whatever tension or distress that may be there. Again, breathe in a calm, peaceful feeling into your pelvis and breathe out whatever discomfort or distress that may be there...Now bring your attention to your abdomen. Breathe in a calm, relaxing feeling into your belly and breathe out whatever tension or discomfort that may be there...do this a few more times...Focus on your chest. Breathe in a relaxed, peaceful feeling into your chest and breathe out whatever tension or tightness may be there...do this a few more times...Now focus on your shoulders, your arms, your hands, and your fingers. Notice if there is any achiness or tightness there. Breathe in a calm, relaxing feeling from your shoulders all the way down to your fingers and breathe out whatever tension or distress may be there...do this a few more times...Now bring your attention to your back...your lower back and your upper back...Breathe in a calm, relaxing feeling into your lower and upper back and all the muscles in your back and breathe out whatever achiness or tightness may be there...Focus on your neck and all the muscles in your neck. Breathe in a calm, relaxing feeling into your neck and breathe out whatever tension or distress may be there...Now bring your attention to your face and head. Notice if there is any tension or discomfort there...Breathe in a calm, peaceful feeling into your face and head and breathe out whatever tension, tightness, or discomfort may be there.

Now become aware of your whole body. Notice what your body feels like. Does it feel heavy or light, numb, or something different? People often sense something as they start to relax, so just notice what your body feels like now. It's possible that as you let your guard down, you may initially feel some angst. Try to let those feelings come and go. Breathe them in and breathe them out. You are fine and safe just as you are in this moment.

If there is a particular part of your body that has been experiencing particular pain or discomfort, you can focus on that part for a longer period of time. You may also visualize your breath bringing a soothing feeling to the painful or uncomfortable area, perhaps seeing a soft color in the painful area.

When you are awakened by your gentle alarm or someone's voice, slowly count to three while beginning to wiggle your fingers and toes. Slowly stretch your arms and legs, move your head easily from side to side, and back and forth, gently rub your hands together and then rub your eyes softly, and then open your eyes slowly.

A Quick Guide to Relaxation or Meditation

Set a timer for the amount of time you want to relax or meditate.
Find a comfortable place to sit or lie down.
Close your eyes.

Choose a Method That Feels Right for You or Try Them All

1. Bring awareness to your breath, whenever your mind wanders away from the breath. Return your attention to your breath again and again and again.
2. Use a word or mantra to repeat to yourself, over and over again.
3. Visualize different parts of your body, from toes to head, and calmly breathe a relaxed, calmer peaceful feeling into them.

See any tension or discomfort leaving your body as you breathe out.
Repeat the method over and over and over again until the timer goes off.

This relaxation method will help you when you are tense. Some people feel a little calmer; others feel very calm. Still others feel more alert. It is best not to expect to feel or hope for any type of feeling but appreciate wherever you are at and what comes up as your brain processes a more optimal way of handling all that you are going through. Regular practice of these exercises will raise your threshold for reactivity to the stressful thoughts or emotions that arise in your life so you can respond more clearly and calmly and thoughtfully. But like all exercises, if you don't do them, you won't see any results. These benefits are much more difficult to see than muscle tone or strength that comes with lifting weights.

Relaxation exercises are best practiced initially at home for 5–30 minutes at a time. I even practice meditation on my daily train commute, with or without a CD to listen to. Individual, conscious breaths can be used for brief de-stressing moments in the doctor's waiting room, in the exam room, in an MRI scan, while getting an IV inserted, on your couch at home, or when visiting your relatives. You don't have to be tense to practice them. In fact, practicing them when you are not in a higher stress situation will facilitate competency in the method so you can call on this relief from your bullpen when you do have higher distress. They will become second nature eventually. These exercises can help your brain create alternate pathways and give you a break from the snowball of worried thoughts. Distressing thoughts can be mischievously familiar and beckoning. They can also be exhausting. Just when you are sure you will zero in on a solution to or clarification of a problem or dilemma, something gets in the way. The best way to handle this predicament is to short-circuit the worry path by trying a different tactic and engaging in one of the relaxation techniques.

Breathing or relaxation exercises can help you engage in the DRAFT process of Emotional Judo, described next, if you feel stuck and unable to enact it. Remember, this helpful technique is not just literally but figuratively right under your nose and at your fingertips all the time, and not just in your comfortable chair at home. In the same way that monotonous repetition of fielding ground balls helps baseball infielders smoothly catch and throw balls under pressure, repeating or practicing the relaxation technique will help make it work when you are feeling distressed out in the real world. Professional athletes use similar techniques to visualize optimal performances when in competition. For instance, while you are home, you can visualize relaxing in an MRI scanner, using the relaxation technique you prefer from the described methods. When you get in the scanner, you will more easily move into your breathing technique and feel more comfortable. These relaxation techniques would also probably help the infielder do better at snagging those balls more efficiently and with less stress and errors.

Here's a Refill

If you cannot find the last prescription for relaxation, or you haven't practiced in awhile, here's a refill. You can always restart, just like you can always become aware of your breath.

Time for A Refill Prescription for Relaxation and Mindfulness

Rx:	Relaxation exercise/mindfulness/meditation
Sig:	One session daily (10–30 minutes) plus brief calming breaths as needed throughout the day
Dispense #:	Unlimited per month (no insurance approval needed)
Refills:	Lifetime supply

Now You Are Ready to Enter the DRAFT with Emotional Judo

Traditional insight-oriented psychotherapy can feel too passive to some men. More active CBT can feel uncomfortable to others who feel they must shine a spotlight on every thought, feeling, or behavior. Just as we reconfigured the gateway to anxious or depressed emotions by using the word *distress*, I have similarly reconceptualized this emotion-thought-behavior-conflict process in a way that has been more acceptable to my patients with prostate cancer. I call this technique Emotional Judo (EJ). I cannot find a specific reference for EJ in the literature that uses these concepts in this way, and it is certainly not a commonly used term in the therapeutic community. There are references to mental karate and mental judo, both of which seem to highlight how a person can get the upper hand over another person, often in negotiating situations, by using mental martial art maneuvers. That is not the purpose here.

I took the term *judo* from my understanding of its martial arts principles, where a person can learn skills to neutralize or overcome a more powerful opponent. If you run away (flight) from the big, bad opponent (i.e., distress, anxiety, or depressive emotions related to cancer or mortality), the adversary will menace you again later or tomorrow. Trying to resist or attack back (fight) could result in your defeat or continuing to feel bad. Learning how to adeptly adjust to or fend off your opponent's attack will cause it to lose balance, reducing its power. Though these are mental maneuvers, the image of an adept judo martial artist deftly flipping his opponent to the ground is striking to me. EJ makes it possible for those under emotional attack to beat apparently stronger opponents. It can help men struggling with prostate cancer to more successfully spar with distressing emotions, situations, thoughts, and behaviors. It is designed to help men feel less victimized by prostate cancer and its sequelae.

Scientific Disclaimer

Emotional Judo has not been studied scientifically. Though its component therapeutic roots of the previously described therapies have gone through rigorous scientific trials by others, the DRAFT EJ combination of these parts has not been studied. What I present here is based on my years of clinical experience caring for men with prostate cancer. I've seen it work, and I've seen it benefit men who would otherwise shy away from psychotherapy.

EJ is an illustrative combination of cognitive-behaviorally oriented therapy with a more active engagement of insight-oriented therapy that takes into account the goal of acceptance and commitment therapy to acknowledge and accept where things are at now, in order to have a better present and future. Along the way, it encourages, meditation and mindfulness in order to facilitate all of the above. EJ focuses on identifying your internal thoughts and emotions and their roots when appropriate, and can succeed in dissolving overwhelming or overpowering feelings or thoughts, which are perceived as formidable opponents, which can feel like invaders living within you. EJ is a way to fight back, to not give into or give up in the face of uncomfortable emotions, but to handle them in a way that (a) recognizes the power and source of the emotions; yet (b) can deftly deflect and reshape them into more accurate thoughts, more manageable emotions, and more appropriate behaviors; and (c) can help you get on to a more satisfactory path of feeling, doing, or thinking. This is an active process. You cannot sleepwalk through this. Like all good learning systems, it usually requires more than just one or two attempts to own and master it.

Earlier I likened the meditative process to a mental exercise or emotional aerobics (E-Robics). If you've ever done strength training, think about lifting dumbbells. A few repetitions of bicep curls over one or two sessions do nothing for muscle tone or strength. If you expected muscle mass and measured progress at this point, you'd quit, disillusioned. A few repetitions done only once or twice give you little tone or muscle. But 8 to 10 reps, two to three sets, two or more times per week over 4–5 weeks: Wow! A few reps, a few days a week, over many weeks, starts to show results, which often encourages more reps and additional exercise. It may even inspire a better diet that further enhances muscle tone and strength. This is a dynamic process that requires that *P* word again. But practice with EJ cannot be done with rote, mindless inattention. There needs to be conscious awareness and tweaking that has to happen over and over again, until you are feeling more comfortable with your situation, your thoughts, your emotions, and your behaviors. You will be working on content and form.

Emotional Judo helps men recognize that emotions, thoughts, and behavior are human and natural, though often uncomfortable, at times self-defeating, and at worst debilitating, especially in the context of external stressors. EJ proposes techniques which, if followed diligently, can decrease the intensity, duration, and impact of anxious, depressed, irritable moods and thoughts, thereby strengthening your ability to be calmer and more content with your life as you live with prostate cancer and whatever lies in its wake.

Some situations bring out more intense or uncomfortable emotions or thoughts. When those distressing emotions, or the thoughts or events that brings out those emotions, are big, bad, and ugly, they can be overwhelming. They are not enemies, though they may feel that way because they make you feel bad, uncomfortable, or threatened and are not always under your immediate control. Irritable reactions can make the people you love appear to be the enemy. Depressed moods can be like bullets that destroy from within. Too much anxiety can paralyze and inhibit healthy behaviors. When not easily contained, your reactions can become destructive to your loved ones and to yourself.

In sports, a draft is a process used to select prospective players (usually from college or high school ranks) for the teams in a league. The DRAFT method proposed here will give you a solid emotional strategy and the resources to put into play as you deal with prostate cancer. DRAFT is the basis and building block of Emotional Judo. It is unlikely that you will go through these phases in a fluid, sequential order. In fact, it may be impossible to do that, given how complicated our thoughts and emotional processes are. However, you can judge where you get oriented or reoriented, using these techniques as a checklist or guide. Then just as with your car's GPS system, recalculate a location or destination as needed. Any time you feel you need to take a breathing break, take it.

The EJ process has five major aspects that will eventually build into a symbolic judo flip. DRAFT stands for **D**etect, **R**ecognize, **A**cknowledge, **F**lip, and **T**ransform.

Enter the DRAFT of Emotional Judo

Detect uncomfortable emotions, thoughts, or behaviors.

Recognize the rational and irrational aspects of the emotions, thoughts, or behaviors.

Acknowledge and accept your current circumstances and the good that still exists and how the irrational aspects of your emotions, thoughts, or behaviors pull you away from what you really want.

Flip your attention away from the distress and back to the present with the *however* statement.

Transform through relaxation, distraction, or quick-list activities to a pleasurable or meaningful activity.

Many of my medical school classmates used mnemonics or acronyms to better understand and remember important, yet complicated concepts; each letter stood for an item or concept or category to remember. Sometimes the sillier or more vivid the mnemonic, the easier it was to remember. I hope that DRAFT will help you remember the steps of EJ so that when you are stressed, you can easily pick up where you need to.

DRAFT: Detect

First, it is important to **D**etect the uncomfortable emotions, thoughts, or behaviors that are acting like culprits or "opponents" out there—or, in reality, in your head—that feel as if they have run amok and seem to paralyze you or just make you feel as if you or life is out of control. You can learn to better detect any or all of the following: anxiety, sadness, depression, preoccupations or ruminations, unfocused or distracted thinking, anger, irritability, loneliness, and fear, which are most likely reactions to some aspect of your cancer or treatment. These reactions may be familiar from previous challenges in your life. Table 4.1 notes the types of uncomfortable emotions, thoughts, or behaviors that may be present for you, whether or not they make sense. Of course, helpful and pleasant emotions, thoughts, or behaviors can and should be detected as well, although they are often overshadowed by the uncomfortable, scary ones. The good ones should not be taken for granted, even though the uncomfortable ones usually take center stage during a crisis.

TABLE 4.1 DETECTING UNCOMFORTABLE, UNHELPFUL EMOTIONS, THOUGHTS, AND BEHAVIORS

Uncomfortable Emotions	Uncomfortable Thoughts	Unhelpful Behaviors
Anxiety	Repetitive, ruminating thought loops	Drinking more alcohol
Fear	Unfocused	Smoking more tobacco, marijuana
Worry	Difficulty concentrating	Not exercising
Panic	Preoccupied	Eating more junk food
Sadness	Forgetful	Using drugs or medicines inappropriately
Depression, unable to enjoy activities	"I'm going to die"	Apathy; decrease in previously pleasurable activities
Demoralized	"Why me?"	Not productive at work
Hopeless	"This is unfair"	Stop planning for the future
Anger	Upset with others who are healthy	Arguing more
Irritability	"It doesn't take much to bring out my temper."	"Just ask anyone who is around me—they'll say I yell more often for little reason."
Loneliness	"Who would want to spend time with me?"	Social withdrawal

The detection antennae are up after a prostate cancer diagnosis, trying to keep surveillance of what is going on emotionally, physically, and cognitively. But unless you tune into them, these feelings and thoughts are not easily decipherable. You might notice them in your head or in restlessness or discomfort in your body or when you yell at someone with far greater intensity or frequency than you might otherwise. Some people know they're angry when they feel their face flush; others tell me they feel the back of their necks get tighter; some feel lightheaded or start pacing when nervous. Different people will detect different emotions in different ways at different times.

D*RAFT: Recognize*

Second, **R**ecognize, understand, and analyze what is going on. **R**ecognize the emotion, thought, or behavior and where it comes from. Did it really just come out of the blue? Was there a trigger? Identify and then try to separate the irrational from the rational, the unreasonable from the reasonable aspects of these thoughts, emotions, or behaviors. Often there is a rational part of an emotion which is helpful to observe:

"I looked at my calendar and noticed that I am scheduled to be at my urologist next Tuesday for my PSA test, and I got scared that the level went up; I started pacing."

"I was watching a TV show where a couple was going to make love and I got angry because I still can't get an erection. I yelled at my wife for not putting gas in the car."

"I got a pain in my back and I thought the cancer was progressing. I got worried that my next doctor's appointment wasn't for another month."

"I thought about the PSA test I had 3 years ago that was fine and the next one I had last month. It was abnormal and I got diagnosed with prostate cancer. I got so angry at myself that I didn't go for a PSA test sooner and kicked a wall. Why didn't my doctor call me back for another test?"

It is vital to **R**ecognize the irrational, illogical, exaggerated, and highly charged or untimely features of your emotion(s); try to determine where they are coming from, and distinguish them from the rational aspects that coincide.

"I understand my anxiety about the next PSA test because I want this ill-
    ness behind me already, but I worry a lot about whether I will get to
    see my 10-year-old granddaughter graduate from college."
"I am really frustrated and embarrassed because my sexual life has
    changed so much. It has really affected my relationship with my wife.
    I don't think we will ever feel really close again."
"I'm pissed off at my Dad. He never gave me anything good, and this
    prostate cancer is one more example of that. I tried to be so different
    from him."

It's important to understand unfamiliar emotional territory and deci-
pher emotions and thoughts that trespass in your mind before you can
deal with them. Pushing yourself to describe what is going on, and putting
all of that into words, will help you get to steps of resolving the tension.
Most of us cannot "just stop thinking that." Emotions and thoughts are
not inherently bad, but you don't want to be tripped up by them unexpectedly. You want to get the lay of the land. Map out a course before you take
off, but a course that is based on actual topography. You need a good guide.

Example

"If my PSA goes up, I'm a dead man."

Where is this disagreeable, exaggerated thought coming from? It is an
anxious, pessimistic thought and emotion. You don't want to die and
are not likely to die anytime soon because of your new diagnosis of
early-stage prostate cancer. But this thought, and the fearful emotions
that quickly follow, lead you to take a few drinks of Scotch to chill out.
Then you yell at your partner for not calling to say he'd be home late from
work or because he was not there for you when you were freaking out.

When you try to recognize where this thought came from and why it feels so strong now, you think about your grandmother who was like a best friend and who was always there for you. You still miss her terribly, though she died 20 years ago from colon cancer. There is a connection, and you can see the detour that the past brings to your present. Recognizing this will help you navigate through your feelings and thoughts, and cope better with what is actually going on now. Once you **R**ecognize the link between your strong emotion and pessimism about your current problem, past, and future, you will be able to discriminate the rational and helpful from the irrational and ineffective; to separate the wheat from the chaff; to distinguish the pertinent for now from what was relevant 20 years ago and which may get in the way of more contentment in your future.

DR**A**FT: *Acknowledge*

Next, it is time to **A**cknowledge and try to accept that things in the present, and potentially in the future, are different because of the cancer. **A**cknowledge your options for forging a new normal and **A**cknowledge the consequences of not doing this. That means taking into account what is good in your life despite the cancer. When you've separated out the irrational aspects of your emotions, thoughts, and behaviors that do not have to be part of your present or future, you can more easily appreciate what *is* here now and then figure out how to make that as good as possible. Realize how those wayward, yet steadfast thoughts and emotional reactions were not conducive to having a better life. Your cancer diagnosis and treatment threatens what you want so much in the future, that you fear will not materialize as you hoped for. There are understandable reasons for these emotions. You are human after all, and were born with the ability to have emotional reactions that can be important reflections of and guides for what is happening around you.

There are also clear consequences of these emotions and thoughts when they are more intense, frequent, and intrusive than the situation calls for. They can become believable and fabricate a different reality upon which you may start acting. You can **A**cknowledge that these emotions, thoughts, and behaviors have you stuck bemoaning the past or dreading the future while you are not fully engaged in your present. You are off the track you want to be on.

Acknowledge your need to get back on track. In the heat of your anxiety, irritability, or sadness, you may not even realize that you have been detoured from what you really want as you continue to refuse to accept that this part of your reality cannot be undone. It is not easy to acknowledge that the cancer and any post-treatment complications are a part of your life now, however transient or chronic, and it may be even more difficult to acknowledge that you can, or will ever really want to adjust to them. Your best strategy is to figure out how to make them part of your *new* normal and to optimize your new baseline. The threat to your future can help you make the best of your present.

Acknowledging gives you a reasonable rationale for making a change—so you do not inadvertently allow your worries to steal away any more of your life than the actual cancer diagnosis or treatment did or will do. You can see how far you have floated downstream from your true intentions and goals. Acknowledging this does not mean giving up or giving in. It means you can now work with tools that will be useful toward making the best of your life and not losing any more of it through wayward jabs or punches thrown at others or yourself. Here's another good time for breathing.

DRA**F**T: *The Flip*

The next phase of EJ, the **F**lip, allows you to get back on track, to recalculate, and to right your course, given your distressing frame of mind, emotions, thoughts, or behaviors. You will use the weight and strength of the distress you have and **F**lip it back to the present in a healthier, more pleasing or productive manner (just as in the martial art judo, here's where you put the intruder in your brain on its butt). The **F**lip is often introduced by the word *however*, as illustrated next.

> I have been feeling nervous and not sleeping well for the last 10 days;
> I felt too tired and nervous to see my granddaughter last weekend.

I understand why I'm so anxious. ***However:*** My anxiety, insomnia, and social withdrawal are getting in the way of what I really want—a better life today and tomorrow. If I don't enjoy my granddaughter today, what good will tomorrow be?

My irritability is pushing my wife away from me, at least as much as the lack of sex. ***However:*** Even with this fucking cancer, I have a lot to be grateful for. I have a lot of good people in my life, especially my wife and my kids. I need to breathe and cool down, and suggest we take a walk together.

If you have trouble with this part, consider whether you have a "Life sucks, and then you die, so what's the point of changing?" perspective. You might be more of a pessimistic, doomsayer person who sees the "glass half-empty" (or at times, all empty). Don't despair. Your life, your relationships, and your peace of mind are worth continuing with the EJ process. The bar of expectations may have been placed so unrealistically high in the past that trying to achieve change in these areas feels impractical and demoralizing. Take small steps, a few drops of "however" at a time. It takes time, incentive, a willing, appropriate mindset, as well as the bio-mental mechanics to overcome the barriers and challenges to a better life in the face of your cancer. DRAFTing with EJ offers a variety of bio-mental mechanical gadgets to help you manage your prostate cancer experience better and live a better life.

DRAF**T**: Transformation

The last phase of EJ is the **T**ransformation. You have to know where to go or what to do with all of this information or else you are just a sitting duck for the discomfort and self-sabotaging thoughts, behaviors, and emotions to return again and again, with a growing feeling of helplessness and potential complacency, and possibly feeling even worse than when you started because you are now more aware of the discrepancy between what you really want and where you are. This phase will **T**ransform the detection, recognition, acknowledgment, and flipping of the unwanted, uncomfortable emotions, thoughts, or behaviors to move toward a more acceptable and meaningful destination. It will bring you from the unhelpful and annoying dimension of emotions, thoughts, and reflexive behavior into the present so you can decide on a different course of feeling and thinking and doing.

This is like your designated hitter (DH) that figuratively resembles the DH in Major League Baseball's American League. The DH may not be a home run slugger, but you count on him more than others to come through and get runs scored in tough situations. Your "go-to" quick list will come in handy now. Another way to think of this is considering the play action pass or the old flea flicker in football. You are running a play that takes account of *your* defenses and *others'* defenses and the irrational, unproductive aspects of your emotions, thoughts, or behavior. This play is designed to fake out those unhelpful emotions, thoughts, and behaviors. But all successful plays, whether trick plays or not, require preparation and planning to carry them out. Following is an example of **T**ransformation:

> Honey, I'm sorry I yelled at you when you asked me to go to the store. I was watching a show. Well, I wasn't even watching the show. I was stuck on seeing myself wearing diapers for the rest of my life after that diaper commercial came on. Let's take a drive together to the store and then go for a walk.

The Complete EJ Playbook

What follows is the complete EJ playbook that puts the five DRAFT phases together with examples of how it is done. But remember, this is a playbook. You need to design the plays on your chalkboard, that fit your life and circumstances, and then get to practice. The more intense the feelings, and the more familiar and "normal" they seem, the harder you may have to work to acknowledge the irrational aspects and eventually **F**lip and **T**ransform them. If this were a physical wound that became infected, a surgeon might have to clean it out (debride) over time, *and* give you antibiotics to bring complete healing. I hope EJ will help you avoid the need for the equivalent of psychiatric antibiotics (professional psychotherapy with or without antianxiety or antidepressant medications). But if it is insufficient to help you reroute, and you do seek professional help, EJ can be a useful supplement.

1—**D**etect

People do not always realize they are anxious or worried or sad or depressed until the uncomfortable emotion has built to such a crescendo or rolling snowball that they want to cover their ears or eyes, or feel the need to jump out of the way of what now feels boulder-sized. Sometimes their inertia leads them to just lie down under the boulder. Unfortunately, the noise, and in some instances the deafening silence, comes from inside the head, and the snowball just keeps rolling on. The first skill in DRAFT is developing an early warning detection system, to know when you are starting to feel stressed and what is causing that distressed feeling; to be aware of when your thoughts are backing you into a corner; or to realize when your behavior is not in tune with what you feel is best for you or those around you.

Have you experienced "beneficial" stress (the kind you may have felt before playing a game of basketball or soccer that gets your adrenalin and motivation going and stimulates your muscles and senses)? Without detecting that there is something to get ready for, you might not play well at all. Maybe you've felt the same feeling before you've given a public presentation, where the energy brings on a better talk. Or did you instead feel so tense, tight, or headachy and have such discomfort that you felt too incapacitated to perform well? If I worry too much about dealing with a patient emergency, I will not be able to help my patient. I can't think clearly, increasing the likelihood that I will fail at my job.

When I was too anxious during a piano recital I feared I would not recall the whole piece; my fingers trembled and my brain did not know which keys to play. I would blank on what I was supposed play now, thinking of the notes I did not want to forget a few bars ahead. I created a self-fulfilling prophecy. But if I had practiced sufficiently with my family as a pretend audience, and felt the adrenalin of wanting to perform as well as I could, I'd worry less about perfection, and perform well enough during the actual recital (assuming my family was a supportive audience that did not stress perfection).

The more frequently you tune into your early warning system, the sooner you will be able to *detect* when anxiety is in your neighborhood and whether it is motivating or threatening your peace of mind and well-being, before it becomes overwhelming.

What you may be thinking. "I am worrying about the PSA test that I have to take next week. Will the level go up since the last one? If it does go up, how high will it go? If it goes up, I am a dead man. How will I survive a life of pain and suffering?"

"Shit. There's another cancer commercial advertising a new treatment for prostate cancer. Am I really getting the best care? Did I make the wrong treatment choice?"

What you may be feeling. You may feel worried, not focused, and unable to enjoy usually pleasurable activities. You may have gastric upset, headaches, or other muscle aches and tension, along with sad or forlorn feelings. You may find your fingers trembling or be at a loss for words.

What you might be doing. Perhaps you're not sleeping well for a few nights, pacing at times during the day, not eating right, and find yourself oversensitive, yelling at others for unimportant reasons. You may not be seeing friends regularly, feeling too preoccupied by your cancer itinerary to participate in some of the fun stuff that used to bring a smile to your face; you may fear that if you did something pleasurable you wouldn't be taking the cancer seriously enough. Maybe you find yourself reviewing old PSA results multiple times and scrutinizing computer charts of PSA levels to forecast whether your next PSA will go up and by what amount. The emotions to look for that may accompany these behaviors are sadness, anxiety, and irritability. The emotions may also be disguised as the previously described physical symptoms or as fatigue, diarrhea, constipation, increased or decreased appetite, or a change in sleep habits.

You need to **D**etect these early signs of distress!

2—*Recognize*

Recognizing and identifying the rational and irrational aspects of your emotions is usually better than trying to block them or giving in to them. It is more fruitful to spar with and ultimately transform the essence of these emotions, thoughts, and behaviors, rather than feel trapped and bound by them as if they were your only reality. You can only sweep so much angst under the rug before you trip on a big mountain of aggravation.

> Of course I am nervous about my PSA test—the PSA test was how I got diagnosed with this cancer in the first place. If it goes up, who knows where it will stop? I could die. That saddens me. That worries me. There's so much more I want to experience in life. And my father who had pancreatic cancer really suffered toward the end of his life. It was painful to watch him; he was like a vegetable. I don't want to get like that or have my family see me like that; I don't want them to have to take care of me like that. And I have read that prostate cancer can be so painful when it gets into your bones—imagine all that suffering—now that really scares me.

Recognize the rational (PSA tests monitor cancer progression but also treatment successes; we will all die; pain is not good) and irrational (the PSA can only go up; a rising PSA means death; pancreatic cancer and prostate cancer are similar; Dad's illness trajectory will be my trajectory) as well as the historical kernels of your reactions, which will help you understand where your brain is coming from when it is in fight-or-flight mode. It is considering all possibilities (though not necessarily likely probabilities) of danger and assessing defenses, and you are starting to hone in on the right ones for the right threats.

3—**A**cknowledge

Giving words or descriptions to your reactions may clarify what is going on. Understanding what's behind the emotions and where they are coming from is useful for you as well as for those around you, who feel as helpless as you do watching your plight. **A**cknowledge the emotions in order to validate them. It can be reassuring for most people to hear that they are not "going crazy" for thinking or feeling *that way*. Most men are surprised and calmed to find out from me just how common these emotions are among men dealing with prostate cancer. It is even more comforting to know that you can rein in these emotions. You can get more control over them and make them more tolerable. But that cannot be done if you are not sure what to rein in or how.

> My granddaughter is only 17 years old now; I feel so bad when I miss her soccer games on a weekend because I don't have the energy to go. I don't want her to see how tired I am. I usually feel elated taking her out to lunch afterward even though it is tiring for me. I'll feel horrible if I don't get to see her graduate from high school next year.

Some men emphatically ask, "Hey, this is my life we are talking about, why should I rein in any of my emotion?" To that I would emphatically respond, "Exactly right. This is your life. But it is important to look at your current and longer-term goals so your future can play out on a winning track for you." We are not trying to ignore or snuff out the emotions of worry, sadness, or anger, or the hope for a healthy future, or longing for the past of more perfect health. If a thief broke into your house and stole irreplaceable family heirlooms, insurance coverage doesn't help very much. You could play the past as a non-stop rerun for the rest of your life, staying angry as hell and remorseful.

Some replay is appropriate. How much replay is appropriate depends on the individual and the circumstances. Too much preoccupation with your stolen heirlooms may sacrifice your future, inviting the intruder to haunt your life forever. You don't want to inadvertently steal too much time from your current life because you are stuck in the past or fearful of the future. Remember, I said these were common, understandable reactions in the here and now. But you don't want the emotions getting in the way of your goals to have a better life now, in your present, or down the road, in your future. Again, PSA is not a test you can study for. If worrying about a PSA test helped the level go down, we would see that worriers may never develop prostate cancer and I would be advocating a program to help men worry *more*. But it does not.

If not being intimate with your partner brought you closer together in some way, I'd advocate celibacy after prostate cancer diagnoses. But it does not.

> I'm scared that I won't be able to get it up if we start kissing. I'll just say that I don't feel well. I don't want to fail or disappoint my partner or me.

Acknowledge where emotional distancing is coming from, as well as some of the faulty logic that goes into it. This will help you perceive what some of the consequences may be. The desire to avoid failing and disappointing may actually lead to a failure of intimacy in your relationship that can have serious downstream costs.

If you can **D**etect, and **R**ecognize, and **A**cknowledge the emotions, thoughts, and behaviors, separate the rational from the irrational, and understand how getting stuck in the past or projected into the future leads you to lose sight of the beneficial aspects of your present, you can eventually accept the cards you are dealt and sculpt an even better new normal. This will allow you to have a more fulfilling present and future. Fuller acceptance will only come with time. The next two phases of EJ, the **F**lip and the **T**ransformation, will facilitate living with what you have, and live better than if you just tried wishing away the present. Let's move on.

4—The **F**lip

The **F**lip is a key aspect of the EJ technique. As in football, you get to the line of scrimmage and you read the defense. You can more clearly recognize the rational and irrational emotions, thoughts, and behaviors;

you can see where they are coming from; and perhaps understand how they keep you from having a more fulfilling life with prostate cancer. It's not what you expected. In fact, you may never have seen this defensive alignment before, yet you see how your usual coping methods just keep getting you thrown for losses and setbacks, regardless of what play is called. You've been playing by history and a game plan, but not by the current circumstances. A quarterback can call a play in the huddle but get to the line of scrimmage only to see that the defensive setup is easily going to thwart the play call. So the quarterback calls an audible (a last-minute change of play at the line of scrimmage by audibly shouting out predetermined disguised signals for a different play): "The situation calls for a pass. They are set up for a pass. This is a great time for a running play. I need to change the play."

Just as a quarterback can call out an audible, so can you—in the form of a conscious thought or softly whispered audible direction to yourself. It can be aided by the words *however* or *hold it*, after you've snowballed and felt flooded by the intense anxious or depressive statements and/ or feelings or unhelpful behaviors for a significant amount of time. Now that you've detected, recognized, and acknowledged that there are irrational aspects to your emotional and behavioral responses, you can see how they are sending you up a path that is not where you want to go. The texture or quality of your life has been deflected by your tunnel-vision focus on quantity and possibly predicted quality of life. In baseball terms, the team in the field realized you always hit to the right side, so they put on a defensive shift to the right side. If you don't adjust, you will likely keep hitting ground balls or pop-outs to the right side. That meatball pitch, likely a mistake by the pitcher, that you could knock out for a home run never seems to come. The **F**lip will further separate the irrational, over-exaggerated, unhelpful, runaway emotional and cognitive detours from the more realistic, rational, and satisfying ways of dealing with and accepting your plight so you can keep hitting the winning pitches.

Hold it. The PSA helped diagnose my cancer—it didn't cause the cancer; the test helped diagnose the cancer earlier than it would have been without it. It has given me a better shot at surviving this thing.

As for my father who died a horrible death from cancer—that was 30 years ago. I am told that not all cancers are alike; and prostate cancers are not all alike either. My father had pancreatic cancer, for which there is no blood test to help with earlier detection. So in a way, I'm lucky…I know that cancer treatments are overall much better today.

As for the pain and suffering from prostate cancer, my doctor did tell me that if it occurs, it won't start soon, like my anxious thoughts lead me to believe. He also said he's very good about treating pain if and when it arises. He won't ignore it. But look at all the emotional pain and suffering I am going through just worrying about what happened 30 years ago and about what hasn't happened and, maybe more importantly, what may never happen.

Use the force of the emotions coming at you to deflect or flip your thoughts. Can you imagine yourself, the Emotional Judo expert, flipping the big, bad opponent?

5—*Transformation: The "Flea Flicker" or Play Action Pass*

This is your chance to pull a fast one on the uncomfortable irrational emotions, thoughts, or behaviors. The **F**lip has set up your new alignment. You can now run that "flea flicker" or play action pass, where the quarterback fakes a running play by starting to give the ball to the running back. He then pulls it back. The aim of the fake handoff is to try to get the defense moving in one direction, and then the quarterback has the option of running in the opposite direction or passing to his running back (or to any other receiver), who now acts as a receiver. It takes forethought. It takes planning; you have **D**etected, **R**ecognized, and **A**cknowledged (and accepted) where the defense (or your automatic thoughts and emotions) has indeed lined up, as opposed to where you wanted them or expected them to be. It's time for the **F**lip. It also takes a temporary belief in the deception by the defense. They were looking for a pass. You saw that. You faked a run. They fell for it. You have the option for run or pass. It may take many rehearsals and adjustments to convincingly pull off a play like this. Your brain and your body have been on automatic pilot for many years. Just saying "no" and rejecting emotions doesn't cut it. You need to have something else in mind in your playbook and believe it can work.

> Overall, I had been feeling pretty well, though I wish I had more energy. I remember Dr. Roth saying that doing something pleasurable but undemanding is a good antidote for this anxiety and sadness.

An important part of the **T**ransformation is having an activity to go to after you've detected, recognized, acknowledged, and flipped the emotions, thoughts, and/or behaviors. Just figuring out the defensive strategy is not sufficient.

Have your quick list of simple and uncomplicated activities handy. Go down your list of "play options" to see what might work or feel right at the moment. When you feel very anxious or sad on your funk treadmill, you will have difficulty contemplating the best activity to help you switch gears that will allow you to feel better. Marsha Linehan, in her skills training manual for treating people with borderline personality disorders, developed a list of pleasurable but easy-to-do activities to detour someone from the repetitive hurtful thoughts or emotions that could be self-destructive—they can apply to all of us in stressful situations. It is amazing to notice how many choices we have for activities that most of us take for granted or that otherwise do not come to mind, especially during tense moments (or hours). These activities are right in front of our eyes, but we fail to take advantage of them because we are blinded by our distress. We are instead remarkably seduced to follow that distress, even if it makes us and those around us feel worse, because we cannot see a more pleasurable or meaningful door to walk through. It's like having a scab that itches—you may find yourself itching and scratching and picking at it, perhaps inadvertently, causing harm to yourself with bleeding and potential infection. When the itch is related to a physical wound, we can visualize it more clearly, though we may not have any better control over it than less visible emotional and cognitive "itches."

Taking a lot of time to figure out how to solve The Problem of prostate cancer allows your anxiety to keep going like a revolving door that does not allow slowing or stopping—it may even feel like there are two of you in one section of the door. You'll get tackled behind the line of scrimmage most times and feel like you are losing yardage. When this anxiety or sadness cycling occurs, it is best to move in a different direction with the ball, or perhaps to pass it. If you are easily inspired by an activity that may be pleasurable, do-able, and distracting, and is not already on your quick list, go for it.

Transform your energy through activity!

Have Your Quick List Handy and Put It into Action

I am going to put on a CD—maybe Mozart, Springsteen, or Sinatra.

I am going to grab my smartphone/tablet/MP3 player and go out for a short walk.

I am going to give one of my kids a call just to talk.

I am going to give one of my kids a call and see if I can take my granddaughter out to breakfast Saturday—if I miss her growing up now (when I have control) what good is it showing up to a graduation or wedding, even if I could make it—it will be an empty celebration that achieves a goal but really misses the boat.

I'm getting my Sudoku/crossword book and doing a few puzzles.

I'm going to play a computer game of chess or solitaire.

I haven't seen Tom since we played golf last fall—I'll call and make a lunch date.

Be Aware of Risky Thought Processes and Behaviors

This section will discuss the good, the bad, and the ugly rational and irrational aspects of our thoughts, emotions, and behaviors that put us in or can get us out of distressing funks and ruts. These ruts often represent half-empty perspectives that drain into half-empty or less fulfilling lives.

It is not easy to demand what thoughts or emotions you will or will not have. But it is possible to reorient your thought processes and even your emotional reactions before they lead you down predictable and familiar paths to high anxiety and higher distress. Men become used to habitual modes of thinking that they believe are natural and inevitable. For instance, the thought, "Well if I didn't have cancer, I wouldn't be thinking this way" is common, but only partially correct and not very relieving. If a catastrophizer foresees and anticipates unwanted doom-and-gloom disasters around every turn that awaits him in life's roads, he will tend to avoid all roads with turns in them. People who think this way are often called pessimists or worriers by loved ones and even by themselves.

However, I see these folks a little differently, with a more optimistic perspective. These men are often successful in their careers that reward prevention of mistakes or quick-fix responses to problems. It is hard to measure how much extra work and money is saved by people who see potential problems a few steps before others. Yet their success comes because they "worry" about and want to prevent disasters. Like a foxhound, they can smell approaching danger and avoid it, or better navigate it before things go badly; they might also catch a problem early so repairs or recovery is less extensive—and isn't that the goal of PSA testing? It is not easy to change a way of thinking that has been rewarded and reinforced in the past by slaps on the back or monetary rewards for a job well done, just because the current situation, a medical situation, requires something different.

A few years ago, I heard Joe Torre, former manager of the New York Yankees and author of a book about what it takes to be a winning manager, give a speech. His talk was enlightening to me. He discussed strategies that he felt were important in managing a baseball team and how they also helped him manage life in general. He noted that it is difficult to control or ensure a win. Essentially, you can prepare to perform at your best, but it is important to acknowledge that another good team will try just as hard to do the same. Outcomes are not guaranteed.

You prepare for your ordeal with prostate cancer by getting baseline information about the cancer and treatments; by choosing a doctor and hospital you trust; by improving your lifestyle with proper diet and exercise; and by doing activities that relieve stress, are enjoyable, and that feel meaningful. Worrying about what your life will be like if the cancer returns or spreads, or trying to find out what the next treatments are in the pharmaceutical pipeline before you need them does not help most men and does not really diminish their anxiety. Watching graphs of your PSA tests on your computer at home, trying to figure out where it might land on the next test like a roulette wheel, also does not help most men. Trying to guess the future with recurrent "what if" questions does not help to control or ensure a "win." These behaviors lead to significant distress, less time spent and less enjoyment with family and friends, less sleep at night, and more worry. This obsessive and often compulsive planning, research, and worry do not help most men handle or cope better with illness. Some feel more in control, but at what price? Are they really in control? Most often, their oncology team, their families, and I conclude "no." You might want to give your "worry proxy" to your doctors and nurses—this is one of the unwritten agreements of a good doctor–patient relationship or "good bedside manner."

Developing new survival skills when you become ill is a formidable challenge. But it can happen over time if the old skills are counterproductive. It is more realistic to try to **D**etect warning signs, **R**ecognize what the signs represent, and **A**cknowledge which are appropriate and which are not, as well as the consequences of and interactions between your emotions, thoughts, and behaviors. With EJ, you can see each of these entities from a different angle and see how they get in the way of what you really want in life, since you cannot make the prostate cancer or repercussions from treatment disappear. Having a guidebook of what is going on, along with suggestions for improvement, can help you move into **F**lipping and **T**ransforming. It is empowering to know that you are not bound to the irrational and unreasonable, even when they seem "right" or "justified" in the moment. Those are thought traps.

The relaxation or meditation exercises we practiced can come in handy at any time along this process. Practicing to more clearly understand your thoughts, labeling them, and seeing how they impact your emotions and behaviors, rather than just believing and expressing them, will help you be more in control of your destiny and what is most important to you. This is important, because thought traps can lead to emotional and behavioral traps as well.

Sample DRAFT Situations

Let's look at some examples of irrational thoughts that come from stressful situations and lead to destructive and overwhelming emotions or behaviors, and how you can counteract or deflect them. The illustrations that follow isolate the process, out of context, to show you how to put the EJ Playbook into action as it relates to prostate cancer. The examples come from experience applying the DRAFT with EJ strategy with men who have prostate cancer. Most begin with classic thought traps that are elucidated with cognitive behavioral therapy, but notice how EJ tries to integrate the various psychotherapies described earlier—cognitive behavioral therapy, acceptance and commitment therapy, insight-oriented therapy, and supportive therapy—to promote freedom from the trap.

Catastrophizing

Catastrophizing thoughts fall into an "all or none" category. There are usually no possible alternative interpretations of what's going on. Therefore, you cannot see alternative solutions out of the dilemma. See how the following statement, "If my first PSA after surgery goes up, I'm a dead man," differs even from "Prepare for the worst and hope for the best," which sounds all or none but leaves room for believable hope.

First scenario

If my first PSA after surgery goes up, I'm a dead man.

Detect the alarm and despair in this statement and the emotional trap it sets for you because you are miscalculating the future. Hear what you are thinking. If you take a moment, you could probably identify that, in addition to despair, the statement also reflects anxiety that your fate is out of your control. Even though most would say that the statement is irrational, or exaggerated, we can all see some logic in it. But the alarm rings "despair" and "anxiety."

Recognize the less logical, less realistic, and exaggerated aspects of the thoughts and emotions implied by the statement: Rising PSAs are worse than falling PSAs. But they are not equated with impending death. Could there be a lab error or can a small increase be within a range of normal? Understand how this all-or-none catastrophic view can lead you down a road of waiting for death and acting as if you will die soon, rather than living more fully until you die, whenever that occurs.

Acknowledge the consequences of what's behind your thought and emotions: After "definitive treatment," can a rising PSA mean that there is no chance of cure? Yes. Does this mean there is an increased likelihood of a shortened life span? Perhaps. But this "shortened" life span is based on whose plan, expectations, or guarantee? It is calculated not by an actuarial table but by the anxiety and frustration of prostate cancer tunnel vision. Yes, you can accept that you have prostate cancer, but no, you don't have to accept a doom-and-gloom forecast inaccurately predicated by each PSA test. Where's the warranty on life? Is it shorter than you planned or hoped for or had expectations about, because of family longevity (for instance, to what age did your parents live)? Will this subjective prediction lead to a self-fulfilling prophecy at least for a less fulfilling and enjoyable life? Likely. Perhaps this prediction leads to more stress, which puts more strain on your cardiovascular system, which can also shorten your life. Possibly. Catastrophizing can seep into every meaningful relationship and situation you encounter. You've just read the defense and it is time to call your "audible," because if you go up the road of your automatic reaction, you'll be thrown for a loss.

The **F**lip: Counter these downstream thoughts and emotions with more logical scenarios:

> Sure I am worried that my PSA will go up. If it goes up that would not be good; however, I know I won't be a dead man anytime soon, unless I start

acting that way prematurely. The whole reason they take PSA tests regularly is to make sure my doctor can catch potential recurrences or progression of disease earlier than without the PSA test, so that something beneficial can be done sooner. Does a rise in my PSA mean I will die sooner? Sooner than I want? Perhaps it could, but it is not likely. Did my (fill in the blank of the last medical illness you, a close friend, or a family member was diagnosed with that was not cancer related, such as hypertension, diabetes, angina) mean I or they were dead? Did I die when my PSA initially rose so I could get diagnosed with this cancer and get treated? I absolutely did not. Did I start to worry about the possibility of death, which I never seriously thought about before? Absolutely.

Transformation: Run the new play you just called in the audible. Rather than expecting death soon, why not get back to living more fully. Pull out your quick list: "I'll tell my wife I'm scared about how the PSA will turn out and ask if she'll take a walk with me."

Second scenario. Three weeks after completing radiation therapy a man states, "My shoulder hurts...the cancer must be spreading...I'm so tired...this is a losing battle."

Detect the possible distressing aspects of this thought that go along with sadness and feeling exhausted—radiation can cause fatigue that lasts weeks after completing the treatment. Fatigue can set the context for more depressing thoughts and sidelined behavior.

Recognize the more and less logical aspects of the thoughts and emotions: Sometimes a sore shoulder is just a sore shoulder; perhaps this man forgot about the heavy box he lifted off of a shelf the day before that might have injured his shoulder. He thinks his painful shoulder means he is losing his battle with cancer; he lives daily with the expectation of a downward spiral into death. He lives waiting for a catastrophe to hit.

Acknowledge what's behind the emotions: It is not unusual soon after a cancer diagnosis and treatment to fear that new aches or pains are signs that the cancer is back or has progressed. This is your internal warning system on overdrive because of your cancer diagnosis. The rug was pulled out from under you when you got diagnosed, when you least expected it; you will not let that happen again. When you recognize that your shoulder hurts because of the box you lifted, you may find a different situation to distress about: "Why the heck did my wife ask me to get that box. Damn her. That's why my shoulder hurts!" In reality, you don't want to act like an invalid for the rest of your life. Sore shoulders and backaches have come and gone before. But you can now give them new, inappropriate meanings in the context of prostate cancer. In fact, given the fatigue you have from the radiation therapy, you may be at more risk of injury from activities that were previously of no concern.

The **F**lip: Your hypervigilance is meant to be protective, so you will not be caught unaware if the cancer were to return. In fact, many men act as if staying on constant guard will prevent the cancer from coming back, almost like an early radar warning system. This reflex of hyper-alertness can be particularly prevalent if there was a delay or error in the initial diagnosis. "My doctor wanted to get another routine PSA test in a year, but he should have been alarmed by even a mildly elevated level. Now, I am alarmed by every potential sign and symptom." Over time, distress decreases with clarifications and reassurances by your doctor or medical team that these aches and pains are not related to cancer recurrence. This will help recalibrate your early warning system. You can assist this distress-relief **F**lip by reassessing and reformulating the catastrophizing statement after detecting it: "Though it is possible that my shoulder pain is related to my prostate cancer, I recall that I moved that heavy box cleaning the garage; additionally, my last PSA was unmeasurable just 3 months ago. The cancer is not likely to come back that quickly with metastasis. I know my doctor is aware of my concerns and is watching me closely."

Transformation: "My shoulder hurts, but that does not mean I am on the disabled list. It's time to do something fun right now! Otherwise I will literally watch my life passing away. Since it's a nice day, I'll garden, or pull out my water colors that I've been meaning to get to."

Generalizing

Third scenario

> I read in the newspaper that a famous politician/actor/athlete died of prostate cancer…there's no hope for me.

Detect the possible exaggerated generalization of this irrational, distressing thought. The emotions you may be feeling are sadness and worry.

Recognize the more reasonable aspects of the thoughts and emotions interspersed with the faulty logic: The patient is generalizing from the celebrity's circumstances to his own. What valid medical information such as overall health, family history, lifestyle behaviors, and cancer specifics does the reader have about the celebrity, other than he died of prostate cancer and his age at death? Are there any details that might allow for relevant comparisons? The more celebrities are diagnosed with and talk about their prostate cancer experiences, the more public notices will be available to compare your circumstances with theirs (however faulty those comparisons may be).

Acknowledge what's behind the emotions: Often men assume, "If bad things can happen to a celebrity, who probably has excellent resources for excellent care, surely these bad things can happen to me." Though there may be some truth to this statement, it is an incomplete truth that leads to a potentially faulty conclusion, undermining the fact that "I have been getting excellent care and I do trust my doctors."

The **F**lip: It is important to remind yourself that each person is unique, that not all prostate cancers are the same, and that people tolerate and respond differently to treatments and medications. Men do die of prostate cancer, just as they die of many other illnesses. We all die of something, sometime. But it is important to recognize that you have done and will continue to do what you can to keep yourself healthy and to keep the cancer at its most minimal state. Many men have told me that they want to live long enough for a better treatment to come along. This does not mean that you will find the fountain of youth and stay alive forever; but the longer you live, the better shot you have of living longer. Yogi

Berra could have said that. It is also good to recall that men who participated in clinical trials for prostate cancer, who have already succumbed
to the disease, were instrumental in adding to the knowledge base that
has kept you and others alive more comfortably and for longer periods
of time than was thought possible even 20 years ago. Though unknown
to you, these men have left a legacy that you benefit from today and that
you may decide to pass forward to others as well.

Transformation: First, stop reading the obituaries that describe who
died of prostate cancer! On the one hand, reading the prostate cancer
obituaries may make you feel less isolated with your cancer and make
you feel like you are part of a group or club. But that's not really the
group or club you want to belong to. Most men reading obituaries come
away feeling more depressed, as they contemplate their own cancer tra-
jectories and life timelines. Consider participating in a clinical trial to
further the knowledge needed to treat prostate cancer for those diagnosed with it in another 20 years. It could help your son, grandson, or a
nephew, or someone you will never know.

Catastrophizing and personalizing about the worst things you hear
about prostate cancer and worrying that they will happen to you leads
to avoidance of important and meaningful life experiences. It can paralyze you as you wait for the worst to happen. Men feel victimized before
there is any actual bad news to receive. After getting blood drawn for
PSA tests, men wait for a call from the oncologist's office to get the *news*,
as opposed to the *results*. This can feel like waiting for a jury to give a
verdict, as if you were on trial. Though no news often means good news,
men are left with anticipatory torment if they don't hear from their doctors or nurses with a reassuring phone call.

Ask the nurse to arrange a time to call for your PSA result. If this were
a business issue, it would make perfect sense to set up a phone appointment, without the feeling that you are bothering someone or that you'd
(hypothetically) rather not get bad news. Some cancer centers now have
the ability for patients to check their lab results online. The ability to get
results close to real time gives many men a sense of increased control
and, if the news is good, fast relief. However, it can also lead to increased
worrying because rising levels do not come with a clinician's interpretation of those results. Do you know what the margin of lab error is so you

know whether a change in your PSA level from the last test is clinically significant? If the results are not completely normal, there is room for unchecked emotional hyperreactivity.

Additional examples of common thought and emotion traps in men with prostate cancer follow; however I will not go into Playbook specifics. For the next few traps, it will be a good exercise for you to DRAFT the EJ Plays yourself.

Trying to Forecast Your Future from Others' Experiences

My friend's PSA went up... I think mine will go up too.

This is similar to the example of the celebrity obituary mentioned earlier. Just as it is easy to make comparisons with others even in the doctor's waiting room ("he looks so much healthier than me"), it is easy to think that all men have the same prostate cancer experience. They do not. It bears repeating that men are diagnosed at different ages, at different levels of general health status, with different family and medical histories, at different stages of disease, with different Gleason scores and different anatomy and physiology, with different tolerance for surgery or radiation early on, or for hormonal or chemotherapy for advanced disease. It is reasonable to note that you feel upset that your friend's PSA went up, but your PSA levels rise because of what is going on in your body and your body only.

I just heard another guy died of prostate cancer... All men seem to die of prostate cancer.

This is quite a broad generalization. First of all, over 200,000 men are diagnosed with prostate cancer every year. A little more than 30,000 die of this cancer each year. Most men who have prostate cancer do not die of it; in fact 2.5 million men diagnosed in the United States with prostate cancer are still alive today. It can, however, impact their lives significantly. If you are diagnosed with early-stage prostate cancer, you do not know and cannot know if you will die of prostate cancer or die with it from another cause, so why not plan to die of something else, unless you have been told otherwise? And if you have been told otherwise, remember doctors do not have a crystal ball to know for sure. I have had the good fortune of treating many men who, at the time of diagnosis, were given life expectancies of 3 months or 6 months, and they were seeing me years later. Unless someone is truly at the end stages of life, physicians are not good at predicting how much longer their patients may live.

My PSA went up last time; I know it will continue to rise.

To some extent, these are also examples of generalizing or forecasting—if something happens once, it will happen all the time. Without any good evidence that your PSA will trend up, you make a forecast anyway. PSA levels may be as unpredictable as the stock market. Remember the fine print disclaimer in a stock portfolio: past performance does not guarantee future results. I don't think I would take bets on whether any particular PSA level will go up or down. Even high PSA levels and high Gleason scores which indicate poorer prognosis or more aggressive tumors cannot predict what will happen in any particular circumstance with different treatments. Remember, what goes up may come down; what goes down may come up. You cannot know for certain, but you can certainly hope for the better option and then learn to accept and live with whatever does happen.

All-or-None Thinking

Either I am cured or I will die.

All-or-none thinking, or seeing things in black and white, cuts down your options for good outcomes considerably. This type of thinking makes it difficult to see a glass even half-full. Again, one must distinguish what it takes to cope with cancer from other life activities, where all-or-none thinking may bring success, such as, "Go for the gold; World Championship or nothing." If you get a cure with absolutely no complications from the treatment, that is wonderful—but it cannot be guaranteed. The adage "all things in moderation" is a reasonable and sustainable principle. It does not mean you cannot hope for the best, but if you get something less, you will be able deal with it; in fact, you *can* still live well with it, if you're willing.

Superstitions and Magical Thinking

> I should have had the same nurse draw my blood. I was so stressed by getting three sticks that it probably increased my PSA. I read somewhere that stress can increase your PSA level.

Just as with the "Why me?" question, men look for reasons to explain what happens in their world, even if it doesn't really make sense. But some explanation can feel better than none. Associations can seem causal rather than just coincidence. Does it really matter if your surgery is scheduled for March 15th, the Ides of March, or any Friday the 13th? If you know someone who went to Colgate University, you know that Friday the 13th is actually considered a good luck day! How does one deal with dueling superstitions? Even if you know that superstitions are just superstitions, that you think twice about them can be distracting. Examine the data. Examine the rationale behind hunches. Keep your eye on the ball.

Changing Perspectives, Changing Your Life

Notice what is going well in your life and what gives your life purpose and substance. And not just in the DRAFT process of EJ when you're feeling horrible or upset. The more you focus on these fundamental realities, the more you will infuse yourself with more hopeful moods and have a higher threshold for copying with stressful events. This can be done in thought, in conversation, in prayer, or in journaling, as in the therapeutic writing discussed earlier.

> This prostate cancer diagnosis is killing me. Well, I'm worried the cancer will kill me. Everyone I know who's had cancer died of it. I am 75. I get tired more easily and I have some pain in my back. I still enjoy working part-time in my law office, and I love visiting with my grandkids even more since the diagnosis.

This sounds pretty good doesn't it? It does if this man looks at the bigger picture, but it may depend on which parts he chooses to zoom in on. As with a telephoto lens, he can see a nice forest with some beautiful trees, or he can just see the withering patches of illness or aging. This is the basis of the homework assignment I will outline and which I give to every new patient I see. We are all susceptible to tunnel vision in our emotional, cognitive, and behavioral experiences and responses. This homework assignment will allow you to reconfigure your perspective on the immediate reality. Changing your perspective will allow you to change your emotional responses and behaviors, or at least your experience of them. This in turn will facilitate changing how you think about your illness and your life. The homework can break you out of a rut by placing a snapshot of your emotional and physical concerns in front of you so you can see them in a different way than you've looked at them previously.

The goal of this homework assignment, rearranging your perspective, reminds me of a newspaper puzzle called Jumble that I love to play. The goal of the puzzle is to unscramble jumbled words to form ordinary words. Looking at the scrambled word could stymie me if I couldn't easily rearrange it in my mind. I found that if I wrote out the letters in a different format, I would see more possible combinations and be able to figure out how to rearrange the letters correctly. For instance, in an example I made up, the letters T-T-S-E-R-P-O-A may be written:

$$
\begin{array}{ccc}
TT & & PO \\
SE & OR & SE \\
RP & & TT \\
OA & & AR
\end{array}
$$

Many other combinations are possible as well. One of them may give me a faster visual clue that the word is PROSTATE.

A Mood/Activity Chart to Change Your Perceptions, Moods, and Activities: Oy, a Homework Assignment

Perhaps the last thing a man expects when coming to a psychiatrist's office is a homework assignment. However, I have seen how much there is to gain from this assignment; even if you do not complete it, you will benefit by understanding the principles, so please read through it.

Waiver 1: If you do not do this assignment, you will not get a failing grade.

Waiver 2: If you do not do this assignment, it doesn't mean you shouldn't read through it. Read it anyway—it will change how you think about what goes on in your mind and body, allow you to see potential patterns and triggers of moods, and hint at ways you can feel better.

Make a chart that will illustrate your activities and moods (Table 4.2). I recommend charting a whole week per page, because I think you can get a nice visual comparison of days, without the chart looking too crowded. Some men like to do a daily chart with one day per page, while others like the idea of a monthly calendar. Still others who hate charts will write in a diary or journal format, or will keep track of these issues on their computers or smartphones. Don't let style get in your way. Just do one—you can always revise later. Each day should be divided into three sections: morning, afternoon, and evening.

Don't feel trapped into compulsively filling out the information minute by minute, throughout the day. Instead, at the end of each segment of the day (i.e., at the end of the morning, or the end of the afternoon) jot down how you felt emotionally and physically, taking into account mood, anxiety, irritability, tearfulness (or any other emotional reactions you had), energy level, pain or discomfort, gastric upset, or nausea (or any other physical symptoms you may have

TABLE 4.2 MOOD/ACTIVITY STATUS CHART

Time	Monday	Tuesday	Wednesday	Thursday	Friday	Saturday	Sunday
Morning							
Mid-day							
Evening							

Indicate:

*Tearfulness, *anxiety, *sleep, *depressed mood, *pain, *energy, *concentration.

*List as "ok" or "not ok," or on a scale of 0–10.

*List possible triggers to problematic symptoms.

Also indicate: good/enjoyable activities.

Instructions for Completing the Mood/Activity Chart

Two to three times per day, jot into each box the presence and intensity (0–10) of emotional and physical issues, as well as good things that happen:

Mood; Anxiety; Tearfulness; Frustrations; Irritability; Energy; Pain; Gastric upset; Hot flashes; Sleep; Appetite; Concentration/ Forgetfulness

Record things you enjoyed: read a book; went to a concert; had dinner with friends; saw granddaughter.

If there is a trigger to any of the above, list it:

Felt anxious: Was thinking about visit to oncologist tomorrow

Frustrated: I had to sit after walking up subway stairs

---

had). Then rate the symptoms. This can be done easily and quickly, yet descriptively. It can be completed with a 0–10 scale, "good" or "bad," "yes" or "no," or with any other scoring system that you find easy and vivid (Table 4.2). Note that a "0" may signify a low point of mood or anxiety so may be construed as negative (depressed) or positive (not anxious) depending on the subject. Similarly, a "10" may be interpreted as positive (great mood) or negative (significant pain). Apart from investigating the potential multidirectional impact of emotions, thoughts, and behaviors, you may become aware of persistent physical or medical issues that your oncologist or primary care doctor can address.

Scoring Your Charted Items

The idea is to take a snapshot of how all that we've been talking about—emotions, thoughts, behaviors, and physical issues—interact in your life. This is not just a chart for the bad stuff in your life. Also chart good experiences, such as "lunch with my wife—enjoyed," "read a book—enjoyed," or "energy improved, enjoyed spending more time with my grandkids." Why should you put positive goings-on into this chart? Most of us don't acknowledge the good things happening in our lives when we are feeling bad, emotionally or physically. Life feels quite out of balance, very much in favor of a glass (or life) being half or more empty. However, if you look back over a week or a month and fully see the good that interfaces with the uncomfortable, you will develop a different feeling about your life. You will hopefully be able to start seeing your glass (and life) as at least half-full, even though you have cancer. You will see a better balance that you could not see when your focus was primarily on feeling anxious, depressed, frustrated or feeling pain or other physical discomfort. For most men, the gloomy overtakes the shine, until they stop and smell the roses that are present, though otherwise taken for granted.

Mood/Activity/Physical Status

This charting exercise is really another way to get into the DRAFT with EJ Playbook. You are identifying the "down" or more negative items in your life (**D**etect, **R**ecognize and **A**cknowledge) as well as the good things that are happening that you may be less cognizant of, and can then use the **F**lip and **T**ransforming plays to change things around in the service of feeling better. A sample table (Table 4.3) depicts identifying emotional and physical symptoms as well as possible triggers. The list in the nearby text box will guide you to short-circuit the worry times and get back to living your life with or after cancer, rather than trying to figure out how to relive your life before cancer or without the real complications from your treatment. This is more than the quick list of go-to activities you developed earlier for use when feeling bombarded by uncomfortable emotions. In fact, some of these suggestions can be used to help you get unstuck from the aggravation about the past or future. Barbara Rubin Wainrib,

**TABLE 4.3 SAMPLE MOOD/ACTIVITY CHART:
GETTING THE SNAPSHOT**

Monday Afternoon	Triggers
Energy 4/10	
Anxiety 3/10	
Felt down	Watching movie on TV. Enjoyed it until an erectile medication commercial came on
Tuesday Afternoon	**Triggers**
Mood is good	Had lunch with spouse
Energy 6/10	
Increased anxiety (7/10) and irritability at night (8/10)	A friend called after dinner and asked, "How are you feeling?" and "When is your next PSA test?"
Wednesday Afternoon	**Triggers**
Felt calmer, inspired, more relaxed and hopeful	Started reading *Managing Prostate Cancer: A Guide to Living Better*

Jack Maguire, and Sandra Haber also suggest a number of activities for couples to do together in *Men, Women, and Prostate Cancer: A Medical and Psychological Guide for Women and the Men They Love*.

DRAFT with EJ Cheat Sheet

Detect current emotion(s).
Recognize their credibility or lack of credibility.
Acknowledge accuracies and inaccuracies for the "here and now."
Flip stuck-in-the-rut statements or viewpoints.
Transform opportunities to shift your focus to the present.
Cope with and live in the present; or keep coming back to the present using distraction, relaxation, meditation, prayer, music, activity, socializing, journaling.
The DRAFT allows to you continue to come back to the here and now.

Be accurate about reporting your physical and emotional symptoms (if only for yourself)—your spouse or partner may want to "correct" your chart as they see you and your activities. If you want to talk it over, that's your business, but it is your chart. Remember to indicate the positive, hopeful, meaningful, and rewarding aspects of your life. It's okay to start with the elementary basics that we often take for granted (i.e., "It is good to be alive"). Once you have noted what you are doing and feeling (or not doing or feeling), consider how you can schedule and pace your activities to optimize your health and sense of worth in your life.

Schedule and Pace Activities

You are more likely to do healthy and fun activities if you schedule them in advance!
Don't wait to see "if you feel like it."
Start low and go slow, but go.
Listen to your body.
Encourage a nurturing attitude toward yourself and your partner.

Engage in Agreeable Activities (you can always expand your quick list)

Hobbies	E-mails, surf the Net (but not about prostate cancer issues)
Journaling	Phone a friend or family member
Read a book	Play cards
Books on tape, CD, electronic device	Take a walk
Go to the park	Go to the mall
Go out to lunch with wife, partner, or friend	Go to a concert
Take a bath	Get a massage
Go to the gym	Take an art, music, literature, or crafts class

Coping with Sleeplessness

This chapter has taken into account the interactive ingredients of emotions, thoughts, and behaviors that blend into anxiety and depression, and the non-medication methods of treating these entities. The last topic to be covered in this nonpharmacological chapter is insomnia, one of the more aggravating aspects of managing prostate cancer. Your sleeplessness may be due to a medical problem or a medication side effect, so it is important to first discuss this problem with your doctor.

What happens when you cannot sleep in the context of your prostate cancer diagnosis, treatment, or after treatment period? Is this a sign of understandable and temporary distress, or is something else getting in the way of your usual sleep architecture? Of course, some of you had poor sleep routines before your cancer diagnosis. This is not a time for anyone to expect a good night's rest, although this is especially true for men who were never good sleepers. Upsetting waking hours make the nights more difficult. Expectations have to be managed and adjusted to account for your present reality. Jobs and even retirement can accommodate for men who have done night shift work and were rarely able to sleep well during usual nighttime sleep hours. But they may not sleep easily at any time now. Doctors' appointments and the angst of medical procedures and tests that have to happen during daytime hours make sleep more difficult to come by.

Distraction can be useful to deal with stress and worry—during the day. Men tell me they feel better emotionally when they can get their minds onto something other than the cancer and treatment. But during "down" times—and there is no better opportunity for down time than the nighttime, when others in the family are asleep, the phone is quiet, and it is just you tossing and turning in bed—your brain will try to wrap itself around problems and try to figure them out. Often your focus is passively attentive to the details and inexplicable transitions from one subject or scene to another. Perhaps that process worked fine for career, work, or family problems before cancer. Problems got resolved, or they were not that important. However, with cancer, trying to figure out the "right treatment," or wish away the potentially rising PSA or the unwanted treatment complication with "if only" thoughts does not speed the arrival of the "right" solution. But your brain marches on, if unwittingly, on a fruitless task. The Emotional Judo DRAFT strategies can help here. There is a DRAFT with EJ sample for sleeplessness at the end of this chapter. You might eventually assure yourself that you have made the best decisions you could. But the intellectual is not always connected to the emotional and physical. After some reasonable amount of time spent on this mental work, you might still be wide awake as the problems continue to linger. You know it is important to rest, but you cannot.

Suggestions for Sleeping Better

Sleep experts suggest techniques that can help you get to sleep and stay asleep more successfully. Certain behaviors and activities detour your way to better sleep. First, are you drinking any caffeine during the day? How much caffeine, and when? How late in the day? After 2 PM? Remember that caffeine comes in many forms: coffee, tea, soda, juices, and desserts. (Tobacco also has a stimulant effect, though it may be calming for some.) Try to cut back on these caffeinated products as much as possible, especially after 1 or 2 o'clock in the afternoon. Change your nighttime goal from "I need to get to sleep" to "I want to relax." It is less demanding and thus less activating and aggravating. Many older men wake up periodically to urinate, because of anatomical or physiological problems related to prostate problems, bladder issues, or aging. But most are able to fall asleep again relatively easily after each awakening, unless there is some underlying sleep problem, anxiety, or depression. The physics of fluid in and fluid out is relevant here. It is important to keep hydrated during the day, especially when you are taking medications, but try to avoid drinking larger amounts of liquids before going to sleep. You can usually meet daily requirements for fluid intake by dinnertime. I have only had one patient who told me that he woke up less often if he drank right before going to sleep. See what is right for you.

Additional rules of sleep hygiene include having a regular time for sleep and for getting up in the morning. Try not to go to sleep too late. Don't eat any heavy or spicy meals or do robust exercise just before bedtime—they usually perk people up. If you have hot flashes that awaken you at night from hormonal therapy, keep the room cooler than usual. This has upset a few wives or partners, but they adapt by adding a blanket to their side of the bed. Don't use alcohol to induce sleep—though a drink or two may help you get to sleep, it is likely to act as a diuretic and make you pee in the middle of the night. At that point, the physiological sedative affect of the alcohol has worn off and you are not just up peeing, you are wide awake again; your brain is in activated mode, as if an internal alarm clock went off telling you to wake up. If you are going to take a daytime nap, do it in the early to mid-afternoon hours, and try not to sleep for more than 30–45 minutes. Your body can only sleep so much in 24 hours. It is also good to get exposure to outside daytime light every day.

If you want to drink or eat something before going to bed, the old favorite of warm milk and cookies, or hot cocoa (yes, even though cocoa has a little caffeine in it) can promote drowsiness and thus, hopefully, sleep. This is because the chemical reaction of the protein in the milk and the sugar in the cookie combine to increase a substance called tryptophan, which causes grogginess. This is the same biochemical reaction we get when we eat turkey and get groggy on Thanksgiving. What about the warmth of the milk? That's probably more psychological.

The bedroom is for sleeping (and sex or snuggling together)—not for computer or work or games. Be dedicated to sleeping. If you tend to look at your digital alarm clock every few minutes that you lie awake, cover it up or turn it around. Minute-by-minute reminders that you are awake will not help you get to sleep; they will get you upset, pushing sleep even further away. Mindfulness meditation has been shown to help people sleep. If the other muscle relaxation, meditation, or breathing techniques described earlier in this chapter, such as progressive muscle relaxation or meditation, are easy to practice or work, use them.

Otherwise, if you are still lying wide awake, try the following relaxation exercise.

A Relaxation Exercise for Sleep (Tried and Tested by Dr. Roth)

A colleague described an easy-to-learn relaxation exercise that I have found handy and useful myself. The only time it has not worked for me is when I was sure I was given caffeinated coffee instead of decaf coffee at a restaurant after dinner. Otherwise, it has been consistently successful.

While you are lying in bed, take a slow breath in, and a slow breath out. Do this a few times, trying to just focus on your breath. After a few breaths, begin to mentally draw a box as you **inhale** and silently count to four (if getting to four takes too long and is uncomfortable you can use a count of two or three). See the nearby illustration. See the line going up on the left, counting "1-2-3-4." Then **hold your breath** as you draw the line along the top to the right, silently counting "hold-2-3-4"; then **exhale** as you draw the line down to the bottom right corner, counting "1-2-3-4." Keep your rhythm as even as possible throughout, and then easily hold your breath as you mentally draw the line back to the starting point on the lower left of your mental screen, and count slowly "hold-2-3-4." You can change the rhythm (1-2-3 or 1-2) if needed so that your breathing feels comfortable. See the box, and continue to draw it over and over again in your mind, as you count to yourself.

Illustration of Sleep Relaxation Technique

For a sleep relaxation technique, follow the steps outlined in Figure 4.2.

If you still do not fall asleep, do not toss and turn in bed for more than 20–30 minutes at a time. If you are not asleep by then and you feel distressed or worried, sleep will not likely come quickly just by demanding or wishing for it. Sleep experts recommend getting out of bed at this point and even out of your room, if possible. Recall that the bedroom is for sleeping only. Pick up a magazine or book; do some other low-energy, non-stimulating monotonous activity such as

Step One: *Inhale with slow count of 2, or 3, or 4 as you Draw the Line Up the Left Side:*

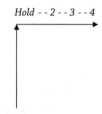

4 - -

3 - -

2 - -

1 - -

Start here

Step Two: *Hold for Count of 4 as You Draw the Line Along the Top to the Right:*

Hold - - 2 - - 3 - - 4

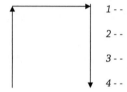

Step Three: *Exhale with slow count of 4 as you Draw Down the Right Side:*

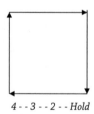

1 - -

2 - -

3 - -

4 - -

Step Four: *Hold for Count of 4 as you Draw Along the Bottom Right to the Left:*

4 - - 3 - - 2 - - Hold

See the Box:

Repeat As Needed and Relax

After a few drawings, visualize your breath moving in and out of the box.

Figure 4.2 Sleep Relaxation Technique.

working a puzzle. Television is not a good tool to help you fall asleep; it can become too enticing for long periods of time. Television screens, just like computers or tablet screens, have white backlights that cause awakening while you are trying to get bleary-eyed for sleep. Kindle readers do not have that white light and are apparently fine for night-time reading. Doing your bills or work projects will likely activate you too much, making it more difficult to get back into sleep mode. Reading a real page-turner novel may also keep you more awake than bring on sleepiness; commit to one chapter or one section only. After about 20–30 minutes of a distracting activity, get back into bed and try to relax again. If after 20–30 minutes you are still not asleep, go through the process again. Try the Box Relaxation Technique (Figure 4.2) again. Continuing to just toss and turn for extended periods of time will usually not accelerate sleepiness.

Too much focus on a goal to achieve can get in the way of accomplishing the task. This is true for sleep. If you tell yourself, "I don't want to stay awake any longer; I need to get to sleep now or I will be exhausted tomorrow," it is almost like saying, "Don't think about a pink elephant for the next 3 minutes." Whether it is a "do" or "don't" command, it becomes almost impossible to accomplish the goal once the idea is suggested. It is activating rather than calming. Change the goal to one that is achievable in smaller increments, leading to ultimate accomplishment of the desired task. Rather than thinking to yourself, "I must get to sleep... it is already 2 in the morning and I will be very tired tomorrow if I do not get to sleep... I hope that sleep comes soon... I'm tired of thinking about this cancer stuff anyway," change the goal. The goal now is "I'd like to relax." If you relax and sleep is needed, sleep is more likely to come. It is easier to achieve a level of relaxation than to leap-frog to sleep. Use either the Box Relaxation Technique or the relaxation breathing techniques described earlier. Again, practicing them during less stressful periods makes them easier to use and more efficient when you are more stressed and really need them. Practice these techniques during the day when there is no sleep goal to be met. The more these exercises are part of your repertoire and *muscle memory*, the easier it will be to use them when crisis or insomnia is present.

Continuous refocusing on your breath is a way to short-circuit your thought-express train. Your breath gives your mind an option for redirection, so it does not have to just follow the thoughts and uncomfortable emotions.

You can find many CDs to listen to that can help you fall asleep (see resources in Appendix). Some are music based, some have gentle natural sounds, and some describe visualization techniques that will lead you on a path to sleep, whether by the ocean, a lake, or in the mountains.

Commonly Suggested Habits for Healthier Sleep

Exercise early in the day rather than late at night.
Decrease caffeine and alcohol consumption, especially at night.
Change goal from "need to sleep" to "want to relax."
Try warm milk and cookies or a light protein and carbohydrate snack.
Practice a relaxation or breathing exercise or use the Box Sleep Relaxation Technique.
Get out of bed if you can't sleep after 20–30 minutes.
Find a low-stimulating and diverting activity like reading.
After 20–30 minutes, get back into bed and try again.
Repeat as needed after 20–30 minutes of not falling asleep.

Nighttime Don'ts—for Better Sleep

Don't toss and turn for more than 20–30 minutes.
Don't eat big meals or exercise vigorously before bed.
Don't watch TV or use your computer in your bedroom.
The bedroom is for sleep (and intimacy) only.
Don't drink caffeine after 2 PM in the afternoon.
Don't use alcohol to get to sleep.
Don't read with a computer or tablet (white backlight is awakening).

DRAFT *with EJ for Insomnia*

> I haven't fallen asleep in 45 minutes. I'm wide awake! If I don't get to sleep now, I never will; tomorrow will be horrible. I'll be tired for my doctor's appointment. This sucks. If I don't fall asleep soon, I'm going to be exhausted tomorrow; I won't be able to ask good questions. If I miss something the doctor says it could kill me.

Detect the distressing aspects of these thoughts, the feelings of frustration and anger, as well as concerns about being tired and not sharp the next day. Notice that you have jumped to expecting a worst-case scenario that leads to more adrenaline flowing and decreases your chances of falling asleep.

Recognize the faulty, irrational logic interspersed with the more reasonable and rational aspects of the thoughts and emotions: "The more I want to fall asleep, the more upset I get, which makes it even less likely that I will get to sleep." Yet it does make sense that you would want to feel sharp for your doctor's appointment. You recognize that that if you miss something your doctor says, it is not likely that you will die.

Acknowledge what's behind the emotions and what makes sense even about the irrational aspects: "I think I overdid it today while walking in the gym and lifting weights. I'm achy; and I have to be in Manhattan early for my doctor's appointment. It is understandable that I want to get some rest. Maybe the pain is keeping me awake. I can take my pain reliever and see if it helps."

The **F**lip: "The harder I try to get to sleep the more frustrated I get." Let me change the goal to "I want to relax," instead of jumping to a foregone conclusion of predicting no sleep. I think this would be a good time to try one of the breathing exercises Dr. Roth described earlier." Even if you get no sleep tonight, tomorrow is not mandated to be horrible. If you miss something the doctor says, it won't kill you. You can call back to clarify. You might be tired, but "becoming horrible" can become a self-fulfilling prophecy. You've been able to focus in the past when tired. You might even tell your doctor that you haven't been sleeping well and that you are tired. Maybe you can acknowledge that your partner/friend will be with you and will assist in hearing what the doctor says, and making sure your questions are asked and answered, and understood. It's good you two decided to go over the list of questions earlier today.

Transformation: "Tomorrow will go like other visits have gone—good news or not, I will figure out what needs to be done so I can stay as healthy as possible. I think I'm just worried about getting bad news. But worrying so much tonight is bringing possible bad news from tomorrow, here tonight. I've been tossing and turning for over 45 minutes. Dr. Roth said no more than 20–30 minutes. First I'll take my pain medicine. Then I'll go in another room and read for 20 minutes; then I'll get back into bed and try to relax again. Maybe I'll have some warm milk and cookies." This strategy can short-circuit the worry wheel and provide you with that emotional reset button. When you get back to bed, try one of the relaxation exercises previously mentioned.

If these techniques do not sufficiently help your sleeplessness, consider asking your doctor if it is safe to take an over-the-counter sleep aid or a prescription medication to help with sleep, if needed. Maybe your pain needs to be treated more optimally. If your overall distress level remains high, consider consulting a therapist or attending a support group. There is a huge barrier to overcome to take this step—the stigma of seeing a mental health professional. But your quality of life, and your mental health, as you and your family go through this cancer process, is worth it. You can ask your oncologist or your general physician for local referrals. Often a social worker or psychologist will be able to bring relief. If not, and a medication is required, you can ask either the therapist or your doctor for a referral to a psychiatrist; or perhaps your oncologist is comfortable prescribing a sleep medication. Chapter 5 will discuss common medications used to relieve anxiety, depression, and insomnia.

Chapter 5

Do I Really Need a Psychiatric Medication to Cope with Prostate Cancer?

It can feel embarrassing and shameful for some men to see a psychiatrist or mental health professional. It can feel outright disgraceful to take a medication to help with mood or sleep, or to relieve anxiety symptoms, even if some have essentially self-medicated for years. In this chapter we will discuss clues about whether anxiety and depressive symptoms are related to physiological or psychological causes. This may give you a clue regarding the extent to which you can fix the problem on your own, or whether you could benefit from psychotherapy or psychiatric medication. I will give you indications for when you might benefit from a medication to treat anxiety, depression, or insomnia, as well what possible side effects to look out for, and how to weigh the balance between potential benefit of medication and potential down sides of side effects.

> Do I really need to take one more medication just because I feel anxious, depressed or cannot sleep? Is this distress related to physical or psychological causes?

My heart was pounding and I was restless and anxious after my neu-roma surgery; I was having a panic attack. I tried to do the breath-ing exercises described in Chapter 4; they helped, but only briefly. This panicky feeling was likely due to a steroid I'd been given to treat a postoperative complication—though this felt "psychological" the cause was physiological. When the panic returned with even more momentum, I asked for an antianxiety medication and got a good night's sleep. When I had pain, I feared drowsiness and constipation from pain medication, but decided it was okay to ask for that med-ication, too. I heard my own advice given to many patients: "High anxiety and pain are not good for anyone or for your recuperation," "Don't worry about addiction," and "You don't need to suffer."

Although anxiety and depression develop in healthy people, they are even more common in the medically ill, especially in those with life-threatening illnesses like cancer. These emotional responses may be relieved by time, will power, a change in circumstances, traditional psy-chotherapy, or the DRAFT with EJ method learned in Chapter 4. If you jumped straight to this chapter on medicine, yet are not convinced that medication is right for you, go back to Chapter 4 and try the self-help DRAFT with EJ techniques. If they do not help sufficiently, you might consider seeing a professional therapist. EJ or talking about your stressors can improve your coping abilities. Psychotherapy can help you decrease your anxiety so you can feel better emotionally. In addi-tion, it may be a good supplemental treatment strategy if you do require an antianxiety medicine or antidepressant. The benefits may kick in sooner or last longer than with no psychotherapy at all.

Intense, frequent, or long-lasting emotional reactions may warrant treatment with medicine. Men wonder if taking a psychiatric medication is "just masking the truth, the real me, so that I won't be ready to handle reality. Will I feel like Alice in the Looking Glass or like in a topsy-turvy world of a Gilbert and Sullivan show?" A number of men have asked me, "Why do you think they call them drugs, doc?"

However, overwhelming anxiety, depression, and insomnia also mask our true strengths and ability to confront reality and cope with stressful situations like prostate cancer. We have already seen how anxiety and depression can distort our versions of reality and lead to more worry and pessimism. When I suggest a medication to help a patient's mood or anxiety, it is not just to help with a little frustration. It is to treat a biochemical syndrome that is a significant deterrent to having a better life as a man deals with prostate cancer, and maybe to help cope better with the cancer as well. More often than not, people taking psychiatric medications feel more like their real selves, being able to live better in general and with illness-related stressors in particular, with less intrusive noise of irrational thoughts or out-of-control feelings. If you don't feel right on a psychiatric medicine for anxiety or depression, it can be stopped. One man told me, "You know, doc, I didn't like the anxiety, but I certainly don't like NOT feeling anything—I didn't feel any emotion on that medicine you gave me." We discontinued the medication and tried another that he tolerated better. He remarked how grateful he was to have his life back. He had not realized how far away he was from his baseline while he was so anxious. He found a balance between concern for what was appropriate without an overabundance of anguish and emotional noise that distracted from his sense of clarity. Most often, people who take medications for sleep, anxiety, or depression feel they handle everyday life better and can get through challenges and struggles more easily. Thus they are able to cope with the more trying crises in their lives. And most people struggling with cancer who take psychiatric medications do not need them for the rest of their lives.

Men tend to shun medications for anxiety, depression, pain, or fatigue for many additional reasons. They fear (usually inaccurately) addiction; even more commonly, they dread side effects. Even though psychiatric symptoms can be quite debilitating, many men put up with emotional suffering rather than risk the possible downsides of these medications. In truth, most of the side effects of antidepressants and antianxiety medications are more benign or less toxic than the potential side effects from medications used to treat medical or cancer conditions. The philosophy of "I don't believe in taking medications" may have worked for many men for colds, headaches, or other minor ailments, as well as mild anxiety and sadness. However, few refuse antibiotics to treat bacterial infections, just as most do not refuse to take treatment for prostate cancer when indicated. When it comes to psychiatric medications or medicines to treat pain or fatigue, men are concerned that the side effects of the medication will outweigh the benefits; many believe they are already on too many medicines that could cause side effects or drug interactions. In general, this is not a bad rule of thumb. If the possible benefits of a medication do not outweigh the possible complications, why would any of us put a pill in our mouths or undergo a medical procedure? But the list of side effects on the pill bottle insert does not predict who will get which ones, how many of them, or even if they will arise for any particular person; and if they do arise, it is hard to know how severe they might be. Your doctor cannot make that prediction for most individual patients. We each have to weigh the benefit–risk ratio and be convinced that it is in favor of the benefit side.

Men with prostate cancer tend to undertreat frustrating physical symptoms like pain and fatigue. Fear of complications and side effects, or a desire to "tough it out" and therefore not treating those physical symptoms, unfortunately has the downstream effect of worsening depression and anxiety that ultimately can worsen physical well-being. This is a prime example of mind–body interdependence. If we can decrease physical pain, or the negative psychological feedback from the physical discomfort, we may be able to short-circuit the repetitive process overall. Many men recuperating from prostate cancer surgery or radiation or undergoing treatment with hormones or other medications cannot accurately predict when or if secondary complications or side effects will be resolved. These men can build up a lingering vulnerability to anxiety. This is especially noticeable when new illness or symptoms raise their ugly heads. It's as if these men had already primed, or kindled, the worry-pump. This entity is similar to post-traumatic stress. These men are hypervigilant, are easily alarmed, and want to avoid certain medical situations. They also re-experience aspects of their cancer struggle, such as hearing their doctor say, "You have cancer," or not wanting to get the next PSA test result. Anxiety or depression levels may be higher than expected for men who have been through "let-downs" or "traumas" before. Managing these symptoms wisely and judiciously leads to improved physical and psychological quality of life now and in the future.

Earlier I reviewed the common, "normal" emotional reactions to a cancer diagnosis, or to news that the cancer, once treated, has returned. Psychiatric medications are used if psychological symptoms interfere with one's ability to function—if non-medication options discussed in Chapter 4 such as psychotherapy are not available, not palatable, or do not bring sufficient relief or are not appropriate, given the current severity or acuteness of the symptoms. But what does "ability to function" mean? Is it your "usual high level of functioning," feeling very productive, easily multitasking with lots of energy? Or does it mean being able to get by and take care of the most important or basic things in your life, given the circumstances of a new diagnosis of and treatment for prostate cancer? For instance, maybe it's *good enough* to get to your job and perform reasonably, even if not ideally. This could pass the "good enough" test for many men. Some jobs require more exacting performance because of safety issues, and going on automatic pilot is not okay. Are you able to get enough sleep so you are not walking around exhausted much of the day? Are you too worried about the cancer or the treatment to focus well enough on your work?

The symptoms of high anxiety or disabling depression are often obvious and profound: major procrastination at work; frequent inattentiveness during conversations; pacing; restlessness; heart palpitations; irritable, fluctuating moods; excessive worry; or irregular bowels. Some men will start drinking alcohol more in order to transiently ease the tension. It is important for your physician to first consider whether the symptoms are due to a medical problem or due to a medication you are taking. Medical or physiological causes of anxiety or depression include electrolyte imbalances such as low calcium, thyroid abnormalities, and vitamin deficiencies (i.e., B12, folic acid); infections; cardiac or respiratory ailments; abnormal glucose levels; pain; and fatigue. Medications used to treat cancer that cause anxiety or depression as side effects include hormonal agents, steroids, some pain medications, and some antibiotics. If anxiety or depression is swallowing you up and preventing you from moving forward, whether the cause is medical or distress about your medical issues, it is time to consider taking medication.

Anxiety Medications

Your general physician can prescribe medications to relieve anxiety, as can your oncologist, a nurse practitioner, or a psychiatrist. These medicines help you get beyond the barriers to good lifestyle behaviors, barriers that anxiety creates in the context of cancer, and are advocated by most reasonable practitioners. The first choice of medications for acute anxiety is from the class of benzodiazepines or minor tranquilizers. These medications give a calm feeling or "take the edge off" the anxiety. Men feel they can face frightening situations or have less intense worry when they take these medicines.

Glossary of Medications Used to Treat Anxiety

Benzodiazepine ~ minor tranquilizer

SSRI/SNRI (serotonin-specific or serotonin-norepinephrine reuptake inhibitors) antidepressants also used to treat anxiety

Antipsychotic ~ major tranquilizer ~ neuroleptic

Popular antianxiety medicines in people with cancer are the benzodiazepines: Valium (diazepam), Xanax (alprazolam), Klonopin (clonazepam), and Ativan (lorazepam). They may relieve panic attacks, which consist of palpitations, restlessness, tremors, and shortness of breath, butterflies in your stomach, a nervous stomach, or diarrhea. Benzodiazepines have similar effects in the brain to those of alcohol. Their calming effects are comparable, as are potential withdrawal effects. But alcohol has other extensive effects on other parts of the body that can be more problematic over time.

A common side effect of these antianxiety medications is sedation (which is not bad if you want help falling sleep at night, but it's not good if you need sharp attention and alertness to work during the day). Again, think alcohol. Some people get headaches from these medicines. These medicines usually carry notices of caution about the danger of using them while operating heavy machinery (i.e., driving a car or using chainsaws or lawnmowers). Again, think alcohol and DUI, or driving under the influence. These medications can cause respiratory slowing at higher doses in some people, so they need to be prescribed with caution if someone already has breathing problems.

These medications are best taken on an *as needed* basis when anxiety and worry are intermittent. Diazepam (Valium) and clonazepam (Klonopin) last longer in your body, so they can be taken once, twice, or at most three times a day (if needed that often). Lorazepam (Ativan) is a moderately long-acting medicine and can be taken two to three times a day, while alprazolam (Xanax) is short-acting and may need to be taken up to four times daily.

There are up sides and down sides to both short- and long-acting medicines. Shorter-acting medicines provide their antianxiety action relatively quickly and don't hang around your body much longer than you need them. There is less likelihood of a hangover effect with shorter-acting medicines once the anxiety is gone. Unfortunately, for many people, shorter-acting antianxiety medications can cause *rebound anxiety*, where the medicine feels like it suddenly leaves the body—that is, you can feel just as nervous, or more so, than before you took the pill. Then you might want to have another dose of the medicine to feel comfortable again. A general rule of thumb is shorter-acting medicines are not useful for those who have more free-floating, generalized anxiety or distress, because the medicines would need to be taken several times a day everyday to keep anxiety levels relatively steady. The down side of longer-acting medicines is that your distressing event may have passed and you do not need the medication any more, yet it is still in your body. This can cause sluggishness and less activity for a longer period of time. But for those who have anxiety most of the day, for a few days at a time, such as the week before a PSA test, longer-acting medications like clonazepam are indicated to give a less bumpy, less roller-coaster-like ride through the day. In fact, if your anxiety is more generalized, lasting for more than a few days, you may do better with a medication like an antidepressant or buspirone (see the next section for more information about more enduring anxiety).

Men tend to fear taking minor tranquilizers because they worry about becoming "addicted" to them. It is the same fear people have about taking narcotics or strong pain medicine. Although addiction is possible with these medications, the fear of addiction is likely overestimated in the cancer population, largely because addiction is misunderstood. The distinction between psychological addiction, physical dependence, and physiological tolerance to these potentially habit-forming medicines is important—however, too many people, including healthcare professionals, use the terms interchangeably and, thus, incorrectly.

Physical dependence is likely in most, if not all, people taking a benzodiazepine daily for a month or longer. Dependence can put someone at risk for life-threatening withdrawal symptoms if the medicine were stopped abruptly (i.e., going cold turkey) or tapered too quickly. Withdrawal symptoms from the minor tranquilizers usually begin 2–3 days after stopping the medicine. Symptoms more commonly include increased anxiety, shakiness, restlessness, panic attacks, palpitations, insomnia, or paranoia, and rare, but sometimes fatal, seizures. This is similar to alcohol withdrawal or delirium tremens, when someone who is dependent on alcohol stops it abruptly.

Another feared consequence of regular use of these antianxiety medications is physical tolerance. *Tolerance* means that patients need a higher dose after a variable amount of time—for some this can happen after daily use of the medication for months, for others it does not happen for a few years. The same dose that gave relief for a few months no longer does so, and a higher dose of the medicine is needed, especially if the anxiety is related to stressors that may continue to worsen. Like dependence, this is a physiological phenomenon, even though it appears to others as "addiction" because someone is requesting more medicine. Unlike dependence, even though this is a physiological phenomenon, it does not happen to everyone, so we cannot predict who will run into this problem. Tolerance may be considered an acceptable price to pay for getting relief and being more able to be compliant with your cancer treatment. However, this potential outcome must be discussed with and understood by patients prior to starting the medicine. This is a good topic to discuss with the physician who is prescribing it. I tell patients that if they require these medications long term because of prolonged stressors, we can eventually taper the medications slowly, down the road, when the pressures ease.

Over time, we might also move from short-acting to longer-acting anti-anxiety medications or add an antidepressant, either a serotonin-specific reuptake inhibitor (SSRI) or a serotonin-norepinephrine reuptake inhibitor (SNRI), which can treat ongoing anxiety even in the absence of the minor tranquilizers. Because of the already mentioned complications with long-term use, the benzodiazepines are often not recommended for people with long-term generalized anxiety (anxiety that predated the cancer and has continued most days for at least 6 months) or free-floating anxiety that is present most days, most of each day.

Lastly, some people who have had addictive tendencies in the past develop compulsive drug-seeking behaviors related to psychological addiction. Addiction refers to a craving for and use of a substance or medicine despite harm. Addictive behaviors are noted by use of larger amounts of the substance than is indicated; having a persistent desire for or making unsuccessful efforts to cut down or control substance use; spending a great deal of time trying to obtain, use, or recover from the substance; and giving up or having problematic social, work, or recreational activities because of substance use. Sometimes patients look like they are addicted when they are not, because their anxiety symptoms are not treated sufficiently. We call this *pseudo-addiction*.

Does this mean you should avoid these medicines altogether? Absolutely not! Men with prostate cancer, and perhaps older men in general, are reluctant to take "extra" medicines that are not directly related to treating the cancer. They even avoid pain medicines and try to put up with significant discomfort and physical debilitation to avoid the uncomfortable side effects of those medicines. Physical and emotional quality of life suffers more than if the pain or anxiety were treated appropriately and side effects addressed. For the most part, when the crisis has lifted and the stressors have decreased and there is less need for these medicines, people can taper off them. But your physician should monitor the medicines, and if you find that your daily or weekly anxiety increases on the same dose, check with your doctor. There is nothing to be ashamed about—remember, tolerance is a physiological phenomenon.

Taking Anxiety Medicines Regularly Does Not Make You an Addict

If you do not understand the differences, you might suffer unnecessarily.

Physical dependence is likely in most if not all people within a month of daily use. This is not addiction. Abrupt cessation can lead to withdrawal symptoms including anxiety, restlessness, insomnia, and, rarely, seizures. There is no reason for withdrawal if you taper the medicine over a week or two.

Physical tolerance: Some people need a higher dose after a few months of daily treatment to obtain the same amount of relief they got with lower doses earlier on; this is physiological and not an addiction.

Psychological and biochemical addiction involves compulsive use of the substance despite harm when the substance is often used in larger amounts than is indicated; there is a persistent desire or unsuccessful efforts to cut down or control substance use. People spend a great deal of time in activities necessary to obtain, use, or recover from the substance, and they give up or have problematic social, occupational, or recreational activities because of substance use. In other words, they use the agent despite harm and not necessarily to relieve physical or psychological discomfort.

An Antidepressant for Anxiety—How Confusing!

Medicines like Lexapro (escitalopram), Zoloft (sertraline), Celexa (citalopram), Prozac (fluoxetine), and Paxil (paroxetine), in the SSRI class of medications, are best known as antidepressants. By increasing the effectiveness of a chemical called *serotonin* in the brain, they are the most common medicines used to treat depression and anxiety today. SNRIs, another popular group of medicines that includes Effexor (venlafaxine) and Cymbalta (duloxetine), increase the efficacy of both norepinephrine and serotonin. Another antidepressant that works primarily on the serotonin system is Remeron (mirtazapine). All of these antidepressants have been found to help people with free-floating, generalized *anxiety* and *panic attacks*. Bupropion (Wellbutrin), an antidepressant also used to treat tobacco addiction, is *not* often used to treat anxiety, since it can be energizing, and if it overshoots, it commonly causes anxiety as a side effect.

The antidepressants differ from the minor tranquilizer/benzodiazepine antianxiety medicines mentioned earlier in many ways. First and foremost, they are *not addictive*. However, antidepressants cannot be taken on an as needed basis. If you are starting to have a panic attack, taking an extra antidepressant pill will not relieve the attack the way a minor tranquilizer like alprazolam, clonazepam, or diazepam might. The same is true for anxiety that starts to build days before a doctor's visit but diminishes considerably after you get your PSA level back—taking an antidepressant for a week won't relieve your anxiety at all. SSRI and SNRI antidepressants need to build up in your body over many weeks (2–5 weeks at any dose level) before they prevent or curtail the anxiety symptoms, just as they need to do when prescribed for depression.

These antianxiety antidepressants are often started together *with* a benzodiazepine so a person can get immediate relief of their distress. After a few weeks, when we expect the antianxiety effects of the antidepressant to have kicked in, the benzodiazepine can be tapered down and eventually stopped, or used on an as needed basis. The most common side effects of the antidepressants include gastric upset, anxiety or insomnia, and daytime grogginess, which often improve within days to a couple of weeks. Antidepressants used for anxiety can be tapered after 9–12 months of treatment. At that time, they should be tapered to prevent a discontinuation syndrome, which may be uncomfortable but not dangerous, as with benzodiazepine withdrawal.

Buspirone (Buspar) is another non-benzodiazepine antianxiety medicine that affects gamma-aminobutyric acid (GABA), a brain neurotransmitter that inhibits excitatory responses in the brain. Like the antidepressants, it does not have the complications of dependence, tolerance, or addiction. But also like the antidepressants, buspirone needs to be taken daily, and there is at least a 2-week medication buildup time until you feel relief. Buspirone does not treat intermittent panic attacks. It is prescribed for more generalized, free-floating anxiety.

Neither You nor Your Doctor Are Crazy If You Get a Major Tranquilizer for Anxiety

Major tranquilizers, also known as antipsychotics or neuroleptics, treat anxiety in the medically ill when the benzodiazepines or antidepressants mentioned earlier do not work, are not tolerated well, or are not appropriate for a particular patient. These medications are also called mood stabilizers. The package inserts for these medications are frightening to read when you are already anxious and not having psychotic symptoms like hallucinations or delusions. Outside of the cancer world, antipsychotic medications are used in higher doses to treat people with schizophrenia and bipolar disorders. But medications like Zyprexa (olanzapine) or Seroquel (quetiapine) are extremely helpful for debilitating anxiety if you cannot tolerate a benzodiazepine, if the anxiety is due to a medication such as a steroid, like dexamethasone or prednisone, if you have shortness of breath, or if you have had a problem with alcohol use in the past. We have found that these antipsychotics often relieve medication-induced or illness-induced anxiety, insomnia, and restlessness better than benzodiazepines when given for short periods of time. Patients sometimes fear and resist these medications; they may have heard about the worrisome side effects of older versions of the anti-psychotic medicines like chlorpromazine (Thorazine) and haloperidol (Haldol) (involuntary muscle movements or "feeling like a zombie"). These problematic side effects are unusual at low doses and with short periods of use, as in cancer related anxiety situations. People also assume incorrectly they must be "really crazy" to need something called an anti-psychotic. Not true. Anxiety related to coping with prostate cancer or as a side effect from another medication you are taking, like a steroid, is not *crazy*. However, understanding why your doctor is prescribing one of these medicines will allow you to get relief without developing undue anxiety. Most of the medications used to treat anxiety in men with prostate cancer are listed in Table 5.1.

TABLE 5.1 A SCOUTING REPORT ON MEDICATIONS TO TREAT ANXIETY

Drug Class Generic Name (Brand Name)	Scouting Report
Benzodiazepines	First-line medications for worry and panic attacks. Commonly used to treat sleep problems. *Can cause drowsiness, unsteadiness, and forgetfulness, and lead to falls.* Your physician should supervise treatment. If taking for more than a month, physical *dependence* can develop. **THIS IS NOT ADDICTION. BUT DO NOT STOP ABRUPTLY!** Taper as directed to avoid life-threatening withdrawal symptoms. Physiological *tolerance* (needing higher doses to achieve the same relief) may develop after a few months. **THIS IS NOT ADDICTION!** *Addiction*, or use despite harm, is rare to originate in this population at this time, but use should be closely monitored in people with histories of addiction to other substances.

TABLE 5.1 CONTINUED

Drug Class Generic Name (Brand Name)	Scouting Report
Alprazolam (Xanax)	Shorter acting; best used as needed for intermittent panic symptoms; increased likelihood of *rebound anxiety*; quick, noticeable onset of action can more easily lead to addiction.
Lorazepam (Ativan)	Moderately long acting; also helps nausea. Good for MRI anxiety.
Diazepam (Valium)	Long acting, despite quick, noticeable onset of action, which can more easily lead to addiction.
Clonazepam (Klonopin)	Long acting—avoids rebound anxiety. Good for panic attacks and sleep. Disintegrating wafer available; no pill swallowing needed.
Antidepressants Citalopram (Celexa) Escitalopram (Lexapro) Fluoxetine (Prozac) Paroxetine (Paxil) Sertraline (Zoloft) Venlafaxine (Effexor)	Useful for generalized anxiety and to prevent panic attacks. Need to be taken daily. Beneficial effects take 2–5 weeks or longer with any dose change. *Common side effects*: anxiety; restlessness; drowsiness; and gastric upset (bloating, diarrhea, or constipation), which often get better over time. There are no life-threatening withdrawal effects, but it should be tapered under physician supervision to avoid discontinuation syndrome. *Treatment range*: 9–12 months. Suicidal ideation is rare for all antidepressants but should be monitored for all antidepressants. May help with hot flashes for those on hormonal treatment.
Mirtazapine (Remeron)	Sedating. Helps with sleep and anxiety. No gastric upset. May increase appetite and cause weight gain.
Duloxetine (Cymbalta)	May also help with neuropathic pain syndromes.
Non-benzodiazepine Non-antidepressant Buspirone (Buspar)	Onset of action/prescribing suggestions similar to those of antidepressants, but does not help depression. Not helpful for panic, or for those used to benzodiazepines.
Neuroleptics/ Antipsychotics Olanzapine (Zyprexa) Quetiapine (Seroquel)	Used when benzodiazepines are not tolerated or effective (respiratory problems). Can cause sedation and unsteadiness. Can cause abnormal sugar control, cardiac rhythms, and weight problems. No dependence; addiction; need to taper.

Depression

In Chapter 4 we reviewed the difficulties in determining whether sad or depressive feelings in a man with prostate cancer who is not engaging in usually pleasant activities is having an understandable reaction to a difficult situation, a complication of a medication or medical treatment, or a severe major depression. Proper assessment and diagnosis of these alternatives will help guide whether you should be treated with an antidepressant. Depressive symptoms caused by medications used to treat the cancer (i.e., steroids, hormones, pain medications) can be resolved by changing the dose or timing of the dosing of the causative medication, by changing the medication altogether, or, when those options are not possible, treating with an antidepressant.

If physical symptoms such as pain, nausea, or fatigue lead to an inability to do or enjoy usual pleasurable activities, men feel frustrated and demoralized and may feel depressed, but they do not necessarily have a depressive disorder that requires treatment with an antidepressant. In these situations, the physical symptoms should be addressed directly. Ask yourself what you would like to see happen in your life, in the near future and way down the road. Do you have any desire to get involved in life if the physical symptoms can be relieved?

How would you answer Dr. Roth if he asked, "If I could give you a pill to take away some or all of your pain or fatigue, what would you want to do?" The answer can sometimes help distinguish a frustrated reaction to physical limitations from a major depressive disorder, where someone doesn't really care about being involved in anything. So an answer like "I don't care; it doesn't matter" likely signifies a significant depression that does require an antidepressant. An answer like "Of course I'd like to get out and garden or to see my children or grandchildren" suggests that you are less likely to benefit from an antidepressant (unless that antidepressant has some energizing or analgesic effects) and more likely to perk up your spirits with further efforts to increase energy or decrease pain.

The ongoing stresses of cancer can kindle a severe major depression for some people. Noteworthy clues suggesting a severe depression in someone with cancer include feelings of worthlessness or helplessness; severe, nagging guilt about being punished for something you did or did not do in your life (this is distinguished from regrets for things we feel we could have done better or not done at all in our lives, which occur to most of us); a sense of hopelessness about the ability to find any meaning, joy, or purpose in life; and constant thoughts of death or dying or the wish to die or take your life. When the symptoms are present most of the day for most days over the course of a couple of weeks, and the symptoms interfere with your ability to carry on with daily life activities and enjoy them, even in the context of cancer, it makes sense to try an antidepressant under the guidance of a physician or nurse practitioner who will monitor for the benefits as well as attend to possible side effects. Be careful, though. People with cancer may understandably, and appropriately, feel less hope about the future and think about dying more than they did before their diagnosis. That is not depression. When you have a cancer, these thoughts may actually be good reality testing. Remember that neurovegetative symptoms such as changes in sleep patterns, appetite, and concentration and energy levels, which are helpful diagnostic patterns of depression in someone *without* cancer, are not as helpful in someone *with* cancer. These signals may be due to the cancer or to medications, and not causally related to the psyche, although, if not addressed, they can certainly lead to hopelessness and a depressive episode.

Distinguishing offhand comments about wanting to die in the future if things get bad enough, from more serious, acute intentions and plans to hurt oneself because things feel bad and hopeless now, is critical in terms of providing appropriate care. A mental health professional should help in that assessment. Your physician and family must take seriously any concrete plan to commit suicide or any intention to hurt yourself. Thoughts like "Maybe I or my family would be better off if I were to die," or "I'd want to die if it gets bad enough in the future" (usually with very personal criteria for what "bad enough" means, such as too much pain, not being able to care for oneself, becoming incapacitated like the aunt who had dementia) are serious. They are also common, often futuristic reflections among cancer patients who agonize over losing a sense of control or putting up with the powerful distress in their lives that they cannot imagine enduring over time. These musings of control over destiny and freedom of "not having to take it anymore" (i.e., the uncertainty, the prognosis, the losses, and the changes) can bring relief to the "here and now." But they should be addressed. Fears of future helplessness and burden can be met with assurances from physicians and families of doing their best to relieve suffering at any time.

Thoughts like "I want to die now," "I can't stand this anymore," or "Please kill me; there is no reason to live anymore," or having a concrete plan about how to commit suicide with the intention to do so is very serious. These individuals need immediate evaluation to maintain safety and to provide help.

So Many Antidepressants . . . Which Is Best for Me?

All antidepressants can be effective; unfortunately, there is no "one size fits all" antidepressant. Some people respond to one class of antide-pressants or one medication in particular and not to others. Some men are more susceptible to certain side effects than others. The good news is that unsafe side effects from antidepressant medications are quite rare. Isn't it amazing, though, that for all medications (psychiatric or not), the list of benefits on a package insert is quite small, yet the list of potential side effects is quite lengthy, often with bold black warning boxes surrounding the most serious of side effects? Yet if it were clear that the potential benefits did not outweigh the potential side effects, who would take any medication? And if the likelihood of developing all side effects were the same for all, would any of us take the chance of get-ting the dangerous, life-threatening ones? But severe complications are rare, and the benefits of antidepressants, when used appropriately, out-weigh the side effects, or they would not be approved for use. As there is still no test to tell us who or what type of depression will respond to which antidepressant, there is still trial, error, and an art to choosing antidepressants.

Ask your doctor why he or she is picking a particular medication for you, and ask about the more common side effects to be aware of. For most antidepressants these include gastric upset, daytime grogginess, possible anxiety, and difficulty sleeping. If someone feels groggy, they should take the medication at night. If they feel energized, they should take it in the morning. These medicines are dosed once daily; as long as you take it around the same time every day, the actual time of day won't impact effectiveness. Other possible side effects to be aware of include dry mouth, changes in appetite or weight, decreased sexual arousal, and delayed orgasm. These medications do not weaken erectile functioning. Your doctor can work with you to see which medication you tolerate best with the least side effects. Depending on the status of your sexual functioning after your prostate cancer treatment, sexual side effects can seem like deal breakers. Men with advanced prostate cancer who are on hormonal therapy may already have similar side effects, so antidepressants do not raise new concerns.

The choice of medication for depression should be based on the patient's medical, physical, and psychiatric condition. I tell all of my patients, and often their family members, about the most common side effects of the particular antidepressant that I am considering prescribing. We try to determine which side effects, should they occur, would be problematic for a particular man. We try to avoid those. We also try to figure out which potential side effects may actually be beneficial (i.e., activating medications for fatigued patients; calming or sedating medications for those with anxiety or insomnia). Your doctor must also consider potential drug interactions, given any other medications you may be receiving for prostate cancer, for other medical illnesses, or for psychiatric conditions.

Just as for anxiety, most antidepressants take 2 to 5 weeks at any particular dose to be effective in treating depression. Therefore, do not stop the medication prematurely if you do not see an immediate benefit without speaking with your doctor first. Some side effects occur within a few days or weeks, though they often diminish or disappear over time. In order to minimize side effects or their impact, the dosing strategy of "start low, go slow, but go" is strongly recommended.

Antidepressants by Class: Looking under the Microscope

Selective Serotonin Reuptake Inhibitors (SSRIs): Escitalopram, Sertraline, Citalopram, Fluoxetine, Paroxetine

This class of antidepressants is the most often prescribed in cancer patients because they are effective and very well tolerated. They are all available as generic medications, so they are not overly expensive and usually covered by prescription insurance plans. These medications treat major depression as well as generalized anxiety disorder, panic disorder, as well as hot flashes caused by hormonal medications taken for advanced prostate cancer. They even help men who have premature ejaculation. SSRIs essentially increase the amount of serotonin that gathers between two brain cells, by not allowing resorption, or reuptake, of unused serotonin for metabolism. When a downstream cell, or neuron, sees more serotonin gathering in the space (the synapse) between the cells, and it doesn't have enough receptors to attach to all the serotonin, it starts to manufacture receptors that will specifically match to the serotonin, causing a lock-and-key connection. When enough serotonin transmitters and matching receptors make contact, conduction is improved and more efficient. Eventually, you will see improved mood and anxiety. After shutting down the resorption of serotonin, it takes only a few days for significant amounts of serotonin to start building up. But increasing the numbers of receptors can take weeks. That's why it is not a good idea to stop an antidepressant too soon if you do not see results. However, common, uncomfortable side effects can happen soon after starting the medication, although they typically decrease with time.

Serotonin-Norepinephrine Reuptake Inhibitors (SNRIs): Venlafaxine and Duloxetine

The SNRIs function similarly to the SSRIs to treat major depression, generalized anxiety, panic, and hot flashes. They increase the amount and efficiency of serotonin and norepinephrine neurotransmitters and receptor conduction in the space (synapse) between specified brain cells and thereby also relieve depression and anxiety symptoms. Venlafaxine and duloxetine have differing ratios of serotonin and norepinephrine effects. They have many of the same side effects as SSRIs. Because of a greater norepinephrine effect, duloxetine, has also been found to be useful to treat neuropathic pain syndromes as well as depression. Venlafaxine can also relieve hot flashes for many men getting androgen deprivation agents.

Additional Antidepressants: Mirtazapine and Bupropion

Mirtazapine works mainly on serotonin receptors like the SSRIs. It relieves both anxiety and depression. Side effects can also be both beneficial and problematic. It has sedating effects at lower doses, so it is dosed at night to decrease daytime sedation. This sedating effect improves sleep. Mirtazapine is the only antidepressant that does not commonly cause gastric problems; it can increase appetite and thus weight, which may be a benefit for many patients. It has even been used to relieve nausea. A medicine that can decrease anxiety, improve mood, improve sleep, improve appetite, and decrease gastric upset? That's a grand slam plus! If daytime grogginess occurs, stopping or adjusting the dose usually brings relief.

Bupropion works primarily on dopamine receptors. Compared to other antidepressants, it has an energizing effect that can improve cancer-related fatigue, but sometimes can make men feel anxious or have trouble sleeping. Bupropion is the only antidepressant that does not cause sexual side effects, so it may be useful in otherwise sexually active men (however, it won't improve libido in those impacted by androgen ablation therapy). Bupropion has also been used to help people stop smoking tobacco.

Patients with a history of seizure disorder or bulimia should not take this medication.

> **Bupropion: Another Psychiatric Four-Bagger**
>
> Improves mood for depressed patients
> Helps stop smoking to improve physical health
> Improves energy for cancer-related fatigue
> No sexual side effects!

Tricyclic Antidepressants (TCAs): Amitriptyline, Imipramine, Desipramine, Nortriptyline

Tricyclic antidepressants (TCAs) were introduced in the 1950s and were the mainstay of the pharmacological treatment of depression until the 1990s when the SSRIs became available. Unfortunately, the uncomfortable and potentially dangerous side effects of TCAs include dry mouth, blurry vision, constipation, difficulty urinating, sedation that often led to falls, cardiac conduction problems, abnormal heart rhythms, as well as blood pressure changes, which make them particularly problematic for medically susceptible adults with cancer. Today, these medications are used to treat chronic neuropathic pain syndromes and occasionally insomnia, but are seldom used as first-line medicines to treat depression. Although SSRIs and SNRIs are used more commonly, TCAs can be helpful in some treatment-resistant patients.

Myth vs. Reality

"I've heard antidepressants can be dangerous. I'm trying to fight cancer—why on earth would I take a medicine that could kill me?" (This future-oriented statement might suggest a man does not have a severe depression and therefore not benefit from an antidepressant anyway, though he might be prescribed an antidepressant as an antianxiety medicine.) Two media-generated fears have frightened some people from trying an antidepressant: first, that antidepressants cause cancer, and second, that antidepressants cause people to kill themselves. I believe both assertions have been overstated and misunderstood.

Can Antidepressants Make Cancer Grow?

Reports many years ago warned that antidepressants could be carcinogenic. Certainly no patient or physician wants to do anything that could promote tumor growth. However, these concerns were not proven in lifelike situations in humans. The studies, completed in rodents, were carried out in ways that do not mimic the way tumors behave in humans. The doses of antidepressant medications were much higher than would be used in treating depression in humans. Additionally, tumors were often implanted into the animals, which does not reflect what happens in men with prostate cancer. Data have not supported this when human subjects were examined. Therefore, prescription of antidepressants is still recommended when needed so patients do not have to suffer both the trauma of the cancer *and* depression.

Will an Antidepressant Make Me Suicidal?

A second more recent concern about antidepressants is whether they cause suicidal ideation in adults. In fact, the U.S. Food and Drug Administration (FDA) has instituted a black-box warning about this potentially deadly side effect. Again, what depressed person would want to take a medication that would cause him to have one of the most severe symptoms of depression, suicidal thinking or behavior? The suicidal concern, though small, is more concerning for pediatric patients. Studies done in adults looking for increased suicidality from antidepressant use have not shown consistent, convincing evidence. However, the worry is there, in a black-and-white warning that finds its way into every discussion when an antidepressant prescription is considered.

Do claims of suicidal thinking come from depression that worsens before there is enough time for an antidepressant to take effect (remember, it can take up to 5 or 6 weeks at any particular dose before we see the benefit of an antidepressant) or from the medication? I believe that these medicines have a rare side effect called *akathisia*, a state of agitation, distress, or restlessness that is subjectively very uncomfortable. People affected often state, "I can't stand this feeling; it's like I am jumping out of my skin." They cannot sit still or even lie in bed without moving constantly. It's like having an internal motor that just won't turn off. When stimulated like this, some feel an impulsive urge to hurt themselves, just to put an end to this inner restless discomfort. Regardless of the cause, rare events can be managed safely when a prescriber provides adequate information beforehand and careful, timely, and appropriate follow-up after prescribing the medicine. Therefore, before a patient starts an antidepressant, I review this rare side effect with him, along with the more common ones mentioned earlier. Patients are instructed to call me if they feel uncomfortable or restless and to stop the medication.

I am not a "medication pusher," but I believe that antidepressants help many men with prostate cancer to live better, since severe depression can kill as well. Many people with cancer are willing to take anti-cancer medications and treatments that are known to more commonly have more severe side effects, yet they hesitate to take a psychiatric medication that may also be life-saving. It is unfortunate that in our society a strong stigma about psychiatric treatment is still in play.

Using Secondary Side Effects in Your Favor

The main goal of antidepressants is to treat depression or anxiety. In addition to avoiding problematic side effects, physicians can use helpful side effects of medicines in a patient's favor. Antidepressants like bupropion or fluoxetine have energizing side effects, and may be helpful if depression is accompanied by significant fatigue, until the primary antidepressive effects of the medication take hold in 2–5 weeks. The energizing side effects of bupropion can also improve cancer-related fatigue or lack of motivation due to radiation therapy, hormonal therapy, pain medicines, or chemotherapy, even if there is no depressive syndrome. Mirtazapine can help those with insomnia and decreased appetite. Venlafaxine can be prescribed to treat hot flashes.

Psychostimulants can boost energy levels; they can also improve concentration and mood in much less time than it takes for an antidepressant to work. These medications are generally known to treat attention deficit-hyperactivity disorder (ADHD) in school-age children. When I suggest a stimulant to men with prostate cancer for fatigue, they wonder, "How can medicines that can calm kids give me more energy?" Attention and ability to focus in children with ADHD improve with these medicines. They concentrate better and can stay still longer. It looks like they have been calmed. In medically ill patients, heightened focus is also accompanied by increased energy. The research on using stimulants for cancer-related symptoms has been mixed, some studies showing no improved outcomes over placebos. Our research group found that methylphenidate, a psychostimulant, was a useful energy boost for many men with prostate cancer who were fatigued from androgen ablation or chemotherapy. Occasionally, unwelcome side effects of this stimulant include increased heart rate and blood pressure. Given the mixed results of the research, I recommend that oncologists consider prescribing these medicines for severe fatigue in men who are cardiologically and neurologically healthy, and continue to monitor pulse and blood pressure for a number of weeks until effective dosages and safety are established for each patient. Stimulants are often used in the early treatment phase of depression in conjunction *with* antidepressants before the antidepressant effects have had time to kick in. The stimulants give more immediate energy and can be stopped after the antidepressant takes effect.

Table 5.2 lists common antidepressants and a scouting report on good-to-know details about them.

TABLE 5.2 A SCOUTING REPORT ON MEDICATIONS TO TREAT DEPRESSION AND FATIGUE

Drug Class Generic Name (Brand Name)	Scouting Report
Antidepressants	Be alert for drug interactions between psychotropics and androgen ablation agents.
Serotonin Specific Reuptake Inhibitors (SSRIs) Citalopram (Celexa) Escitalopram (Lexapro) Fluoxetine (Prozac) Paroxetine (Paxil) Sertraline (Zoloft)	Varying degrees of gastric distress, nausea, headache, insomnia, sweating, increased anxiety, and sexual dysfunction. In general, sertraline, citalopram, and escitalopram produce the least drug–drug interactions. In addition to treating depression, these medications are used for anxiety and panic syndromes as well as "off-label" for hot flashes.
Serotonin Norepinephrine Reuptake Inhibitors (SNRIs) Venlafaxine (Effexor) Duloxetine (Cymbalta)	In addition to treating depression, these medications treat anxiety and panic syndromes as well as "off-label" hot flashes. Duloxetine may help with neuropathic pain syndromes and fibromyalgia. Side effects include varying degrees of activation, gastric distress, nausea, anxiety, sedation, sweating. Venlafaxine can cause hypertension.
Other Antidepressants	
Mirtazapine (Remeron)	No gastric side effects. Can improve sleep and appetite but if overshoots may cause unwanted daytime sedation or weight gain. Dissolvable tablet form available—no swallowing needed.
Buspirone (Wellbutrin)	Activating: helps fatigue but can overshoot, causing anxiety, restlessness, or insomnia. May cause seizures if predisposed. **NO SEXUAL SIDE EFFECTS** Also helps with smoking cessation.
Psychostimulants *Methylphenidate* (Ritalin; Metadate; Concerta; Focalin) *Amphetamine* (Adderall; Vyvanse)	Can improve mood, energy, concentration, and appetite. *Side effects:* possible cardiac rhythm complications or hypertension; seizures if predisposed; agitation, restlessness, anxiety, insomnia, tics can occur.
Modafinil, Armodafinil (Provigil; Nuvigil)	Wakefulness agents. Usually well tolerated. Improve energy, mood, and focus. Not covered by many prescription plans. *Side effects:* nausea, anxiety, insomnia, and increased heart rate.

Sleep Medications

Sleep can be hard to come by because of anxiety or worry. Sleeplessness may also become the cause of anxiety—the boundaries are not often clear. It is not unmanly to take a medication to decrease distress or to promote grogginess and sleep if distraction, relaxation exercises, meditation, and the other sleep hygiene recommendations mentioned in Chapter 4 or the warm milk and cookies remedy are not enough to bring on sleep. Sleep medications are thought of as short-term remedies over the course of a few weeks, or while a crisis is still brewing, to break the cycle of insomnia and to promote healthy sleep structure. Keep all of your doctors in the loop about what medicines you try, whether over the counter (OTC) or prescription for sleep, anxiety, or depression. They all need to know what you are taking in case there are side effects or possible drug interactions that could be dangerous or negate the potential benefit of the medication they are prescribing. Regardless of which medication you try for sleep, remember they are sedating medications. That means that if you do wake up in the middle of the night, your body and mind might feel hazy. Try to get in the habit of sitting on the edge of your bed before standing up. Make sure you have your physical and mental sea legs to prevent falling. Have a nightlight in the room so you can see where you are walking, as a darkened room increases the likelihood of falls. If you are living with someone, let them know you are taking a sleep medication (especially in the early stages of taking the medication) so they can have their antenna more alert for any nighttime awakenings when you may not be 100%.

OTC medications for sleep often contain diphenhydramine (Benadryl), a common allergy medicine, which helps many men sleep better. But these medications also have side effects that include confusion, a hangover–groggy-like feeling the next day, and urinary retention. Some people experience a contrary awakening effect instead of a sedating effect. As-needed dosing (not every night) of a prescribed sleep-inducing medicine such as zolpidem, zaleplon, eszopiclone, or ramelteon, or sedating antidepressants such as mirtazapine, trazodone, or doxepin can be helpful. Ask your doctor if you can safely take melatonin or magnesium sulfate, two other OTC medicines that help with sleep.

Most sleep medicines work best for people who are having difficulty falling asleep; they are not as helpful for those who fall asleep early but cannot stay asleep through the night. Those men who awaken frequently to urinate or because they have other physical discomfort but who get back to sleep without a significant lag period still feel well rested in the morning. These men are probably better off not taking a sleep medicine. Your bladder and urinary sphincter, the gatekeepers to maintaining nighttime urinary control, often let down their vigilant watch in the presence of sleep medications. You can therefore be at increased risk for urinary accidents as you sleep through the "need to urinate" internal alarm signal. More than one of my patients has awakened irritatingly and shamefully with a wet mattress. But here, too, up-front information is important. You do not necessarily have to avoid these sleep medicines. But be forewarned and know what to look for, so you can make an appropriate choice for you. Take the lowest dose of the sleep medicine that works for you. Ask your urologist if there is a medication to control your nighttime urination. For reassurance, put a waterproof cloth on top of your mattress.

The usual first-line prescription medicines for sleep are the non-benzodiazepines such as **z**olpidem (Ambien), **z**aleplon (Sonata), or es**z**opiclone (Lunesta). Did you notice they all have z's in them? These medications have been referred to as the *Z drugs*.

The upside of these medicines is that they are usually not habit forming and do not cause next-day hangover effects. They often work soon after taking. The downside is that these medicines may not give a full night's sleep (though there is a new longer-acting version of zolpidem (Ambien-CR) that allows many to sleep longer through the night). Eszopiclone may cause a metallic, unpleasant taste in the mouth for some men.

Ramelteon is a melatonin-like medication that resets a person's dysregulated sleep wake cycle over the course of a few weeks. People may not get immediate results of improved sleep, but they may experience better snoozing after consistent nightly use.

If these medicines do not work well enough to address sleep issues, the next step might be a sedating antidepressant, or a trial of a benzodiazepine such as temazepam, lorazepam, or clonazepam. Minor tranquilizers such as lorazepam, clonazepam, or diazepam are helpful to take the edge off of problematic anxiety and bring on sleep without sedating you too much the next day; they are reviewed earlier in this chapter. In addition, these antianxiety medicines can help prevent losing sleep while waiting for test results such as PSA tests, biopsies, or MRI scans, or over

TABLE 5.3 A SCOUTING REPORT ON MEDICATIONS TO TREAT INSOMNIA

Drug Class Generic Name (Brand Name)	Scouting Report
Non-benzodiazepine Hypnotics (Z-Drugs) Zolipdem (Ambien) Zaleplon (Sonata) (Es)Zopliclone (Lunesta) (Metallic taste for some is problematic)	Rare physical dependence, tolerance, and addiction are possible; best taken for short-term use, and ultimately on an as-needed basis. Rare but recently publicized side effects include hallucinations, forgetfulness, and sleepwalking. Try to protect against potential falls if awakened at night—have a nightlight; leave a light in the bathroom; have handrails.
Melatonin-Based Ramelteon (Rozerem)	Binds to melatonin receptors. Check with oncologist to make sure this will not interfere with your cancer treatment.
Benzodiazepines Temazepam (Restoril)—for sleep only Clonazepam (Klonopin) Lorazepam (Ativan) Diazepam (Valium)	Benzodiazepines are the most likely sleep medicines to lead to tolerance and dependence, as mentioned in the Antianxiety section in this chapter. If anxiety is a prominent deterrent to sleep, a benzodiazepine (i.e., clonazepam, lorazepam) may help more than a hypnotic, which will only produce drowsiness. When used for sleep, these medications are also best used on as-needed basis, for short periods of time.

worrying about upcoming doctor appointments. Sometimes benzodiaz-epines interfere with memory, just as alcohol can. So if you want your attention sharp the next day, consider avoiding these medications on nights before doctor visits. Again, it is good to consider potential ben-efits and side effects before taking them. It is not a bad idea to try one of these medications on a night when there is no significant meeting or event the next day, so you can see how your body and mind react. A short-acting tranquilizer such as alprazolam won't leave a hangover but may also be too short-acting to help you sleep throughout the night. Again, the best way to use these medicines is on an as-needed (not every night) basis or for short-term use, so tolerance and physical dependence do not develop. During the course of a crisis (finding out about a new diagnosis or recurrence of disease or that a treatment did not work), it is fine to take one of these medicines on a nightly basis, but after a week or two or three, try to cut back when your normal sleep architecture is likely to be back to a baseline level, so you do not become reliant on the medi-cation. See the list of possible medicines to help you sleep in Table 5.3.

If you still have sleep difficulties after trying different sleep medi-cines, ask your doctor that you be tested in a sleep lab. Many men do not know that they have mild to severe sleep apnea. This can be aggravated in the presence of other medical illnesses and medications. The classic characteristics of a man with sleep apnea include being overweight and snoring when he does sleep. These men do not feel rested even if they do sleep at night. But even thin men who do not snore can have sleep inter-rupted by sleep apnea. Get tested. You may get to sleep better without having to take another medication.

Chapter 6

Keeping the Flames
of Intimacy Alive

Among men, sex sometimes results in intimacy; among women, intimacy sometimes results in sex.

Barbara Cartland

What would a book on prostate cancer be without a chapter on sex?

Erectile dysfunction (ED) is one of the most dreaded complications of prostate cancer. This chapter guides men and their partners to come to terms with temporary and long-term complications of erectile dysfunction and to think about the unthinkable: how to reset goals, thoughts, and behaviors when it comes to sex. These issues are important to heterosexual and gay couples, as well as to single, divorced, and widowed men. Unfortunately, there are no easy remedies for all. Managing expectations by reassessing needs, priorities, realities, possibilities, and probabilities are key to maximizing intimacy in your life. In order to maintain healthy relationships, it is vital that you not discard or ignore physical and emotional intimacy when erections are not rigid enough for intercourse. Though you may feel as if you've lost your manhood or masculine identity if you cannot get a rigid erection, you risk losing even more—the closeness with your partner or spouse, or the potential of romantic intimacy with others if you are not currently involved in an intimate relationship.

A new area of urology called *penile rehabilitation* has developed around these issues. No, this is not a 12-step program for sex addicts; it is a physiologically oriented plan to optimize erections after primary prostate cancer treatment. Regardless of the physical success of rehabilitation, communication techniques need to be addressed to discuss and accommodate for sexual changes and challenges that arise—whether you are partnered, single, widowed, or divorced, and thinking about intimacy or dating with a different sex-pack than you've been used to all of your life.

Worries Men Have about Sex after Prostate Cancer

I fear that I will lose my manhood.

What good am I if I won't be able to get an erection after treatment?

What's the point of physical intimacy if I can't have sex like I have had all my life?

Can sex be good if you have to think about it?

Sorry, honey, we cannot have any physical intimacy until my erections are back.

Will my spouse/partner leave me if I can't get an erection?

Will I just feel like a tool if I just help my partner come and I cannot?

Sexuality plays a prominent role in a man's life when he is younger and in good health. When the machinery is working well and the going is good, there is rare questioning about whether to make adjustments, other than the media-promulgated male insecurity about whether a guy is big enough, has enough testosterone, can get it up as often and whenever he wants to, or can go longer than other guys. A comfortable sexual relationship before prostate cancer might encounter brief conversations about satisfaction for both partners. Guys may question: "Do I use a condom or not? Is birth control or protection from sexually transmitted diseases with condoms necessary in this relationship?" Before prostate cancer, a man with sexual problems such as premature ejaculation or ED might have difficulty both from an individual and couple's perspective, regardless of the security or longevity or "permanence" of the relationship. Erectile difficulty after prostatectomy and radiation therapy may be more of a problem for those who had erectile difficulty prior to their treatment.

Understanding the distinction between physiological and psychological causes of these difficulties is not easy and may require a medical or urological examination and investigation to clarify. A rough rule of thumb is that if a man can get an erection while sleeping or when he awakens in the morning (this is called penile tumescence), erectile issues are thought to be more likely of psychological origin. But when prostate cancer is in the picture, all of this becomes even more confusing, upsetting, and challenging. Sexual functioning can be problematic for many aging men, even without prostate cancer, because of other medical issues such as hypertension, high cholesterol, diabetes, and a natural decrease in testosterone.

After a prostate cancer diagnosis and treatment, men wonder whether sexual changes brought on by the illness or treatment will be temporary or permanent. Many are also preoccupied with how long is a long-enough recuperation time after treatment before giving up the wait for a return to their old baseline. They wonder if they'll have a new, perhaps inadequate or unsatisfying baseline. Will they be able to adjust to that new baseline? It may go without saying, but men who are able to have better erectile functioning after prostate cancer seem to have less distress, although some are dissatisfied with anything less than their pre-cancer sexuality. Men who do have substantial changes with erections usually have even more difficulty adjusting.

Your physician likely gave you a time frame by which your erections might return after your treatment is completed. Depending on the type and length of treatment, up to 50% of men after radiation therapy and 40–70% of men who had prostatectomy will not return to baseline erections 2 years after treatment, and may have difficulty maintaining or achieving an erection. Erections are impacted sooner after prostatectomy and improve over the following year or two, whereas erections after radiation therapy are usually stronger initially but may be adversely affected after a few years. If men are told that erections could return after 7 to 24 months after surgery, many hear "7 months" and start getting distressed after a few months if there are still no signs of erections returning; they start to worry whether they will ever have an erection again. When something so integral and natural to your life disappears (even transiently), it understandably brings on worry and upset. The void that is left for many men is all-encompassing, the silence deafening. Though your brain doesn't "intend" to make you feel worse, extended and extensive emotional reactions of anger and sadness are not welcome. Most men want to be optimistic. They want to get back to their best functioning as early as possible. Unfortunately, the time frame most men have for overly optimistic expectations is unrealistic. Subsequent dashed hopes lead to more frustration.

My advice deviates from those who say it is crucial to have positive thoughts all of the time to get through your cancer experience, or any life hardship for that matter. For most men, trying to be positive about not having erections is much easier said than done; the pursuit of attaining and maintaining positivity disturbingly brings up more distress and suffering for many. If your doctor does not give a time range by which your erections might improve, ask for one; then look toward the far end of the range as the more likely target. This is a time when preparing for the worst and hoping for the best makes sense. If you regain good functioning sooner than the predicted range, fantastic; but there will be much less agonizing if recuperation is delayed than if you are counting on significant improvement by the earliest part of the time range.

Erectile dysfunction, likely the most feared complication of treatment, can occur from any combination of the following: aging, the cancer itself, surgery, radiation, or hormonal therapy. After treatment, if erectile dysfunction is prolonged, men begin to wonder WHEN or IF they will be able to have sex again. Some men leak urine during intercourse after prostatectomy, while others have blood in their ejaculates after radiation therapy. These known biological complications can be unnerving. Neither of these developments is harmful to you or your partner; urine is sterile. However, these changes can feel embarrassing, awkward, bizarre, dirty, or tainted. They may loom large in your fears, though perhaps not a major concern for your partner. These situations are best dealt with openly with your partner. Regarding urine leakage, voiding before sexual activity can minimize the symptom.

Doctors and patients can mean different things while using the same words. For instance, "having erections again" may be understood as having a rigid penis that is just as hard as it was before treatment. On the other hand, urologists and radiation oncologists may mean "an erection that is sufficient for penetration." This can feel quite different from your pretreatment erection, and take more stimulation to keep erect. A less than rigid erection often leads to frustration and embarrassment for men. So it makes sense to clarify what your doctor means by "having erections again."

One theme that is not different from pre–prostate cancer erections and sex is that if you think or worry about the quality of your erection too much, there is a greater likelihood of earlier fading or no erection at all. This is similar to performance anxiety, where worry feeds back on itself to worsen functioning, which then heightens anxiety even more. A crude analogy is "the watched pot that doesn't boil." With time and practice, the natural inclination to focus only on the quality of your erections will fade, giving yourself the best shot at having the best-quality erections and the most pleasurable intimacy you can achieve.

When erectile functioning is threatened by prostate cancer, most men focus on missing intercourse. The adage "It's not whether you win or lose; it's how you play the game" does not apply to them. It's "erection or nothing"; "intercourse or nothing"; "ejaculate or nothing." Review the "all or nothing" thought trap in Chapter 4 and see how that can spiral into more worries and aggravation. However, it does not need to put your life or relationship completely on hold while waiting for some bodily function to normalize. Though orgasms are possible after prostatectomy, they are dry orgasms without ejaculate. For many couples, ejaculate is part of the sexual turn-on and intimacy of having sex, and another loss to be grieved for. Most agree that orgasm now feels different, less powerful. The ability to masturbate, often a pleasurable, relaxing endeavor for men, can be compromised after treatment as well.

Discussions They Don't Cover in Sex Education

Can there be intimacy without sex? How about intimacy without intercourse?

What does rigidity that is "hard enough for penetration" really mean?

Can you prepare for sex with medications/injections and not ruin the romance?

Is this the last time I'll be able to have intercourse?

Are there different sex positions to make sex easier after prostate cancer?

Ultimately, adjustment and adaptation lead to accepting a sexual "new normal" or new baseline. It can happen for sexual complications, just as for other changes you have to adjust to after your cancer treatment. Most men resist resetting goals and expectations. They like familiarity and shun uncertainty. If expected goals are not attained, men feel failure. Many men would like to reboot their body computer to deliver them back to their initial settings. There are new "bugs" in the system. However, if the hardware cannot be upgraded, the software may need to be reconfigured. Computer-savvy people speak of "workarounds"—how to get similar results by taking a different route. It may take longer, it may not be as scenic, and it may not be as efficient or pleasurable. But you and your partner will be much more content trying workarounds instead of groaning about the lost paradise of sex you had prior to prostate cancer. Otherwise, you risk getting stuck here, leading to a new, often silent calamity of a "couple's cancer": intimacy lost.

These workarounds will be the focus this chapter. To the question, "If all was good before, why would I settle for something less?" the brief, yet initially unsatisfying answer is, because it is better than not looking for a satisfying "new normal" and risking losing intimacy as your life continues along. With intimacy, something is a lot better than nothing; unfortunately, too many couples wind up living with close to nothing.

Your relationship does not have to suffer if you cannot get erections hard enough for intercourse. But it is not easy to change a lifetime of reinforcement and male socialization that intercourse is the "be all and end all" of sex. Statements men use to describe themselves with erectile problems after prostate cancer treatment include "failure," "poor performer," "so different from before," "not a man anymore," and "wimp." This feels even truer if your sex life was active, enjoyable, and rewarding before cancer. There is a special connection with another person that is often portrayed as "magical," "unique," "sublime," "fantastic," "divine," "spiritual," or "indescribable." Men feel a lot of shame and embarrassment about ED, even though their prostate cancer treatment was medically justified and perhaps life-saving. Communication about sexual issues is not simple even when there are no medical or erectile problems. It is not uncommon for supportive spouses and partners to inadvertently conspire with their partners not to discuss sex or to try alternatives, hoping to avoid pressuring their partner or making him feel challenged.

Attitude Adjustments

There are many ways of approaching and coping with changes in sexual functioning. Your spouse or partner may have different ways of coping with these changes that may be at odds with your attempts. On the other hand, many can be helpful:

> The night before my husband had his prostate surgery, we had "good-bye sex"; we laughed about a "goodbye fuck," said a wife romantically as she thought about her husband of 40 years. We knew this could be the last time we would have "natural" intercourse. We had enjoyed sex for so many years that it felt appropriate to have a ritual goodbye. As it turns out, my husband needs an injection in order for us to have intercourse now. We make playful jokes about it, as we are waiting for the medicine to take effect and watch the erection develop, but I know it hurts him emotionally.

This spouse had the ability to accept the changes and losses that she and her husband were dealt, yet was also able to welcome a new level of functioning. She understood and expressed the emotional aspects of what she was facing, but did not let them paralyze her.

Leslie Schover, a psychologist at MD Anderson Cancer Center, found that using the Masters and Johnson approach of sensate focus helped many couples find a new baseline in pleasurable and sensual activities after cancer treatment. Its implementation in the world of prostate cancer is highlighted in a booklet prepared by the American Cancer Society: *Sexual Functioning for the Man Who Has Cancer and His Partner*. Dr. Schover's book, *Sexuality and Fertility after Cancer*, suggests many coping techniques regarding sex after cancer and treatment. Sexual behavior adjustments require a major paradigm shift in men's thought processes. The objective of sensate focus therapy is to take the pressure off of the step-wise, goal-oriented, and performance-focused past, caricatured as, get interested, get excited, get hard, have a little foreplay, have intercourse, have an orgasm, (repeat if desired—since this book is about cancer, no lighting up of cigarettes recommended). Though oral or manual stimulation, ultimately to orgasm, is okay, in that scenario it is likely not the chief objective. Sensate focus therapy encourages reconnecting with your wife or partner, initially with non-erotic physical touching and, over time, with erotic play or fun, short of intercourse.

Often, both men and women become so fixated on what is not going right sexually that they lose sight of opportunities for pleasurable, romantic moments and for physical and emotional enjoyment. Too much focus is placed on physical factors, such as quality of an erection, the estimated time until orgasm, and the vigor and length of an orgasm, and not enough on the degree of lubrication or discomfort, or whether a partner is satisfied sufficiently. Sensate focus therapy takes the microscope off of the intercourse component of sex and shifts it to the overriding physical and emotional nature of an intimate connection. Couples are instructed to get to know each other's bodies in an affectionate, loving, physically close fashion. This was not likely your cup of tea or primary urge when you were younger, more impulsive, and maybe just looking to get laid. But these modifications are essential for aging adults and couples in whom sexual response times may be slowed or dormant. The idea of non-erotic foreplay, which does not presume an orgasmic, or even sexual, outcome, is at the heart of sensate focus. Sounds dull and non-passionate? Exactly. However, this may be the route to eventual satisfying intimacy and sexual relations. Discuss this plan with your partner beforehand. If she or he knows the goal is not about erections or orgasm but just intimacy, the plan will get more careful effort from both of you.

Let's Take a Play from the DRAFT with EJ Playbook

If I cannot get a good erection it makes no sense to get physically intimate with my partner—we'll both be frustrated.
  Intimacy without intercourse? Really?

Detect the frustration and the all-or-none thoughts that go from "no erections" to "no intimacy."

Recognize that the thoughts are reflective of having to cope with changes you didn't ask for, although certainly, neither did your wife or partner. Intimacy without intercourse will be new for both of you, which means there will be a learning curve and there will be a need for patience. You may be thinking that the "awkwardness of making love" is for young people.

Acknowledge that your thoughts and emotions have some basis of truth and reality to them, yet also are magnified to the point of worsening the suffering you and your partner might go through by pushing you further apart. Acknowledge that you are also assuming that your partner feels the same way—that you'll both be frustrated if you try to be intimate without intercourse.

Flip the situation by taking a deep breath and recognizing the bind you are in. Damned if you do and damned if you don't.

If we don't stay close in physical ways, we might move apart emotionally as well—that can't be good or fun. I can't let the cancer screw my life up *even more than it has. There are a lot of ways we can stay close. Maybe if this sensate focus stuff works, we really can try those penile injections which I've been dreading. I want to figure out how to spend time together.*

Transformation: tell your partner you'd like to go out on a date.

When we get back, I'll light a candle and put on that piano music we both like, just like we used to do. But, let's just keep it light for now. Just some hugging, and maybe give each other neck and foot massages . . . like Dr. Roth mentioned about that sensate focus stuff.

That's right; start out by having a date. Yes, call it a "date" even if it's the same as "just like we've been going out to the movies or dinner for the last 25 years." Go out for dinner (no double dates with couple friends are suggested for this date). You can add a movie or concert or play if you both want, and if you don't think you will be too tired when you get home. Have a glass of wine at dinner if you're allowed medically and if it won't cause you to fall asleep. Too much alcohol will cause dullness and get in the way of sexual arousal (and erectile functioning) when the time comes.

An important guideline in the initial stage of sensate focus is NO GENITALIA TOUCHING. So, when you get back from your date, light the candle and put on the music. Try a foot massage, neck massage, or head massage. The idea is to get to know your partner's body (again) without sexualizing the moments. Use massage oils or aromatic candles. It's okay to kiss, but that's it! You're only allowed to get to "first base" in tonight's game. This is a great exercise, regardless of how long you've been together. These intimate, non-goal-directed behaviors are more natural for women. But try it. Try it for a few dates. Try it for a closer connection with your partner. Try it, with a goal of trying to enrich your relationship.

The second phase of sensate focus allows touching of genitalia, but also from a "getting to know you again" perspective. In the baseball/ dating analogy, you're allowed to get to "second base." Orgasms are not allowed. Performance and outcome are not to be measured or analyzed.

There is no grading system—not good/bad; not A, B, C, D or F; not success/failure. There are no strikes or outs. There are no penalty flags during or after the play (unless you start going for orgasm and quit in frustration). The process and practice outweigh any product. These sexual, yet non-orgasmic, encounters will lead to more romantic emotions, not to mention more caring and support. This is a nice blend of intimacy and sexuality—you can call it intima-sex.

The last phase of sensate focus allows for orgasm, while using the romantic and intimate skills you've developed in the last stages. Yes, this is "getting to third base" or even "a home run" when you were younger. If you are not able to get an erection easily, remember that getting to third base for you might be a home run for your partner. It is helpful to have already prepared for any pre-erection medications. See the section on when and how to take an erectile-stimulating medication later in this chapter. You have to take the medication at least an hour before trying to have sex, and you can't have eaten right before taking it. You should avoid alcohol and fatty meals to allow better medication absorption. Let your partner know if you are going to use a penile injection so you can do it before you are too engaged in the romance; maybe you can both be creative and figure out how to make it part of the romance. Without sensate focus, you may have found no reason to play the intimacy game at all. Don't rush it. Take breaks if you need to. Communicate about your needs and wants, and listen to your partner's as well.

Find Physical Intimacy and Pleasure in Sex Again

Part One

Set up a time to go on a date—don't wait for the right moment. When you are back at home:

Put on some music; light an aromatic candle.

Take a bath or shower together.

No genitalia touching, no orgasms allowed.

Give each other head, neck, back, or foot massages.
Hold hands.
Yes, that's all!

Part Two

Go on a date—It's OK to hold hands and act like you really are on a date.
If you will be using an erectile aid medication later:
No fatty foods with dinner.
No food an hour or so before taking the medication.
A glass of wine is fine, but not more.
Take the pill at least an hour before intimacy.
When you are back at home:
Watch a movie together (sometimes movies with sexually oriented content help arousal).
If you are using a penile injection, decide on a time before massaging and kissing.
Put on some music; light an aromatic candle.
Touching genitalia is allowed. Orgasm is not!
Take a bath or shower together.
Massage, kiss, and caress.

Part Three

Go on a date.
Take the erectile medication or penile injection as directed before physical intimacy starts.
Use the same lead-in steps as above.
See this as a process of intimacy rather than a goal of intercourse or orgasm.
Touching genitalia is OK. See what feels comfortable. Have patience.
If frustration starts to build because there is no erection, focus on your partner.
It is not selfless to help your partner reach orgasm. Your relationship endures.

As couples age, women have natural or medically related physiological changes that can interfere with more pleasurable sex. Sexual arousal may be slower or occur in different ways than when they are younger. Insufficient vaginal lubrication can lead to more painful intercourse. Using lubricants help. Her doctor or gynecologist can recommend lubricants that are safe and effective. It may take different types of stimulation, or there may be changes in how long it takes her to reach orgasm. Have patience. In the short and long run, it will be worth it for both of you.

Gay couples also benefit from exploring alternative, pleasurable sexual and intimacy satisfaction. They can learn how to enhance intimacy with the new conditions presented by prostate cancer. *A Gay Man's Guide to Prostate Cancer*, edited by Gerald Perlman and Jack Drescher, discusses coping with complications of prostate cancer treatment, including sexuality, from the particular perspective of gay men. The book illuminates the effects of prostate cancer on long-term relationships, dating, and intimacy. The importance of good communication between partners is germane to both gay and heterosexual couples, though the subject matter and methods may vary. The stigma of discussing these concerns with an oncologist or oncology nurse may feel even greater for gay men, with concerns of medical caregiver prejudice, indifference, or lack of knowledge. The effects of weaker-than-baseline erections, the loss of the prostate, and a loss of ejaculate can have a significant impact on the ability to enjoy sex as usual or derive satisfactory pleasure as in the past. Physical changes can lead gay men to avoid sex and intimacy if they and/or their partners are not willing or able to make adjustments.

Experimenting with different positions during sex may also be helpful. Though it may be difficult to believe, there really is a more satisfactory sex life available if you can accept differences from life before the cancer and be flexible and patient. There are many self-help books available that can be excellent references for how to deal with the physiological effects of prostate cancer, including the sexual side effects.

Sex therapy with a counselor who is aware of the nuances of prostate cancer can help you cope with the feelings brought on by this problem, and also help a couple learn alternative ways of sharing sexual and physical intimacy and finding pleasure. A golfer whose power and distance may be compromised can maintain his game by improving accuracy—sometimes with straightening his shots or working on his slices, fades, or hooks. Sometimes he'll focus on his short game approaches to the green. My Uncle Ben became legally blind in his 70s, yet had enviable golf scores (with a generous handicap) by hitting balls as straight as an arrow—as long as he got help locating the ball and the direction to the flag. Consultation for a spouse with a gynecologist who specializes in female sexual dysfunction can be helpful if she has natural, physiological, or medical changes of aging that interfere with pleasurable intercourse, such as decreased vaginal lubrication. Together, a couple can learn how to maintain intimacy in their relationship, even when the physicality of their closeness has changed.

Penile Rehabilitation: Restoration and Reintegration of Erections after Prostate Cancer

Penile rehabilitation is not a program for sex predators. It is a relatively new urological specialty recommended by many urologists, medical oncologists, and radiation oncologists to their patients. John Mulhall, a urologist at Memorial Sloan Kettering Cancer Center who specializes in male erectile problems, has reported that a penile rehabilitation program helps more men achieve better erections after prostate cancer treatment. In addition to focusing on the physiological issues of erectile dysfunction, Dr. Mulhall's program has a psychologist, Dr. Christian Nelson, who specializes in sexual therapy for men that includes emotionally supportive techniques to overcome the physiological and psychological barriers for both the man and his partner. Dr. Nelson has done groundbreaking work to help men improve sexuality after prostate cancer. He developed and is studying the benefits of a particular type of acceptance and commitment therapy, a program to improve men's use of injection therapy to improve sexual satisfaction after prostatectomy.

Recommendations are to start erection-enhancing medications prior to, during, or soon after radiation therapy or prostatectomy, to more rapidly bring about better erections after treatment than if there were no intervention. Phosphodiesterase type 5 (PDE-5) inhibitors (i.e., tadalafil, sildenafil vardenafil) are the erectile medications recommended. As of this writing, there are better data supporting these findings in animal models than in humans. Penile rehabilitation programs propose that the sooner treatment is started, the less permanent damage will develop from venous leakage development. If there is no response to the PDE-5 inhibitors, urologists recommend penile injections to keep the tissues viable. Age at the time of treatment and pre-treatment functioning likely play a role in the success of the program. Early on, low doses of the medication, insufficient to cause an erection, are recommended. Higher doses of the medication are suggested inter-mittently, which could conceivably bring about an erection. Even nerves "spared" during prostatectomies can take many months to heal, some-times up to 2 years or longer after surgery. While healing, these nerves may not secrete sufficient amounts of a chemical called nitric oxide, dis-abling the mechanism of action of the oral erectogenic medications like sildenafil, tadalafil, and vardenafil.

Some men try the PDE-5 inhibitor medications soon after treatment, but discontinue them prematurely because they don't get adequate erections. Because the nerves are still healing and not producing the nitric oxide, these medications cannot produce erections yet. Other men may not be taught how to use these medications correctly or at sufficient dosages. For instance, sildenafil is best taken on an empty stomach a couple of hours before one is planning on having sex. Patients are not always told that it is best to take these medications on an empty stomach and not with a fatty meal, which reduces absorption, or not with alcohol, which can also inhibit erectile activity. Tadalafil has a very long half-life and can therefore maintain its effectiveness for up to 36 hours. It may help relieve the awkwardness of breaking up the romantic moment by not having to take a pill right before sex and then have to wait for some action. It is important to note that these medicines require manual penile or psychosexual stimulation in order to work.

The adage "If you don't use it, you'll lose it" appears to be true here. Men who use prophylactic penile injection therapy immediately following radical prostatectomy may be more likely to have a return of spontane-ous erections at 6 months after surgery than those who do not use the low-dose daily "vitamin." Men who have had a successful nerve-sparing prostatectomy and don't use the medication regularly or give up using it or penile injections too soon after surgery may unknowingly short-change themselves. Trying the medication again after more healing can take place may lead to better success. Continual use of the medicines in low doses may lead to earlier return of erections. Ultimately, the nerves and blood vessels need to be healed and healthy for the pills to work.

What If You Weren't Told to Rehab or It Doesn't Produce Adequate Natural Erections?

If you think your ED is going on too long, don't be ashamed to ask your urologist about what's causing the problem and whether anything can be done to remedy the issue. When erectile problems have been identified, and the PDE-5 inhibitor medications are not working well enough, there are a number of mechanical means of achieving erections that can be tried. However, most men are not comfortable even hearing about a less natural or just-swallow-a-pill method—penile injections, vacutainers, penile suppositories, or penile prostheses—let alone trying one. These alternative routes to erections are reviewed in this chapter. Knowing something about the pros and cons of these different approaches, rather than dismissing them out of hand, makes sense. Discussing these options with your partner and whether any might be beneficial for your sexual lives takes initiative and courage. A supportive spouse or partner who understands and accepts interruptions in "the romantic moment" or changes from the old familiar routines to new comfortable intimate activities is to be valued and appreciated, and not taken for granted.

"You Want Me to Stick a Needle Down There?"

Penile injections are one of the most reliable ways to achieve an erection after treatment for prostate cancer. Medications such as alprostadil, or a mixture of papavarine, phentolamine, and alprostadil, which dilate blood vessels in the penis, are used for these injections. If you ask men without prostate cancer what they think about sticking a needle into their penis for a better erection, most would wince and say "uch" or "ouch" and then refuse the treatment. Well, it is no different after getting treated for prostate cancer. It feels barbaric and deviant to most men. It will hurt somewhat; the injection is usually described as being similar to a mosquito bite, but it is in a place that most men associate with pleasure and manhood, and not mosquito bites. Those men and couples willing to try this can improve their sexual connections and pleasure.

Another drawback to injections is that they take work and preparation, and can get in the way of or are not conducive to a romantic moment. Taking the time and effort to give an injection can feel less like an interruption if the couple works the mechanical aide into their romantic routine, much the same way other couples allow for placement of birth control devices such as diaphragms or condoms.

Penile injection therapy is not free of problems. Multiple injections in the same site over a long period of time can lead to fibrosis or scarring, which can cause discomfort or a malformation or curvature of the penis, referred to as Peyronie's disease. Thus men are instructed to rotate the injection sites. Regardless, this curvature occurs in a small percentage of men after a prostatectomy.

Injections are not likely to work for men who have an internal venous leak after surgery; escape of blood weakens the ability to keep a penis erect.

The Pump

Some men prefer to use a *vacutainer,* or *penile pump*, to avoid an injection. The pump promotes an erection by pumping air out of a cylinder that is placed around the penis. The vacuum created draws blood into the penis shaft, causing it to swell and become erect. A retaining band is then placed at the base of the penis to keep it erect, so blood does not flow out again after being pumped in.

This device feels cumbersome to many men. The resulting erections are rigid but may not look or feel normal; the rigidity may decrease over time. Again, with a supportive partner and inclusion into the intimate routine, the pump can be seen as the aid that it is: not natural and less romantic, but necessary and sufficient to allow a sexually intimate liaison to occur.

Suppositories

Erectile suppositories fit inside the opening of the penis to allow delivery of a medication similar to the injection that causes dilation of the penile blood vessels and, ultimately, erections. The suppository eliminates the need for painful injections or large mechanical devices; however, the medicine itself can cause burning and pain. There are inconsistent results and, like the other mechanical methods, can significantly interfere with the passionate moment. After insertion of the suppository, the penis needs to be massaged while standing until an erection develops. Sometimes, men lose the erection when they lie down.

Penile Implants

Because these methods have to be used each time you want to have sex, some men opt for a penile implant or prosthesis. Prostheses will quickly lead to an erection with either a quick unfolding or a pumping action. With an implant or prosthesis, the decision to have assistance with attaining an erection is made only once, before insertion of the erectile device. Implants require a separate surgical procedure unless placed during the initial prostatectomy. Ask your urologist about the benefits and complications of prosthetic options.

Erections, and ultimate intercourse with implants, do not always feel the same to a man or his partner as before prostate cancer treatment. And without ejaculation, the whole process may feel very different to a man and his partner. Hopefully, though, intimacy and sexual renewal fall into the "good enough" category to facilitate sexual or romantic intimacy. Some men with implants complain that they can have penetration for extended periods of time (something they may have wished for before prostate cancer); however, they are frustrated by less than a satisfactory release.

Erectile Assists

PDE-5 inhibitors: sildenafil, tadalafil, vardenafil. Following correct instructions is important.

Penile suppositories

Penile injections: alprostadil, or a mixture of papavarine, phentolamine, and alprostadil

Penile implants:

Flip-up—need to adapt to having a constant erection

Inflatable—two- or three-piece options

Can You Get Some Satisfaction?

As noted earlier, sexual satisfaction after prostate cancer treatment is in the eye of the beholder; it does not necessarily mean achieving the same erection you had when you were a teen or in your twenties or thirties. "Success" may be an erection firm enough for penetration to allow for intercourse or masturbation. In fact, many men can achieve orgasm even without attaining an erection and feel some satisfaction. But for all-or-none thinkers, or those who are stuck comparing the present with the past, it is difficult to accept a new baseline, or new normal, and some gratification.

I want to emphasize the importance of a supportive, understanding partner who can facilitate all of these sexual and intimacy enhancement methods. Unfortunately, for a number of reasons, this is not easily accomplished, even when it comes to people who have been in long-term marriages and relationships. "Long term" is not necessarily synonymous with "supportive and understanding"; and sexual differences, conflicts, and tension can exist in supportive and understanding relationships as well. Couples counseling can improve the ability of a couple to cope with and communicate better together about many intimate issues brought up by the cancer.

Not for Couples Only

Imagine how much more challenging it might be for a man with a new erectile condition who is not already in a committed relationship. The next section is addressed to those men who are not currently married or partnered and who've been happy to have flexibility and variability in dating and sexual practices. It is also for those who are without a partner because of marital separation, divorce, or widowhood, and who are thinking about dating. It will deal with a wide variety of dating challenges.

The Singles Scene and Dating

Many single men avoid dating altogether after prostate cancer treatment. They get stuck in the same "all or none" and catastrophic thinking as some men do about injections. Many never had to develop an elaborate language (verbal or physical) for relationship intimacy that did not involve reflex-excitement sexual intercourse and orgasm. Sexual and relationship issues are complicated for men with prostate cancer who do not have regular companions. They wonder if, how, or when they should bring up the issue of their cancer or sexual difficulties when they go on a date. Some men avoid dating altogether after their cancer treatment. Psychotherapy, and support groups in particular, to address these issues and perhaps to rehearse different scenarios and scripts may help alleviate some of the anxiety and fears these men have.

Was Dating Always This Complicated?

Kiss and Tell? Or Tell and Kiss?

Do I tell her/him that I have prostate cancer or that I had treatment for prostate cancer?

When do I tell?

How will I know when to take my medication for an erection?

When do I mention that I can't easily get an erection, or that I need to use a needle or some other device to get hard?

I never had to discuss this stuff, and I don't want to start now. Who wants to date a guy like me? No more dating for me!

If I tell a man, "If the relationship feels right enough to have sex, then that person will understand and be supportive about the erectile issues," my statement is usually met with raised eyebrows, disbelief, and often an irritated response. They either wonder when was the last time I went out on a date or which naïve planet I grew up on—the world of some 1950s or 1960s perfect family TV show? (Disclaimer: I did grow up in that era, and I think there are aspects of that reality that are achievable even today.) Finding a happy medium between a celibate, platonic relationship and sexually fulfilling bliss is not easy if a man does not care much about romantic intimacy and his interest in relationships have been characterized more by having "good sex" or "getting laid." Erections on demand, with minimal visual, verbal, or physical stimulation, may be gone. Some or all aspects of carefree "natural" sex may be lost and grieved for. With or without the erectile assist medications, longer penile stimulation may be required to achieve the firmness needed for penetration or for orgasm.

Support groups attended by other men going through similar experiences can provide safety to discuss these issues, normalize an uncomfortable situation, hear what has worked for others and, perhaps just as importantly, what has not worked, and hopefully provide relief of stress. For all the reasons men can benefit from talking with others, many don't want to. It is uncomfortable; they don't want to compare themselves to others when they know they can be on the *down* side; it can be embarrassing not just to talk about erectile problems but to also discuss one's private sexual interests. It's a club no one wants to be a part of. But for many men, exploring and giving voice to frustration, loneliness, anger, a lost sense of omnipotence, confused male identity and body image, sadness, concerns about commitment and rejection, and the task of experimenting with new routines can be validating, relieving, and helpful in figuring out how to move on. Acceptance and transitioning forward along a new and unplanned-for trajectory may require guidance, support, and encouragement to keep trying, even in the face of unsuccessful attempts.

The New "Petit Mort" (the New Little Death)

The French term *le petit mort* often refers to having an orgasm and the feeling of bliss one feels afterward. Some use the term metaphorically to describe the sense of spiritual transformation after any extraordinary experience. A number of men literally equate their sex lives with life itself. "Doc, it really is not worth living anymore if I cannot do what has given me the most satisfaction in my life. You wouldn't believe how many people I dated and had sex with." This can sound harsh and shallow to some, but it is what gives this man and the partners he's been with meaning and mutual pleasure.

Death and loss go hand in hand. We will discuss loss and grief in more detail in Chapter 10. However, on some level, loss and grief are experienced throughout your prostate cancer experience, and perhaps in no more stark fashion than with sexuality. The death of someone we love is one of the deepest injuries humans can suffer and among the toughest wounds to heal. A large part of psychotherapy with men who have prostate cancer is devoted to coping with loss. A paradigm shift or mindset flip of a different yet acceptable life after loss is explored and encouraged, as well as how to reach and land safely on that new plateau. The loss, as well as reactions to and ramifications of loss, has to be detected, recognized, and acknowledged, and then worked through. Psychotherapy in general often helps people deal with the various losses in their lives—the tangible and intangible mishaps, hurts, and casualties—that they experience in school, jobs, careers, relationships, and health. The slights and perceived slights, the unattained goals and hopes, dashed expectations, and even the envy we have for what others have or what they have not lost, can be understood and often flipped and transformed satisfactorily.

But acceptance of today's reality may only come about when you've mourned for what you've lost. Grieving may be needed in order to conceive of a new potential and suitable reality to fill the emotional, physical, and cognitive void of what was lost. This is different than trying to replace what was lost. There are no logical arguments to convince a man that life could ever be as good or that some meaningful replacement is possible for sexual intercourse when he has taken considerable pleasure in a particular lifestyle and sexual style. What was so fundamental and satisfying previously, and the emotions of anger and frustration that grow in their absence, may have to be explored or addressed before he can see that there are indeed other roads open to him. The potential of new roads may not feel sufficient, especially when viewed from a vista that is looking backward. But they may be necessary in order to find satisfaction again. Don't be held back from some pleasure in the present and future because it does not meet your expectations from the past. These paths can reach a "good enough" level of contentment to keep life interesting and purposeful and, therefore, worth living.

C'mon doc; do you think any woman can see me as a man and can feel satisfied, if I can't get an EOD (erection on demand)?

This is when we are likely to talk about the book *Men Are from Mars and Women Are from Venus*, by Dr. John Gray. Time and time again I have seen that the answer to this question (which seems beforehand a rhetorical, categorical, and self-evident "No" to the man) is a "Yes!" Menopausal or postmenopausal women may indeed be looking for a break from the intercourse = intimacy equation that men grow up with. They do enjoy other types of physical closeness and affection. They do enjoy caressing and endearing conversation. They do feel secure and satisfied, understanding that intimacy is not just about getting erections, having intercourse, and coming. That's a maturation milestone. One virile patient told me he looked forward to his libido catching up (or down) with his poor erections, and living out the rest of his life unconcerned with sex.

If there is hesitation in making these changes, and the thought-changing and behavior-changing methods of the DRAFT with Emotional Judo (EJ) Playbook are not working sufficiently, it's time to figure out what is getting in the way of thinking about and making these changes with a professional therapist. Insights into how your unique patterns of relationships, attitudes, and behaviors developed over the course of your life, and what distinctive reactions you have about the inability to get an erection, or ultimately to dying, may be vital to overcoming the struggle to move forward with major attitude and behavioral changes that will allow you to experience satisfying relationships and an improved life. Are there old grievances you still carry with you? What needs were satisfied in your sexual life? What was unfulfilled? What left your partner(s) feeling distanced?

Researchers (Prochaska et al., 2007) have identified five stages most people go through when trying to make difficult habitual or behavioral changes, such as addictive behaviors like smoking, drinking alcohol, or gambling, or even when spending too much time surfing the Internet. These stages are probably true for ordinary habits that are just difficult to modify, like exercise or diet. Putting in effort to modify how you think about and behave around sex does not mean that you were addicted; however, your thoughts, behaviors, cues, and associations can be so ingrained and reinforced over so many years that they can be as difficult to change as an addictive behavior—not to mention the hormonal and other genetic influences that go into sexual thoughts and behaviors. So I think the analogy can be helpful here as well.

The first phase of change is *pre-contemplation*. At this point, people are not even thinking about changing the behavior—for instance, avoiding physical intimacy with your partner because you can't get an erection, or refusing to use a penile injection in order to achieve an erection. A non-tangible behavior (avoidance) can be more difficult to challenge than an active, purposeful one, like pulling out a cigarette and lighting it up or pouring a drink and downing it. You may be aware of the behavior and possibly some of its downsides, but you are not even considering a need to change it, perhaps you are not even sure what it would take to change it. Perhaps by now, your partner has assured you that less or no intimacy is fine, so neither of you really feels pressured to make a change.

The second stage, called *contemplation*, is motivated by wanting, or seeing, a need to change something, at least some of the time. Maybe others point it out to you. Maybe you experience it by feeling socially isolated, or increasingly irritable or lonely even if you are not alone. If you see no problems or consequences from the thoughts or behavior, why change? What might be a problem for your partner may not be viewed as a problem for you, or vice versa. You may ultimately suffer if your relationship suffers, but you may never see the link. But when you start to sense the potential benefits of change, you will think about it more. You may even go back and forth about the potential pros and cons of making a change and about what it may take to change that behavior.

You haven't done anything appreciable yet to change your thinking or behavior, but you may have gotten over the biggest hurdle.

A therapist joke that you may have heard is appropriate here:

Question: How many therapists does it take to change a light bulb?
Answer: One. But the light bulb has to want to change.

But without awareness, there is usually no desire for change.

The third phase of change is *preparation*. You make a plan to change the behavior. If you are single, you might think about going on a date with someone and letting friends know you're ready to date again. You'll start to think about how to deal with the sexuality questions in case they arise. If you have a partner, you might discuss setting up a time to give each other a massage and choose a definite time to begin. If it's left hazy, it is much less likely to happen, just as we discussed in starting to exercise. Alternatively, you and your partner might discuss using a medication or some other aid to help with erections, and how to create a romantic environment while the medication is taking effect, such as listening to music or watching a movie. Maybe the discussion revolves around the need to get professional help from a sex or couples therapist.

The next stage is taking *action*. It is time to put your new, innovative thoughts, words, and plan into practice to replace the unproductive, less satisfying, or destructive ones you've been stuck with. Set a time to begin. Try out the new behavior. Rehearse your new set of attitudes or behaviors. If you're single, set up a date to go to the movies or dinner with someone you'd like to get to know better. Ask friends for thoughts on potential date companions. Your action might be getting into therapy or a self-help group. It could take months of trying to own the new behavior until it feels like it is working and an acceptable "new normal" is achieved. For those of you in committed relationships, go on a date with your partner and plan to spend time together. Rent a room in a nice hotel for a weekend getaway or make time in your own bedroom with a lit candle and music playing. Get some aromatic massage oil and give each other neck, back, and/or foot massages. Again, get your partner on board first. It will be better to talk this over before you start, and then fine-tune your strategy once you get started. In particular, seriously consider the goals of sensate focus to de-eroticize the date, but don't sacrifice physical closeness.

The fifth and last stage is *reinforcing and maintaining* the new behavior—keep going, keep juggling, keep innovating, keep tweaking, and keep discussing with your partner. Make the time and effort to deal with any disappointments or frustrations that arise. Persevere and keep trying. Take note of the frustrations, roadblocks, and resentments. But also be aware of the small successes and pleasures. If there is relapse to the old behaviors (avoidance) or there are disappointments, try, try again. That means if the changed behavior or attitude doesn't work out as hoped, or doesn't feel so comfortable, keep trying, or put your innovation hat on and consider a different approach.

Changing Sexual and Intimacy Attitudes and Behaviors
Does Not Happen Overnight

Pre-contemplation: If there is a problem, you don't recognize it or the need for change

Contemplation: Awareness of the challenge and thinking about taking action to change

Preparation: Making a plan or plans with your partner to carry out changes

Action: Following through on the plan and tweaking as needed

Reinforce and maintain: Keep tweaking and innovating. Be mindful of success.

This is a great opportunity to use the DRAFT with Emotional Judo (EJ) strategies learned in Chapter 4 if you feel bombarded by pessimistic thoughts, inaction, or hopeless or angry feelings. EJ can help you deflect the thoughts of being "less than a man" or having feelings of failure, and recognize what most partners are looking for—emotional closeness and intimacy. One single man initially told me he was never "into commitment" and he didn't care about "just talking" or "too many sweet nothings whispered without fucking." Eventually he talked about loneliness and the discomfort of not having someone else to count on, even though he wasn't sure he wanted to be the person someone else might hope to lean on for ongoing support. With all the sex he had had in his life, he was actually very much a loner. He eventually started dating, and enjoyed making less erotic, yet more fulfilling, connections. He accepted a new phase and enjoyed it without looking over his shoulder into his past very often. His EJ Playbook consisted of **D**etecting, **R**ecognizing, and **A**cknowledging his anger and grief at the good and the bad of what was lost, and the real and irrational fears of isolation and commitment as he got older. He was able to **F**lip the remorse of loss of his old male identity, which was always dressed in sexuality to a more fulfilling and intimate here and now, and **T**ransform himself into a new and more content male identity.

Another man said,

> I tried the sensate focus but felt embarrassed and like a failure. I wanted to perform well, feel normal, and got pissed off at myself. It didn't feel believable when my wife said, "The erection doesn't matter—I'm just glad you're with me and holding me and kissing me." I thought she couldn't really believe that. I know how much fun it was to have intercourse, and how much she used to enjoy it. So I got pissed off at her. Then I thought to myself that the angry guy was the old me; we had been having a good time until I started getting stuck on the erection. I took a little time out and a few breaths. I asked her to repeat what she said again, and really heard it without editorializing it. We actually wound up having a lot of fun. Yes, it was different, but it was still good. I'm glad I didn't throw away this opportunity to be closer.

It can be easier to hold onto understandable anger or sadness, accepting the pity of others and rationalizing your own self-pity and anger about how much you have been wronged by this illness, than to let those emotions go. I have treated a number of men whose prostate cancer diagnosis came within a few years of a second marriage ceremony. These men had either divorced or were widowed before their cancer diagnosis, but were able to find another partner. Meeting another mate was easy for some and more difficult for others. But disclosing information about a new cancer with possible sexual problems related to treatment can feel unfair. For a divorcee, it might have been tough enough explaining what went wrong in the previous marriage. For a widower, it could have been difficult to let go of the romantic memories of a deceased wife or partner. There may be pressure from well-meaning friends or family—even your adult children—who encourage you to get into a new relationship and move on with your life. There may be others who discourage this, describing new romances as a betrayal of your dead partner. When you declare your new prostate cancer diagnosis, there may be subtle or shrewd pressure from your partner's friends or family—even from your partner's adult children—to encourage your partner to get out of the relationship before you get too sick, and move on to yet another new life that does not have cancer in it. Some spouses hear adult children from first marriages say, "What do you need this for? You just took care of Dad until he died, and that depressed you and took a lot out of you." Many are genuinely concerned about their parent, while some may be thinking about their parents' financial legacy. Their recommendations are sometimes for their mothers to cut and run, and to try their luck with yet a third spouse. Of course, these children have an outsider's perspective on the marriage, even if they are speaking with the good intentions of not wanting to see their parent "suffer any more anguish."

You may feel as if the playing field is different now and you don't know what the rules are. There are few, if any, clear and helpful guidelines or instructions. Your new prostate cancer diagnosis can frighten and irritate you. It may feel the same way to your current spouse or partner. This may be especially true if there were difficult health issues (or even cancer) in your current wife's or partner's previous marriage or relationship. If she or he was widowed before, your spouse may be thinking about having to care for yet another partner who may die; and if the sexual relationship in your new marriage has been good or even better than the first, your spouse may feel as if she or he has been cheated yet again. You may both feel undeserved guilt and even wonder if finally finding satisfying sex brought on this sexually oriented cancer.

By the way, sex does not cause prostate cancer, but that doesn't stop your brain from coming up with rationalizations for any unwanted or unpredictable events that pop up in your life. Whatever we may think about selfishness, feelings of self-pity, self-remorse, or commitment to "til death do us part" in marriage vows, there are unquestionably trials and tribulations of prostate cancer, regardless of outcome, that a couple, new or seasoned, is in for. The new couple will also need to grieve for their loss of how good things had been, and the hopes they had for the future they envisioned.

This is one of many opportunities to heed the findings of George Vaillant, a psychiatrist and researcher from Harvard University, who, in his book, *Aging Well*, discovered which people are more likely to grow older successfully. He suggests that one important ingredient for healthier aging was how people viewed and then dealt with adversity in life. Essentially, when life hands you a lemon, make the best of it; make lemonade. Don't just try to wish the problem away or run away from it. It sounds like EJ. Maybe it is just another truism, but it is nice to know that there is scientific backup.

Interestingly, this concept is also an aspect of the Serenity Prayer that has helped so many people with addictions. It is important to recognize what cannot be changed, understanding what can be changed, and to know the difference. Try it. You'll fare far better than those who steadfastly fight to undo what is unchangeable.

Chapter 7

Urinary, Bowel, and Energy Leaks

This Wasn't Supposed to Happen to Me

You have to pitch your way through errors.

Baseball aphorism

Physical complications from prostate cancer treatment go beyond compromised sexual functioning. In fact, urinary or bowel complications or ongoing fatigue can be quite demoralizing, even though they are known and common complications of prostate cancer treatment. They only seem like errors, as in the epigraph, in men's minds because those snags "weren't supposed to happen to me!" But whether common or rare, temporary or long term, anticipated or an error in expectations, these changes are not easy to live with. For some men, urinary and bowel problems were the definite deal breakers when they were choosing primary treatments up front. There are some practical and pharmacological techniques that can ease the course of recuperating from or coping with these all-too-common difficulties, whether or not they are short term for you.

If you develop complications, you want them fixed—now. But this is not just a parts replacement process. It is very hard to have patience when there is no clear timetable for recuperation. For those of you who've never gone through surgery or major medical procedures previously, it may feel like you've entered the twilight zone. It is impossible to see your cells recovering and making all the necessary connections for better health after things have gone awry. Remember to ask your doctor for timetable ranges for recuperation, and then focus on the far end of that range. If recuperation happens sooner, cool. But you won't feel like you are watching what feels like an unmovable clock if you look long term.

I fell into this trap when I was recovering from the surgery to remove my acoustic neuroma. I developed a facial paralysis that I was told would be temporary. In fact, most times these nerve palsies resolve within 3 months. I had to do facial exercises as part of my physical therapy. I practiced these exercises about 75% of the time I was supposed to. Every day I would look in the mirror and observe my droopy face. Though my doctor told me that most people recover within 3 months, I did not hear him also say it can take a year or more for others and sometimes it doesn't fully heal. I didn't hear anything past 3 months. By the 80th day, I knew it would take a miracle to recover in another 10 days. I was almost fully recovered in 6 months. That period between 3 and 6 months was extremely difficult for me emotionally. I was angry with my body for not being as resilient as those belonging to the recovered-by-3-month group. I was angry with my doctor for not predicting exactly what was going to happen to me, for not reading the crystal ball accurately. I was depressed. At times, I had catastrophic thinking, dejectedly believing that my face would never recover. Despite all of my psychiatric training and helping others with similar situations, I had a hard time practicing what I preached. I thought of my patients who practiced Kegel exercises regularly, and some not so regularly, and how hard those exercises must be to do when you do not see quick results. Who would get help from, and be able to continue to look at, a therapist with a droopy face who was half deaf? Now that is catastrophizing!

Penny Wise and Pound Foolish

It is important to be accurate about reporting any symptoms or side effects you are experiencing to your doctor or nurse during follow-up visits after treatment or for ongoing treatment. Doctors usually ask their patients, "How are you doing?" It is incredible how often a man says, "Just fine"; if his spouse or partner is in the exam room, his or her head is shaking from side to side indicating, "no he is not." Why do men do this? Sometimes they feel a desire to try to make their doctors feel better: "The doctor doesn't have much time with me anyway. If I start complaining we could be here a long time and that will really slow down the clinic." Sometimes men are just used to giving this socially accepted response, because "who really wants to hear all of my complaints anyway; and if I start describing how I really feel, I will become even more upset." Some men hesitate to describe how they are really feeling, especially when they are not feeling well. They are afraid of Pandora's Box: they fear that the cancer is back, the treatment they got didn't work, or, even worse, if they haven't yet started their treatment or are in the middle of it, they fear their doctor will say they cannot continue to get the life-saving treatment because they can't tolerate the stress well enough.

Your doctor does not need you to make him or her feel better or to help him or her have an easier or better day. Your doctor should not be angry with you because the treatment won't or did not work as well as everyone hoped or if there are complications. If the doctor gets angry at you, it may be time for you to find another doctor. Sometimes you may hear a doctor say, "You failed the treatment." You cannot fail a treatment. It may not work, but that's not your fault. Men don't feel well for many reasons, often having nothing to do with the cancer or the cancer treatment, yet which may be easily understood and remedied. But if your doctor does not have an accurate picture, it is difficult to come up with a correct solution.

Concerns about quality-of-life issues such as erectile dysfunction, urinary control, and bowel problems after cancer treatment are common and understandable. Unfortunately, if these fluctuating or inconsistent symptoms occur, they become major distractions to your ability to feel good and whole again or to achieve your "new normal." The effort to cope with these challenges zaps energy, which contributes to mental and physical fatigue and leads to uncomfortable and unpredictable moods, anxiety, and irritability. Patients, spouses and partners, and other family members usually cope better if they can discuss how these changes affect everyone's activities. All can be reassured that if seen as a family issue, a team effort of understanding and support eases everyone's sense of suffering. But these discussions are difficult and challenging. They can feel intimidating and guilt inducing.

I have found that acknowledgment of and trying to work through these frustrating, unpleasant, and complicated issues allows for better coping than trying to ignore or wish them away. However, adjustment does not happen quickly or easily for most people, and may not happen at all in families that have communication weaknesses and perhaps ambivalent commitment. It takes time, as well as conscious, persistent effort.

Urinary Incontinence

> I will not go to a party or to the movies if I have to wear diapers or urinary pads. I can smell the urine even if no one else does. I can feel the moisture in my underwear even if I'm not leaking a lot. It makes me sick and embarrassed and angry. Am I a baby? I cannot see living a life like this.

There is understandable fear of urinary leakage or having a smell if there is urinary incontinence; coping with the many manifestations of this complication can be very difficult and challenging. It is reminiscent of the loss of control and random victimization one feels with the prostate cancer itself. Though it took most of us a few years to get our urination under control when we were infants and toddlers, adult men lose patience quickly when trying to recover their urinary control after prostate cancer treatment. It was not then and cannot be now an all-or-none process. To get through this period as an adult, even an accelerated phase of recuperation can feel regressive and embarrassing. Some men were not told clearly enough by their urologists, or do not remember being told, that full urinary recovery and maximum control after definitive prostate cancer treatment can take 6 months to a year or longer. Just as with erectile functioning, if you are like most men, when the urologist said after your prostatectomy your urinary catheter should be out in 1 to 3 weeks, you heard "1 week." If you were told that your urinary function could return to baseline in 6 to 9 months, you may have heard "6 months." And you started watching the clock on how wet or dry urinary pads were 4 or 5 weeks after surgery. After a few months, and sometimes after only a few weeks, men begin to fear the worst outcome and become anxious and disillusioned. Getting to the far range of the forecast is scary and depressing. Accepting that your urination will not get back to normal on its own will take some getting used to.

I have always been impressed by and respectful of those men who take on the challenge of the hand life has dealt them by making accommodations to old habits so they can continue living a fuller life despite losses. They "take the bull by the horns." They adapt and create new routines. They would rather be at a concert, dancing, or at a grandchild's sporting event, prepared for a urinary accident, than sitting at home moping about how unfair life is and missing important events because of older age or physical problems. When men become socially withdrawn and stop doing activities that used to give them pleasure, others see them as depressed. Certainly, they are at risk for depression. Moods and activity levels would soar for most men if their urinary problems could be magically fixed. Mild depression caused by a stressful situation does not usually warrant treatment with an antidepressant medication.

The man who can see his incontinence in the context of life's continuum through aging, illness or treatment, or life's hard knocks, rather than as a flaw of manly invincibility, may be able to accept this drawback with fortitude and be a role model for others. When given a lemon, try to make lemonade.

You can get back on track and live with urinary incontinence. Strategies to decrease the physical aspects of urinary accidents include noninvasive techniques, medications, and surgical intervention. Remember those Kegel exercises the surgeon recommended? Kegel and other behavioral methods like biofeedback techniques can help you achieve better urinary control, though they may take time to learn and fully incorporate into your life. These exercises not only strengthen the pelvic floor muscles, they also help retrain the muscles to learn when to squeeze. Take charge of this symptom, rather than letting it be in charge of you, even if urinary control is not successful yet. Relaxation and behavioral and biofeedback techniques help improve urinary control and manage the psychological, anxiety-related aspects of incontinence. A therapist can help a man handle this twist in life so he doesn't look back years from now feeling even angrier because he was cheated twice—once by the nature of his illness and treatment, and once by his emotions. Or worse, he feels so distraught now that he does not want to get to a point down the road when he looks back.

> I am so worried that I won't be able to regain control over my urine that I don't practice the Kegel exercises my urologist suggested. What if they don't work? What if I'm not doing them correctly? Why did this have to happen to me at all?

This patient was so worried he would never regain control of his urine that he could not practice the exercises that would enhance urinary control and ultimately decrease his anxiety. He was paralyzed by his emotions, while his pelvic floor muscles stayed dormant and weak. You have to keep trying until urinary control is attained.

Kegel exercises recruit and strengthen muscles that improve urinary control. These exercises are relatively simple to perform; however, men are not used to isolating the muscles involved, as they are not easily visualized. One way to identify which muscles to contract is to intentionally stop urinating in mid-stream. The pelvic floor muscles, and in particular your pubococcygeus muscle, are the ones you'll be focusing on. Surf the Internet for a picture of the muscles involved that can guide your focus while you are practicing. Once you get the feel of how the muscle contracts, practice squeezing when you are not urinating. That's the whole exercise. **Start these exercises before you need them—that means before your surgery or radiation therapy. If you did not do them**

before your treatment, it is better late than never. Practice the exercises when you are sitting, but also in motion, as you rise up or sit down—strengthen them for real-life proficiency.

But it is important to start slowly and not overdo these contractions—too much strain in any exercise is not good. If you are experiencing pain or discomfort, you are pushing yourself too hard, and you can aggravate the problem. Take a break. Ask your doctor about any discomfort. Also ask how long to hold each contraction (they are usually held for 3–5 seconds). Relax for 5–10 seconds and repeat. Start with easy contractions and ask your doctor how many sets to do per day and how many repetitions per set to start with and build up to. Without early feedback that the method is working, it is difficult to continue on faith alone. But continue anyway! You may benefit from biofeedback to help understand your muscle physiology better and gain more voluntary muscular control over urination.

A Prescription for Kegel Exercises

Rx: Kegel exercises
Sig*: As directed by your urologist
Dispense: A few minutes throughout the day
Note: Keep doing them even without seeing results

---

*Sig: Signa—directions for frequncy and amount per dose.

Carrying around extra pads or diapers, and perhaps an extra pair of light pants, in a bag or briefcase brings the practical relief of preparedness and reassurance in case a leak does occur. Some men who are embarrassed about leaking while awaiting fuller recovery use clamps to decrease urinary dribbling, or urinary flow devices to guide urine to an attached pouch. Sometimes a surgical procedure to fix sphincter control or to implant an artificial urinary sphincter is a magical solution. Check with your urologist to see what device is most practical and safe for you.

Taking Control of Urinary Incontinence

Do Kegel exercises as directed by your doctor.

Prepare in advance for outside activities: bring extra pads and diapers.

Depending on how much leakage you get, consider bringing a change of pants.

Ask your doctor if a urinary flow device or clamp is right for you.

Try one of the breathing exercises—heightened focus may enable better control.

I'm not sure what is wrong, but I can't keep the brakes on long enough to get to the toilet. Just seeing the toilet from across the bathroom causes me to lose my urine.

This gentleman was aware of a stimulus–response pattern that had been inadvertently set up between his eyes, his brain, his toilet, and his urinary control. He could hold his urine for ever-increasing lengths of time while driving his car or sitting through a concert (though he carried extra pads and diapers for minor leakages). He knew he would not have a major accident while outside, but as soon as he got to the bathroom, "almost like a child who cannot contain himself and is overwhelmed with relief at having his target in sight, I start to feel the diapers getting wetter, very fast." He was reluctant to have a second urological procedure to strengthen his sphincter control. We worked on practical issues, like leaving shorter time intervals between bathroom visits. He also used a distraction technique to suppress the "see the toilet—drop the urine" reaction. We practiced a relaxation technique that he used to distract himself when he saw the bathroom door and felt the urge to urinate. He carried a little "worry rock" with him that he could squeeze as he neared the bathroom to distract him from his worry so he could target his groin muscles and start to Kegel. Initially, I feared whether a relaxation technique would lead him to have the opposite reaction, and relax his bladder control muscles as well. However, these techniques heightened his focus and resolve, and relieved some of the psychological, anxiety-related aspects of his incontinence, and he got significant relief.

Radiation cystitis is a rare complication after radiation therapy. It is so rare that I thought of not writing about it. However, when it does occur, it causes significant distress, and I have helped men cope better. Cystitis, or inflammation of the bladder, can cause bladder irritation and discomfort, bleeding with urination, or the inability of the bladder to function well. The scope of the problem has decreased with improved radiation delivery methods used to try to avoid inadvertently targeting nearby bladder tissue. If symptoms are severe, hyperbaric oxygen (HBO) therapy is used to try to control bleeding and bladder spasms. Manual catheterization is sometimes required to prevent or resolve blood clots. As with complications in general, those that occur rarely, or those that are more serious, can be more upsetting to cope with emotionally. Less severe symptoms are treated with urinary irrigation or medications to control symptoms. Sometimes cystoscopy or other surgical interventions may be required. The greater the frequency, intensity, or severity of symptoms, the more aggravating this is to deal with.

It is difficult to find solace and appreciation for the many previous years of good health—without cancer and without urinary problems—or even for current good news—that your cancer may be gone now. An uncommon, negative event brings up the "why me" question again. Quality-of-life setbacks like these can radically impact your thoughts about life. One man joked that having to deal with bleeding when he urinates was a real "pain in the ass." Clots can impair the ability to urinate, leading to an uncomfortable bloated bladder. This may require catheterization, and sometimes repeated self-catheterization, to keep urine flowing and to prevent clotting. If you recall the discomfort you may have had just thinking about having a urinary catheter placed painlessly while under anesthesia for a prostatectomy that stays in place for only a week or so, consider the degree of distress felt about having a catheter placed while you are awake and, perhaps even more distressing, having to catheterize yourself. I don't know if men are more averse to penile self-injections

or self-catheterizations, though injections for erections are more voli-
tional; urination is mandatory.

I recently heard someone use the word *worrier*. Since my hearing loss,
I sometimes have to place in a more correct context what is really said
during a conversation in a noisy room. I think what the person really said
was the word *warrior*. But it struck me how these descriptions, though
seemingly on opposite ends of a spectrum, are not mutually exclusive. In
fact, they can go hand in hand. I have found this to be true with men I've
helped cope with radiation-induced bladder cystitis who transitioned
their "worrier" mentality into a "warrior" approach—a little like Clark
Kent transforming into Superman. A backed-up bladder is uncomfortable and can lead to urinary tract infections, dysfunctional contraction
of the bladder, and potential kidney disease. Unlike penile injections,
you cannot opt out of a "no pain–no gain" game plan here.

How do you go to work in an office if you can't pee or have to
self-catheterize during the day? How do you go out for dinner or the
movies? How do you visit friends or family? How do you take a long car
ride or a weekend vacation? How do you fly for pleasure or business if
you risk your health by not self-catheterizing? It seems impossible if
you've never done this before, let alone ever thought about it before. But
it can be done! I've seen the men who courageously do it.

If there is a problem that cannot be surgically improved with ure-
thral or bladder fixes, self-catheterization prevents needing your bladder
removed. You will have to think about and prepare to self-catheterize
outside the comfort of your own home if you don't want to become a
hermit. You'll need to learn from the urology nurses how to do this
safely and cleanly. You'll require the equipment—a sufficient number
of catheters—to match the length of time you expect to be away from
home. You'll want to practice at home before you hit the road. Rarely, a
bladder will need to be surgically removed. It is not easy to move forward
with that decision, as one of a few types of urinary diversion apparatuses
will have to be put in place. Some will tell me "I had no choice." But they
do have a choice about how they move forward after this surgery. That
decision will make a tremendous difference in how good a life they have
after the surgery.

Bowel Problems

Radiation proctitis is also a rare complication of radiation therapy for prostate cancer. Diarrhea, an uncontrolled need to defecate, and occasional bleeding may occur. Here, too, it is easier said than done to "expect the worst before radiation and hope for the best." Though individual men try to balance quality of life against longevity when choosing among different treatments for prostate cancer, most men cannot really imagine what this one would be like, or the likelihood of this complication occurring.

Bill is a 75-year-old man who had prostate cancer diagnosed 4 years ago. He was told at the time of diagnosis that his age and other medical problems prevented him from being a good candidate for a prostatectomy. All of the physicians he consulted agreed that radiation was the best treatment for him. However, Bill was reluctant to have radiation. His cousin had undergone the procedure 10 years earlier and suffered frequent bowel movements and severe rectal bleeding from radiation proctitis. According to Bill, his cousin underwent multiple cauterizations and surgical procedures to control the bleeding but had been left "a social cripple." Bill initially considered watchful waiting, but he reconsidered that option, as it would significantly worsen his prognosis. He understood that even with treatment, the cancer could get out of hand. He did not want that to happen without a fight, so he opted for radiation therapy. He felt a little more comfortable about the procedure when he was told about and read about the advances in radiation therapy over the previous decade, and that the incidence of radiation proctitis was significantly reduced.

When Bill developed proctitis 2 years after his treatment he was both angry and sad. He was upset that the right treatment decision didn't work out the way he wanted. He reduced his social activities significantly, yet spent a lot of time going to various medical specialists to treat his bowel symptoms and his other health problems. Each doctor visit included a ride on the subway that entailed the risk of a bowel accident. Thus each visit required preparation beforehand, thinking through where he could find a bathroom, if needed. He wore diapers just in case. He had backups if needed. Initially, he regretted his treatment decision and wished he had had no treatment at all. He wondered how much worse it could have been even if the cancer grew on its own. He became depressed and anxious and agreed to see me.

Bowel debilitation such as rectal urgency, intermittent bleeding, or rectal leakage due to radiation therapy is indeed more unusual today because of advances in radiation therapy. However, if these complications occur, they are extremely distressing. Regular rectal bleeding or multiple trips to the bathroom for frequent bowel movements is upsetting and embarrassing. These symptoms can lead men to withdraw socially. Work with a gastroenterologist or nutritionist who is familiar with this syndrome to find effective treatment, confidence, and relief in dealing with these symptoms. Fiber or Metamucil added to a diet can improve rectal urgency and leakage. Stool softeners, high-fiber diets, and sitz baths can decrease rectal bleeding. Anti-inflammatory medications such as steroids are also used to decrease bleeding. Persistent bleeding may warrant a colonoscopy and sometimes procedures for correction.

Bill could not seem to get enough emotional comfort from very supportive physicians or friends. Psychotherapy sessions included validating angry emotional reactions, and encouragement to continue to seek help to improve the symptoms. Therapy also included discussions about practical planning to maximize his leisure time when he was feeling better. His friends supported him and hoped, as he did, that this could be fixed easily so he could get over it and move on. Again, this was easier said than done. It was very important for Bill to have his friends hang in there with him. It was also essential for him to get support and suggestions in therapy to develop a "roll with the punches" attitude and to continue to seek and ask for remedies. Initially, Bill got stuck in a self-pity mode for days at a time. But he kept trying. An antianxiety medicine helped decrease his worry about socializing and helped him sleep better at night. An antidepressant helped put a floor to the depth of his mood drops. When he realized the repetitive nature and catalysts of his moods and anxiety symptoms, he felt much more control and much more satisfaction in his life.

Fatigue

"I'm just too tired to do the things that I used to enjoy."

Feeling tired from your cancer or treatment is upsetting and can be demoralizing, especially when you are used to being an active person socially and at work. Men say their cancer-related fatigue is different from tiredness before their cancer when they had a poor night's sleep or a stressful period at work. It is easy to get into a rut, feeling sorry for yourself, and be adamant that you can't do your usual routines because you don't feel like you have the same energy levels needed to accomplish those activities in the past. In fact, it can be quite alluring and seductive to just stay in bed, or to go back to bed, rather than push against your sense of inertia and fatigue. Fatigue can have a number of causes when you have prostate cancer: cancer treatment side effects (after surgery, radiation therapy, and certainly from hormonal treatments and chemotherapy for advanced cancer), as well as effects from any non-cancer-related medicines you might be taking. Just as physical issues can cause fatigue, psychological distress, worry, and depression can also contribute to a sense of weariness. Whether these emotions have a clear focus ("I am afraid this cancer will kill me"), are based on actual fact or fear ("I am so depressed that I will not get to see my daughter's wedding"), or are vague ("I feel so tired I don't feel like doing anything; please leave me alone"), uncomfortable emotions can yield to pessimistic convictions about whether things can get better, which can further deplete mental and bodily energy. On the other hand, to ignore the symptoms or to "just have a positive attitude" about a situation that doesn't feel very good can paradoxically demoralize and, psychologically as well as physically, exhaust many men.

Possible Causes of Fatigue

Recuperation period after prostatectomy
Radiation therapy possibly lasting weeks or months after
    treatment
Physical symptoms of pain and nausea

Other Medical or Psychiatric Conditions

Infections
Cardiac or blood pressure irregularities
Anemia
A sluggish or hyperactive thyroid
Pain syndromes
Severe insomnia, anxiety or depression

Medications

Antibiotics
Antihistamines
Antianxiety medication and antidepressants
Sleep medications (over-the-counter and prescription)
Cardiovascular medications
Pain medications
Hormonal, antiandrogen ablation medications
Steroid medications (they can energize and cause fatigue)
Chemotherapy

Physical recuperation from surgery can be tiring, though energy levels do return to baseline weeks to months after the procedure. Radiation therapy can drain energy levels during the treatment and for weeks or months afterward. Fatigue is complication of many treatments;

it makes sense to ask about a time range for recovery. For my own surgery, I was instructed to double the amount of time I was initially told it would take to regain my energy. Infections, cardiac or blood pressure irregularities, anemia, a sluggish thyroid (hypothyroidism), insomnia, various medications (including antibiotics, antihistamines, antianxiety medications, antidepressants, sleep medications, and cardiovascular medications), and hormonal, steroidal, and chemotherapy agents for prostate cancer can cause varying degrees of lethargy. Pain and the medications used to relieve pain can drain energy. Insomnia can cause daytime sleepiness. When fatigue is present, it is important to tell your doctor about it. In fact, all physical symptoms, including pain, insomnia, fatigue, and mood symptoms, as well as all medications (prescribed and over the counter, traditional and herbal supplements) should be reported to and reviewed and addressed by your physician. Expert medical and psychiatric collaboration regarding these symptoms will lead to more appropriate and successful remedies.

Changing Perspectives, Changing Your Life

In Chapter 4, I described a system for identifying daily patterns of energy, moods, anxiety, pain, and irritability, using a mood and activity chart. This tool gives you a graphic representation of all that happens physically and emotionally on a daily basis. In terms of fatigue in particular, it can help you see patterns that allow you to take advantage of higher-energy, less symptom-laden times and avoid higher-energy-requiring activities during lower-energy, higher-burden periods. Table 7.1 is a replica of that chart, with the instructions of how to complete it. Fill it out over the next week if you haven't done so already, and see how the emotional and physical stressors in your life are connected or, perhaps, not linked at all. Make sure to include activities you enjoy doing as well.

You may see how the physical and psychological features of your life influence each other and how they can add up to more than the sum of their parts in terms of your overall well-being and zest for living while you are feeling fatigued. With the help of the mood/activity

TABLE 7.1 MOOD/ACTIVITY CHART

	Monday	Tuesday	Wednesday	Thursday	Friday	Saturday	Sunday
Morning							
Afternoon							
Evening							

Instructions for completing the mood/activity chart:

2–3 times per day, jot the presence and intensity of emotional and physical issues as well as good things that happen, into each box. A 0–10 scale will work fine.

Issues to include:

Mood; Anxiety; Tearfulness; Irritability; Energy; Pain; Gastric upset; Hot flashes; Sleep; Appetite; Concentration; Urinary accidents/catheterizations; Bowel problems.

Also note potential triggers of the emotional or physical issues. Include enjoyable events: read a book; went to a concert; dinner with friends.

chart, identify times of the day when your energy is better or worse, and what impact timing of particular activities or medications has on subsequent energy levels. Understand that fatigue begets fatigue. The less you feel like doing activities because you are tired, the less you will do; the less you do, the more your muscles will weaken; the more your muscles weaken and the less nutritional intake you require, the more tired you will feel, the less you will feel like doing, and the less you will eat, and on and on. Exercise programs do not cause problematic increases in testosterone or risks for recurrence of disease, as some men with prostate cancer worry about. In fact, regular walking exercise helps relieve fatigue, concentration fogginess, and psychological distress. If you can add easy muscle-strengthening exercises, you'll feel the advantages in all of these areas over a few weeks or months.

Try to refocus your perspective, by seeing how each symptom impacts another and affects your overall well-being. The chart, or some version of it, will help you get acquainted with your new body rhythms. Hopefully, a shift in perspective and potential shifts in activities will help illuminate a path to a more rewarding life. Think about the veteran baseball catcher whose knees are getting older and achier, but who can still hit home runs. He can be reincarnated into a first baseman, where there is less crouching and running for painful legs, and less frequent throwing for a tired arm.

Even mild improvement or lightening the load of one symptom can be sufficient to make other disappointments more bearable. Finding alternative activities to match energy levels is strongly encouraged. Brainstorming with friends or family about what other activities you can do, even with low energy, can widen the tunnel vision caused by anger and frustration and lead to a more pleasurable lifestyle. For instance, if you find it too exhausting to focus on reading a book, try a book-on-tape, CD, or computer. Though this is a more passive activity, it might seem more enjoyable than lying on the couch doing nothing in particular. One spouse started reading to her husband and it reminded them fondly of when they were dating. If you find that your energy is higher in the morning or another time of day, then that is the time to schedule more energy-consuming activities, such as taking a walk or doing easy exercise, or attempting to do some paperwork or paying bills. If you feel like you are stuck at home and cannot get away, think creatively or outside your traditional box of vacations. Couples who used to travel may be frustrated if fatigue prevents the same kinds of exuberance for long journeys or vigorous touring. Long, yet local, weekends away can allow for sufficient rest periods from driving. Cruises require less effort and have options of walking around a port city or staying aboard ship.

Review all the medications you are taking with your doctor to see if any might cause fatigue or mood symptoms. If so, ask if any can be changed to either lower doses or to substitute medications that you might tolerate better. Then discuss non-medication interventions you can begin that do not come with a long package insert of potential worrisome side effects.

Prearranged and sufficient (but not too much) rest during the day as well as mild exercise can help improve energy. Proper hydration and calorie intake, even with health shakes, can improve energy. Proper rest, diet, and exercise? Sounds like rocket science, huh? Adjusting diet, rest, and activity levels for your current health status may sound as impossible as sending someone to the moon, especially when you are ill and your energy is down. But all of these can improve your get-up-and-go at various stages of prostate cancer and treatment. You may be thinking about how much time you'll need to spend in a gym and are already turned off by this idea, given your current energy level. But "starting low and going slowly" is appropriate here, just as with most new activities you try. How about 10–15 minutes of easy walking? A light yoga or tai chi class? Maybe even a chair aerobics class or video?

Remember the stages of behavior change described in the last chapter. These stages apply not only to sexual behaviors. They also apply to many of the behaviors, including non-behaviors, that impede our well-being. Hopefully, many topics discussed in this book will address behaviors that with change can improve your life. If fatigue that leads to less activity leads to more fatigue, it can be helpful to figure out how to reverse that trend. I often tell patients, "When you don't feel like *doing* anything, and there is no medical reason you cannot *do* something, remember the Nike saying and "Just do it," even a little bit. That line has inspired me to accomplish much in my life, including running marathons, recuperating and getting back on track after treatment for my acoustic neuroma, and writing this book. It has helped many men get off the couch during or after prostate cancer treatment and gotten them to start walking and feeling better.

Ask your doctor what exercises or exercise regimens are appropriate and which you could tolerate before you start any exercise program. Your situation is comparable to an athlete coming back from an injury—doing too much or too fast can bring on reinjury or a new injury because the muscles are not used to working out in their usual ways. So even though it's your prostate that's injured, and not a knee or hamstring, think about setting up a reasonable "rehab" program. This is not the time for a weekend warrior (or worrier) mindset. This is even truer if you are new to exercising. Get tips from a physical therapist who has an understanding of your medical condition; those tips can be priceless in allaying fear.

Get into E-Motion: Exercise to Improve Emotion

Many recent studies show that easy exercise routines, like walking or easy aerobic workouts, or isometric or low-resistance muscle strengthening programs can improve energy levels and mood. Getting into physical motion will help you emotionally. So get into *E-motion, exercise to improve emotion*. In one study, 6 to 12 weeks of walking relieved fatigue and improved psychological well-being in cancer patients receiving chemotherapy compared to those who did not walk or exercise. You can build up to 20–30 minutes of walking most days of the week. We're not talking about "power walking" here. What you viewed as a short, slow walk 2 years ago can feel almost impossible when your energy has been depleted by cancer treatment. Aerobic and simple strength-training routines help men after radiation therapy for prostate cancer as well as those receiving hormonal therapy that otherwise causes muscle weakness and fatigue. Some studies now show that cognitive behavioral therapy, with its many thought, emotional, and lifestyle tweaks I described earlier, and mindfulness meditation also improve energy and mood levels.

Doctor's Order: Get Active, Stay Active

Rx:	Walking and easy strength-training exercises
Sig:	Start low, go slow, as directed by your doctor
Dispense:	Daily; progress slowly each week for 6–12 weeks
Return:	2–4 weeks for activity and mood maintenance

It is also important to ensure that your diet is adequate to provide the necessary nutrients to rebuild your muscle and vasculature tissue. Changes in taste and appetite can occur with cancer treatment. Trying to get sufficient fluid and nutrients even from dietary supplements may help provide the calories needed for more energy. A consultation with a dietician or nutritionist knowledgeable about cancer may help identify alternative food regimens to maintain energy levels. Carry around a thermos or small bottle of water for frequent hydration breaks, especially in warmer, more humid weather. Keep topping off your tank.

Identifying and correcting medical and psychiatric causes of fatigue can be helpful; however, that still might be insufficient. Treating fatigue directly is then called for. Physicians have found that low doses of steroid medications such as prednisone or dexamethasone may provide improved vigor. However, these positive effects are often not long-lasting. The long-term use of steroid medication may have other harmful consequences. Adjusting the doses of medications like blood pressure medications or sleep agents that can also cause fatigue, or changing to better-tolerated alternative medications, if feasible, may improve energy and stamina.

Low doses of psychostimulant medications as discussed in Chapter 5, such as methylphenidate and modafinil, have been recommended in fatigue practice guidelines to decrease fatigue, increase energy and counter the sedation of pain medications. These stimulant medications may also improve appetite, improve motivation, enhance a sense of well-being, and improve mood in cancer patients and others with significant medical illnesses and fatigue. Unfortunately, when I mention psychostimulants to some of my patients, they roll their eyes and think about one of their children or grandchildren treated with a stimulant for attention deficit-hyperactivity disorder. They express their distrust, asking appropriately, "Why would you give me a medication that helps calm children down when I am already too tired and passive?" As noted earlier, I explain that these medications do not "calm" kids down. They heighten focus and extend attention spans, so that a child who previously could not sit still for more than a few minutes because he is easily distracted will sit for longer periods of time, focusing better on one activity. The child will appear to be calmer. These medicines can improve your focus and attention as well, and improve your energy and mood.

Men with preexisting seizure disorders or cardiac rhythm problems, such as atrial fibrillation or uncontrolled hypertension, should not take these medicines without clear permission from their medical specialists. But it makes sense to ask your doctor. Over time, stimulants seem to add real benefit to energy leaks. Our research team completed a small study using the psychostimulant methylphenidate (Ritalin) to treat fatigue in men with prostate cancer. We found a placebo effect as is common with many medicines, but that effect disappeared after a few weeks, and the psychostimulant continued to enhance energy levels in many men. Some men developed increased blood pressure or increased pulse rates during the study period; however, there were no serious adverse events. Men burdened by significant fatigue should have the opportunity to enhance their energy and mood with one of these medications, as long as they do not have problematic preexisting medical complications and their physician monitors for increased blood pressure and heart rate over time. Modafinil (Provigil) and Nuvigil (Armodafinil) are gentler stimulants that are more tolerable than methylphenidate in more men, without the risk of seizures and with less impact on blood pressure and cardiac rhythm regularities.

If a psychostimulant cannot be tolerated, activating antidepressants such as bupropion (Wellbutrin) or fluoxetine (Prozac) may also enhance energy and mood. Bupropion would not be recommended for anyone with a preexisting seizure disorder, but is safe for people with cardiac problems.

Suggestions to Energize Fatigue of Body and Mind

Get sufficient, but not too much, rest during the day.
Plan activities around higher daily energy patterns.
E-Motion: Easy aerobic and strength training exercises.
Mindfulness meditation and cognitive behavioral therapy can help.
Ask a dietitian to help you avoid "fatiguing foods" and eat
  "energizers."

Stimulating Medications

Energizing antidepressants
Psychostimulants

Chapter 8

Not for Patients Only

Spouses or Partners Can Manage
Prostate Cancer Better Too

For better or for worse...in sickness and in health...until death do
us part.

When a star player in any sport is slumping, some believe he just needs
to play his way out of the slump; after awhile, most agree that a rest
helps. But over time, he and his team may feel his decreased contribu-
tions as he keeps trying to play at his usual level and expectations are
dashed daily. Of course, the game will be tougher when someone you
usually count on is on the sideline or not performing well. Teammates
can "pick *him* up," and everyone else's spirits as well, by upping their
play. This extra effort propels the team forward for a while. The slumping player recognizes that the game does not rest on his weary shoulders
alone, easing the pressure. This can inspire a good player back to great-
ness. Isn't this what a good team does when they care about each other
and want the best possible outcome for all?

Spouses and partners, this section is for you especially (but men, you
will get a lot out of it, so please read it as well). You can become even more
frightened, distressed, and demoralized than the men in your life who
have prostate cancer. You can benefit from the same coping strategies

mentioned throughout this book. Even though your partner has cancer, you may both feel like patients. This is particularly true if your relationship was already frayed at the edges before prostate cancer arrived. It can then implode from the added pressures of prostate cancer. But your relationship can also mend tattered threads. Healing of relationships happens for many reasons: for the sake of peace and hope; for the sake of better health of both partners; for the sake of pity and compassion; and, very often, for the sake of children, grandchildren, or other family members. I've also seen good, healthy relationships stumble in the face of cancer because of fears of the worst that might happen: death. People have been known to suffer "death anxiety" even when there is no life-threatening illness in the picture—it is even more plausible that its presence is felt when cancer is present, regardless of how good the prognosis may be. Spouses and partners are concerned about enduring future trials and losses, perhaps alone, as well as dreading potentially shattered expectations of plans and wishes that may not come "as advertised." This can be destabilizing and disheartening. Communication often falters; subsequently, uncomfortable emotions and suboptimal behaviors follow. You can find yourself sensing a domino effect of poor communication and arguments. You both may feel overwhelmed and isolated.

But this downward spiral for you or your relationship is not inevitable. You too can use the DRAFT with Emotional Judo (EJ) techniques! It is helpful to **D**etect and **R**ecognize these emotional, thought, or behavioral dominoes and how easy it can be to fall into their traps. **A**cknowledge whatever legitimacy they may have and what is not appropriate, exaggerated, all-or-none, or catastrophizing. You may need to learn new strategies to deal with the stress of a loved one who is ill. You, too, may feel cheated by prostate cancer and have to deal with real and indefinable losses and the fear of mortality. Your partner's vulnerability to death, as well as your own, will move front and center, even though you are not the one with cancer. You can **F**lip these dominoes and **T**ransform your thinking to figure out how to live a fuller life with and beyond the cancer even when the going gets tough. It may not be easy to maintain contacts with friends, to schedule social or fun time away from illness activities and doctors' appointments and caregiving, or to focus on work if you're not retired yet, as well as do all the things necessary to take care of your health and your partner. But it is possible.

Communication and the Tension of Good Intentions

Even if communication has been optimally open and honest between spouses or partners who have been together for many years, it is confronted and challenged in the face of a life-threatening illness like prostate cancer that is intrusive, foreign, burdensome, and distracting from your life plans. Although it is here, it feels like it doesn't belong. Communication often fails and may paradoxically be at its worst because of the stress of this situation. Some men are uncomfortable identifying and sharing emotions. A cancer diagnosis can make men feel inept and weak, as the protective armor seems more penetrable, undermining the role as protector and provider for the family.

Couples find themselves arguing more; perhaps, even worse, many stop talking about charged issues. This develops from what I call "the tension of good intentions." One partner or the other, and frequently both, avoid talking about or asking about issues related to illness, life, coping, or the future. They fear they will upset or pressure the other by bringing up an issue they assume the other doesn't want to deal with. This communication traffic jam can lead to a congested two-way street. The unspoken thoughts and emotions may fester and the couple finds they are bickering more than usual. They may feel more in the doldrums as their sense of isolation, helplessness, and fear of the unknown mounts. This unintended communication gap occurs with the best intentions, but with potential consequences.

On the one hand, avoiding discussions with your spouse about pertinent topics is not helpful. On the other hand, arguing about things that are important or not is not pleasant either. Thankfully, there is a large middle ground. A good communication guide for couples I see who are arguing too much is to "strike when the iron is cold." Trying to make your points when either of you is upset will more likely lead to an offensive attack, or will be met by a defensive comeback that turns into an offensive attack. The escalation has begun and the argument will become more heated. Acknowledging that the discussion is getting too heated to continue now and that you will revisit the topic when both of you are calmer can help. Taking an adult "time out" to chill out is not shameful. In fact, it may keep more peace in your household.

Patient:

> I really don't want to worry my family, so I just don't talk about how nervous I am about that next PSA test.

Partner:

> I know he is worried about the cancer coming back. He sees every new pain as the cancer spreading. For weeks before his PSA tests he doesn't sleep. I know what he's thinking about. I've learned not to ask how he's feeling. I don't tell him "not to worry" anymore—I got yelled at for that. So I make believe everything is fine. I keep the routine going, but the routine is already different. I can tell how upset he is, especially when he starts yelling at me.

An alternative response:

Start the discussion with an acknowledgment or validation of the emotions that your partner has after you are both feeling calmer. You may not think they are accurate or valid, but they are emotions.

> I can understand how the increased PSA test, the new pain, and the recommendation of another MRI scan are making you worried and upset. But when you don't answer me, I have no idea if you didn't hear, if you are distracted by your worries, or if you don't care. When I get yelled at, I stop listening and then I don't feel like helping you, even though I want to.

Men do not hide their emotions very well, except perhaps from themselves by not detecting or recognizing how upset they are inside. It is often the spouse or partner who alerts the urologist or oncologist that their partner has been depressed or anxious or so irritable that it is tough to have reasonable conversations now, or that he just doesn't talk very much at all.

The down side of this "don't ask, don't tell" policy is that emotions fester. Misunderstood and misdirected feelings come out in the wrong ways. More sleep is lost. Arguments become more frequent. Men and their spouses and partners eventually become even more vulnerable to higher anxiety, lower or more irritable moods, and distance from a life partner, rather than finding closeness and comfort between them that can ease a stressful time of their lives.

It is not uncommon for men newly referred by their oncologists or nurses to come to my office with their spouse or partner. I go into the waiting room and call the man's name. Two people stand up. I introduce myself to the patient, and sometimes receive an introduction to the partner. With or without an introduction, both start walking with me to my office. I stop and clarify with the patient whether he wants the partner in the session, sometimes seeing a questioning, quizzical look on the patient's face or an angry one on the partner's. Most of the time he will say, "Yes; she's the reason I'm seeing you; I have no secrets." Sometimes you do things just because you know it will make your partner happier, knowing that the downstream effect will be for you to have a happier life too. Maybe your oncologist or urologist encouraged you to seek psychological support because your spouse or partner mentioned your moodiness; physicians also want to ease the burden couples struggle with because of the cancer, as they understand this can make treating the cancer easier. Men are relieved when I tell them their partners may join us for some or all of the session. Sometimes they'll join us for many sessions.

Cancer diagnosed in an individual has wide-reaching affects on a family. Sometimes the best route to help the individual patient is through his family. I get to see the tensions, the disagreements, the different coping styles, the grief, and sometimes the avoidance of relevant issues firsthand, right there in my office. The customary focus of individual psychotherapy is to discuss issues with the patient only. Whether with insight-oriented therapy or cognitive behavioral therapy, it is hoped that the patient will be able to enact changes that will have a beneficial effect on both himself and the rest of his life, including his partner. However, for a couple struggling in the stressful world of prostate cancer, this is like a coach (the therapist) sending a player or messenger (the patient) into a football huddle (home) to transmit the next play, a new play that the other players (spouse or partner or other family members) have never heard or practiced before. He might know the words to say, and can even draw diagrams on the ground or whiteboard, but his spouse or partner has not rehearsed from the same playbook. When the spouse or partner is present in the therapy session, everyone is part of designing and practicing the strategy and plan together in the office. A therapy session really can be a microcosm for the larger world that the patient and his family live in. At times, the spouse or partner is so overwhelmed psychologically or angry with the patient or medical situation, that it is useful for him or her to get separate individual counseling with a different therapist.

A patient once told me,

> My wife has an important and busy job. I didn't want her getting distracted by this prostate cancer stuff and worrying about my cancer diagnosis until I was sure of what was going on. I needed to collect enough information to help her eventually understand and cope better. So I didn't tell her about the symptoms I was having, the PSA tests or the biopsy. I thought she would freak out.

Good intentions? Yes. Good results? No. Self-fulfilling prophecy? Absolutely! This patient didn't tell his wife about the cancer diagnosis until after a confirmed positive biopsy report, shortly before they went to an oncologist's office for a second opinion. She felt blindsided. She was upset; she was feeling the burden of horrible news that had just been sprung on her. It's like hearing the ending without reading the book. It felt like a *punch*-line: "I had no opportunity to prepare. I had no time to learn about or start coping with the illness." Instead, she felt as if she was presented with a fait accompli or verdict without realizing that her life too was on trial. She was frustrated, scared, and angry. The diagnosis and her emotional reactions felt like a bomb had hit. She thought getting the information over time, as it unfolded, would have provided her the ability to digest and understand each fragment of the situation, from urinary symptoms to elevated PSA test, to biopsy preparation and biopsy, to waiting for biopsy results and, ultimately, getting the diagnosis. What her husband went through over 2–3 months, she had to absorb in a few days. On the one hand, my patient thought he was doing his wife a favor by protecting her from needless worry in case there was no cancer diagnosis. However, by managing to keep all of these details to himself, he inadvertently created a difficult situation in which his wife felt like she "read the sensationalist headlines" instead of "getting the full story": "I felt like I got hit with a ton of bricks; though my husband may have felt the same ton of bricks, we were starting from different places, and he had more time to develop a thicker skin."

The psychologist Alice Kornblith conducted a study while she was at Memorial Sloan Kettering Cancer Center about the emotional and physical quality of life of patients with prostate cancer and their spouses and partners. The men in the study had all stages of early and advanced prostate cancer. The female spouses and partners were tenser, more worried, and more depressed than the men. These findings have been replicated in other studies as well. Spouses and partners as well as patients may need more information and support than they can get from this book and may benefit from professional individual psychotherapy, couples therapy focused on prostate cancer issues, support groups, and possibly psychiatric medication.

When it comes to cancer issues, there are differences in how the genders cope. Women, as spouses or as patients with their own cancers, are usually more willing to participate in individual and group psychotherapy and to share their worries and concerns with friends and family; they make themselves available to get support. Many men do not share their feelings easily with others, though there are now many prostate cancer support groups around the country that many men (and their partners) benefit from. A non-exhaustive list of support groups can be found at the back of this book. When I am asked if I think a support group can be useful, I answer, "Yes, groups can be very helpful. But groups work for some and not for others. The only way to know, despite any preconceived notions you may have about a group, is to try it—you might like it. And if you don't like it, you don't have to go back." This last sentence often brings a frustrated frown to a spouse or partner's face. They are hoping that there is a place and other people a patient can share his strife with, but the patient feels relief hearing he is not being sentenced to jail.

Men tend to refuse to accept help for emotional distress for many reasons. A common reason is a "grin and bear it" or "pick yourself up from your bootstraps" macho attitude. Interestingly, this resistance may also come out of a victim's sense of helplessness. Men think there is little tangible benefit achieved by "just by talking about it." They feel that "merely talking" is a waste of time and energy since it cannot cure the cancer or improve the prognosis; "Talking doesn't fix anything." They do not believe in the process and see little potential gain or change in the end result. They cannot appreciate how information and support from others might be beneficial and bring clear, immediate, or measurable positive outcomes. Spouses and partners suggest groups or individual therapy because they feel helpless when they are not able to find ways to relieve sadness or stress for their husbands. But many men do try groups out. Many find useful questions to ask their doctors; tips on how to manage certain dilemmas; and feel a better sense of control and less isolation.

I noted earlier that it is not always easy to get men with prostate cancer to see me or any therapist for counseling, even when the signs of distress are clear to the attendant in the parking garage of the hospital. This is due in part to the same stigma felt by anyone seeing a mental health professional. Men think that if they have to get mental health help, they are not able to handle problems on their own, the way they did before the cancer arrived. It is also related to not viewing psychiatry (or any type of emotional counseling) as scientific enough. Unfortunately, this attitude is shared by many in our society, including some medical practitioners and health insurance companies, who do not offer adequate mental health coverage on a par with coverage for medical illnesses. Men can find all kinds of excuses and reasons not to see a therapist. But the recommendation that comes from the physician entrusted to fight the cancer carries a considerable amount of weight. It is difficult to trust that after your cancer diagnosis your body will be as resilient and as consistently healthy as it was in the past. It may be even more difficult to fear that your psyche is weakening as well. Sometimes you feel anger, and sometimes the fear of anger. The statement "If I start to let my feelings out, I might destroy someone or something" may reflect how much you feel cancer has destroyed your life. But practically speaking, when there is no appropriate culprit and no one to blame for the spot you're in, you might feel "what's the point of talking." Exactly! Therapy helps men live with what does not make sense and deal with the guilt about feeling angry with loved ones when they know their loved ones are not responsible for the cancer either. Therapy helps couples cope with *their* cancer and *their* losses and *their* lives. That is why so many partners and spouses encourage therapy and want to join in.

Men may have difficulty speaking about how they are feeling. They are ashamed of their cancer, for feeling physically weak, and for feeling emotionally frail. Remember the "why me" question? Many men think they should have seen the cancer coming and prevented or avoided it; this thinking leads to guilt feelings. Some feel that God should have intervened or had a different plan. One man asked me, "How could God forget me?" They feel ashamed about their predicament and then about feeling ashamed. They are angry and often cannot describe those emotions calmly. Discussions about these issues in general are not easy and maybe even more difficult when trying to talk about the specific problems of sex, urinary leaks, other physical symptoms, or the lack of motivation or energy to live life pleasurably. There is often defensiveness about how they are feeling or acting. Many men drift away from socializing because they are embarrassed about not feeling well and whole; they don't want to talk about their illness or their symptoms when they see friends who are healthier. Those experiences make them feel more vulnerable. So they tell their spouses or partners, "Don't make any plans" and "I don't want to talk about it." Though they don't like making comparisons with healthier friends, they can't easily sidestep the turn their lives have taken, which many see as a guidepost toward death.

Communication Comes in Many Forms

The Many Shades of Bob

A patient in his seventies was referred to me for depression and anxiety. He had seen horrific things when he was in the Korean War and was left with a sense of vulnerability and guilt. Before prostate cancer, this was not easily recognized by any but his closest family members. Everyone saw Bob as a macho guy; he talked tough in his New York accent, and did whatever it took to make sure that his family, his friends, and the plumbing business he started 35 years ago thrived. Those who knew Bob well knew he could be sweet as sugar just as quickly as he could become hard as nails, depending on what the situation called for. But at night, feeling alone in bed while his wife slept, Bob stared up at the ceiling, feeling internally agitated and anxious. When he did sleep he had nightmares about the many dead bodies he had seen in Korea. Though horrified by these nightmares, he curiously felt compelled to watch old combat movies. Although Bob knew that the combat movies led to more angst and irritability while awake, and more vivid nightmares while asleep, he felt drawn to watch them, as he also felt a strange familiarity.

He was happy to be alive, but at the same time felt survivor's guilt, given how many of his combat buddies had died. He hoped that watching these old Hollywood films would help him come up with better images for himself, or remake his memories. His wife could not understand much of what was happening, since life was so much different before the cancer. She told Bob not to watch the movies, but he did it anyway. The movies did not seem to bother Bob as much before his cancer. She tried to understand what made him so irritable, but he couldn't explain it sufficiently. When he was around others, he didn't talk about Korea or his traumatic military experiences. He tried to keep his emotions and thoughts about combat buried, as he was uncomfortable and unable to explain why he survived when many others did not. He had post-traumatic stress disorder that was reawakened by his cancer and sense of looming mortality. Yet Bob's military experience gave him a sense of the preciousness of life that was the basis of his relationships with all who came to know him—he would go the extra mile for family, a friend, a business client, and even for a stranger.

When Bob was diagnosed with prostate cancer, he had to start taking hormones to treat the cancer. These medications zapped his physical prowess and machismo. He felt tired much of the time. The invisible barriers that kept the combat and its horrors at a distance had been breached by this new trauma. He was scared, and at times he felt like he was in battle again. He was hyperaware of every potential threat to himself and his family. He became more irritable, argumentative, and depressed. He loved his family tremendously, so no one could understand why he seemed to pick fights with them.

His wife first tried to change the "new Bob" with his fragile, unpredictable moods, and then tried to accept the "new Bob," although this was not a "new normal" she wanted to get used to, but neither worked. She was embarrassed when he'd argue with Little League referees, umpires, or coaches at his grandchildren's recreation sports games. He would turn up for family gatherings, stay around for a little while, give his opinions on what everyone was doing wrong with their lives or their kids' lives, and inevitably walk away in a huff, spending hours in bed, moping. He would sincerely ask his wife, "Why don't they love me anymore. I'm just trying to be a concerned dad and grandfather." His wife reached her limit and insisted Bob see a psychiatrist. Bob was willing to see me only after his oncologist gave a strong recommendation, and only if his wife came too.

I recall the first session with Bob and his wife. It was a hot summer day, and Bob did not take off his sunglasses (shades), an image that stuck with me for awhile. His wife clearly described what had been going on, at first feeling as if she was telling secrets, but Bob was actually grateful that she could talk about the things he was doing that he couldn't fully understand and that he was embarrassed about.

After a couple of months of psychotherapy and medication that targeted his anxiety, insomnia, and moodiness, it became clear that much of his behavior was borne out of fear and guilt, about the blending of past, present, and future in the context of hormone therapy priming his emotions. (The impact of hormonal therapy on mood and physical well-being is described in Chapter 9.) This was helpful for both Bob and his wife to understand. The bravery and skillfulness he exhibited in battle seemed canceled out by the fear he felt underneath and the enormity of the dangers he survived that many of his fellow soldiers did not. He had been so traumatized by his combat experiences that he experienced his cancer diagnosis as a dagger in his back that would not only kill him, but would kill him soon. He became frustrated that he could not "protect myself or my family" from the cancer tragedy. He inadvertently punished himself and them. He speculated during one session whether spending less time with his family, and unintentionally pushing them away, was aimed at trying to help his family get used to his not being around in the future. Bob could see through the veneer of this "protectiveness," and eventually saw how this "strategy" actually had an opposite effect.

After a number of sessions, the episodes of pushing away his family and arguing with them decreased significantly. Both he and his wife saw our therapy as a success. Though we did not eliminate the symptoms altogether, they were confined to smaller, more discrete periods of time—only the week before the PSA test instead of a month or more before the test. This led to much less aggravation on the one hand, and much more understanding, support, and contentment on the other, for both the patient and his family.

Bob pulled out his sunglasses in the middle of one session, smiled a wide grin, put the shades on, and was happy about how far he had come over a few months. Bob also learned that he could tell his wife when he was feeling scared and what brought on his desire to flee, rather than actually fleeing, so that they could spend more meaningful time together, as a couple and with their family and friends. Bob's family felt valuable providing appropriate support for him, rather than just getting frustrated, angry, and distant.

"When He Plays the Piano I Know He Is Still Alive and in My Life"

A few years ago, I evaluated a 75-year-old man with prostate cancer for depression. He had retired from his office manager job about 10 years earlier. He enjoyed retirement with his wife of 50 years, until his cancer diagnosis. When I met Joe, he said, "I'm not depressed." He was frustrated by the fatigue caused by his medications, which also left him feeling apathetic about engaging in anything but low-energy activities. He did not want to go out socially with his friends, and did not spend much time with his grandchildren when they were visiting. He was upset by being asked to do more than he felt capable of, and frankly was upset by our meeting. His wife Sarah had asked the oncologist for the psychiatric consultation, thinking Joe was depressed.

Sarah came into our consultation toward the end of the session. I asked her about her concerns, given Joe's denial of feeling depressed. She quite warmly explained that she understood Joe not wanting to go out socially, and not wanting to be around noisy, active grandchildren for very long. However, one of the special qualities that attracted Sarah to Joe over 50 years ago was his joy and enthusiasm of playing the piano. He learned how to play as a child. As an adult, he only practiced sporadically, given work and family obligations. He continued to play a few times per week after his retirement. He enjoyed playing songs from Broadway musicals for friends and family, who sang along at social gatherings. He stopped practicing after he became fatigued from his prostate cancer treatment. "He doesn't play piano anymore. I think he's lost his will to live. He must be depressed." Joe tiredly responded, "I wasn't playing up to my standards. It didn't sound good." Sarah quickly chimed in:

> "You know, you were never a Mozart…but I loved to hear you play. You could make me smile and cry and I'd get chills down my spine because of how you played with such great emotion. I never told you this, but when I would hear you play, I would feel more alive and more connected to you—it was almost as good as sex." Joe frowned and then had a sarcastic grin on his face, as if to say "Really?" "I don't care how you sound now. I don't know how much longer either of us is going to live and I would love to hear you play so I can enjoy you while we are still together."

Joe did not get treated for depression. Our marker for starting an antidepressant was whether or not he would be able to find the interest and energy to play the piano. He did.

Another Homework Assignment: Hold Hands in the Bus

"Since we started having our children over 25 years ago, we haven't been very romantic," said Sherry.

> I guess neither of us missed it with busy lives—raising children and working. But I feel very alone since Bert's cancer diagnosis. I remember taking long walks when we were dating and holding hands. We used to love to go dancing. But that stopped with the kids. I guess I didn't miss touching that much while we were so busy, but I miss it now, especially as I get older myself. I worry about being alone and I worry about my own death. I think it would just be nice to feel close to someone you've loved for so many years, even though I know he cares about me and loves me.

Bert didn't argue that this was the case. It felt unnatural and like an imposition to have to think about holding his wife's hand. He didn't feel the impulse to do this spontaneously like he did when they were dating. I had them hold hands in the consultation room. I am sure it felt as awkward for them as it looked to me. But embarrassed smiles spontaneously appeared on both of their faces. Since they came to our sessions together on the bus, I suggested that when they travel home that day, they hold hands for a minute or two while sitting on the bus. At the next session, they reported they had completed their homework, and it felt nice, though a little embarrassing at the same time. But they agreed to try to practice this more at home.

Sex Is Not Just about the Sex

> He doesn't get it. For me, sex was not just about the sex. It was feeling a closeness that didn't need words. It was a way to communicate what was indescribable. Sure, I enjoy having orgasms and would love to have him continue to arouse me. However, I realize how upsetting and difficult that is for him. His libido is low, since he needs a pill or an injection to get an erection. I know it doesn't feel the same for him or me, but I like having him in me. There is a union, even though less natural, that is still special for me.

Communication and intimacy can come in many forms and is vital in different ways at different times in any relationship: verbally, sexually, tactilely, aurally, visually, musically, aromatically, silently, and spiritually. Different couples may enjoy one of these varieties or assorted combinations of them at different points in their relationships. Intimacy, too, can also come in many flavors. But being up close and intimate with someone often means acknowledging not just the attractiveness of another but also dealing with vulnerabilities. Some flavors that were pleasing years ago may still be potent today, while others may not be. A key to breaking the isolation and challenges that many couples feel going into their older years is to learn how to accommodate to current circumstances.

Guidelines for Engagement and Improved Communication

Not communicating is communicating (often the wrong things).

Communication is not just verbal; caring can be expressed by holding.

"Strike when the iron is cold"—wait until anger cools before beginning tough discussions.

Don't just say something; sit there (and listen).

Validate what your partner is feeling (scared, angry, sad, etc.): It means you heard, even if you don't agree or cannot fix it.

Suggest different types of activities to do together.

Part One of this book has provided many suggestions for individuals and couples to improve communication, intimacy, and activities after a prostate cancer diagnosis enters their lives and treatment impacts quality of life. My advice to those of you living with prostate cancer is to engage in discussion and experimentation with your partner for the greater good of your partner and your relationship. Push outside your comfort zone and you might find great payback.

Try it; you might like it.

All of this information is useful for those dealing with early- and advanced-stage cancer. Many with early-stage disease will not want to go on to the second part of the book. Though you don't need to, you can try it—you might like it. The next two chapters deal with coping with recurrence of disease and handling practical and existential matters integral to more advanced disease.

Later-Stage Disease
and Recurrence
of Disease

Chapter 9

Coping with Recurrence of Cancer If the "Definitive" Treatment Doesn't Work

Going Hormonal

"Holy shit! I never expected the cancer to come back."

Inaccurate forecasting or unwanted, unexpected occurrences in the world of prostate cancer occur for many reasons. Maybe the surgeon or the radiation oncologist told the patient, "We got it all, no need for worry." Maybe that is what the patient heard. Maybe after months or even years of test results showing no measurable amount of PSA, the patient decided to go with "the glass is full" stance. He assumed the cancer was behind him for good, and he could move on with his life. After all, that's what "cure" is all about. Perhaps he says, "I was willing to put up with the side effects (ED or urinary or bowel problems) for a cure. But not on top of unending cancer!" It is as if he forged a private, inner contract entitled "Complications Remain, Assume Perpetual cure" (CRAP), which now seems null and void.

When the cancer comes back after "definitive" treatment, it feels like the rug has been pulled out from under you, *again*, just as it felt with the initial diagnosis. You don't recall anyone saying your treatment was definitive treatment *intended*. Even though you knew theoretically that recurrence could happen, and you were vigilant about your PSA tests, you prayed and hoped it could not happen to you. In your heart of hearts, you did not expect this cancer to come back, because you did not want it back. You may be angry, frustrated, sad, in disbelief, with an uncertainty about what and who you can believe and trust about your future. These may be similar feelings you experienced when you were first diagnosed. You might have been expecting to "die with your boots on" from something other than prostate cancer, and now you foresee dying a debilitating death from prostate cancer. It is another shock to your system that you never thought could be shocked again, as badly as it was when you first heard you had prostate cancer. It takes a while to regain or re-form new sea legs.

Some men become very angry with their doctors. It doesn't matter whether the cancer comes back in a few years or after ten. The psychological work is to figure out how you can trust your original physician or any other physician again, through the next phases of coping with observation or treatment for recurrent prostate cancer.

> A 50-year-old man, who had undergone a prostatectomy 3 years earlier, has had consistent elevations in his last few PSA tests. He is diagnosed with a biochemical recurrence of his prostate cancer. In our first session he said, "I thought I was done with this cancer and now I have to worry about less than a 50% chance of cure again if I have radiation. I wanted to live into my 80s like my parents did. How can I trust any doctor again?"

Part Two of this book is for those men who have recurrence of their prostate cancer, either biochemical or with progressive or metastatic disease, or those who are newly diagnosed with advanced cancer. Many of these men give up hope for a better life regardless of the stage of cancer, degree of progression, or chronicity of illness, because they now have no chance of cure. The death sentence writing is on the wall again. Men imagine a scenario into the future that is much worse than their reality right now. Their minds conjure up presumed images of what end-stage disease will look like for them: suffering, with pain and with multiple disabilities that seem to lurk just around the corner. They fear a last stage of life that includes poor physical and mental health. Although this distorted carnival-mirror image is not likely to happen soon and perhaps not at all, with or even from prostate cancer, it is where men's minds wander with new bad news. They feel they are on a precipice between life and death. This image does not allow for the *tincture of time* that incorporates adaptation and acceptance of a situation that transforms slowly and that allows a life to be well-lived before death.

Whether the recurrence of prostate cancer is documented by a significant trend of rising PSA levels or if it is already metastatic as indicated by bone, PET, or MRI scans and possibly by pain or other physical complaints, it can take time to adjust to this paradigm shift in your life perspective and get to a point of accepting it and moving on. At least as of the writing of this book, a biochemical recurrence after primary treatment significantly decreases the ultimate likelihood of cure. The presence of metastases does imply no further chance of cure, but does not mean impending death. Recurrence of cancer or the presence of advanced disease leads men and their partners to feel betrayed by life, by God, or by the medical community. They have a sense that their lives are doomed, now for a second time since the initial diagnosis. Many inaccurately imagine the end is near, even if they will live for many years, and be headed downhill because they have suddenly been launched on a different trajectory than they had anticipated, hoped, or planned for.

With recurrence, men often see each PSA test as a marker announcing they are a step closer to death: "The higher my PSA goes, the closer I get to the grave." Each test is viewed and anticipated with great angst, often with a sense that the test, like a psychic (with an accurate crystal ball), prophesizes whether they will live and how they will die.

This chapter will help men live better with recurrence of the cancer or if they are being diagnosed initially with advanced prostate cancer that is unlikely to be cured. Losing the possibility of a cure turns another spotlight onto mortality. Confrontations of mortality are often accompanied by a feeling that time is counting down, rather than counting onward. This can be true for spouses and partners as well. Recurrence of the cancer dashes hopes of a future uncluttered by medical procedures, treatments, and worsening illness, regardless of what the reality would be without a prostate cancer diagnosis. A partner more succinctly thinks about being left alone, whenever death comes along. Accepting that a cure is no longer an option and learning to live with prostate cancer as a chronic illness takes time and psychological adjustment, even though men with recurrent prostate cancer can live many years. Yogi Berra's phrase, "It ain't over 'til it's over," may depend here on how we identify "it's over." In the world of prostate cancer, is it the end of life? Is it the end of life known before cancer? Is it the end of a vision of happy and healthy living until death that is based more on idealistic hopes and wishes rather than on whatever reality will bring?

In Chapter 3 we discussed coping with the anticipatory worries of active surveillance treatment after initial prostate cancer diagnosis. Active surveillance may also be the treatment recommended by your urologist or oncologist when there is an increasing PSA biochemical recurrence after definitive treatment but no tangible signs of progression of disease on imaging tests. Your PSA levels will be monitored regularly and you will have periodic MRI and/or other scans to check for disease progression. Living from PSA test to PSA test can be tormenting, as it was for Bob and his family described in the last chapter. Yet many men handle the psychological aspects of active surveillance well when they engage in adequate education and counseling from their oncology team. Those who are anxious before prostate cancer are likely to be more anxious with an active surveillance regimen. All of the techniques described in Chapters 4 and 5, including cognitive behaviorally oriented therapeutic techniques, DRAFTing with Emotional Judo (EJ), relaxation techniques and meditation, exercise, proper nutrition, and, if needed, medications (antianxiety medications or antidepressants) can be used to relieve distress so you can enjoy your life while you are alive. In fact, they may be even more necessary now, given what feels like increased stakes.

Some research has shown that men who have more anxiety with a biochemical recurrence are more likely to get started on androgen deprivation therapy (ADT) earlier than those who are less anxious. Treatment of anxiety is encouraged in these men to see if they can cope with a "no active treatment" phase, given the impact on quality of life and an unclear benefit for longevity or medical outcome for those on ADT.

The range of emotions felt after recurrence of prostate cancer mimics the new diagnosis phase. Emotional recuperation strategies will need to address whatever emotions arise again or show up for the first time each time a treatment stops working or does not work at all. Strong emotions may need to be addressed again if you hear that there are no further active treatments for your cancer, and your doctor is recommending comfort care. After the initial shock about recurrence, painful feelings gradually subside as you hear what the next treatment strategy is. Sadness, anxiety, and anger can be foreign and awkward for many men. Once again, you have to reacquaint yourself with mortality, even though imminent death is not likely on the radar screen. There are some "troupers" who say, "Just bring it on, I can handle anything." As much as most people would like to have this gutsy attitude, it is not common. How your spouse or partner handles the information will affect your own reactions: do you both have a fighting spirit ("We'll fight this recurrence together, with our best shots") or a pessimistic one ("We are doomed; what's the point of more treatment if quality of life can become so bad? Let's stop now."). It may not be stated so succinctly, but this is often the atmosphere that exists and the message that is communicated because a couple feels so frightened and helpless. If the good-faith bubble burst when you got the initial diagnosis, a recurrence can completely decimate whatever rebuilding of confidence and faith that was able to take place. The same issues of disbelief, denial, anger, sadness, and anxiety may be present. You had "definitive" treatment for a cure; now you have to get used to the idea that there is likely no cure. At best you can look forward to controlling a chronic illness, hopefully for a very long time. This is now a cancer to live with. Winning is no longer defined by the complete elimination of the prostate cancer, but perhaps by remissions or keeping the cancer stable. This takes getting used to. This prognosis would have been fantastic news to any man diagnosed with advanced prostate cancer 30 years ago. Today, much more is expected.

Recurrence of the cancer is perhaps one of the biggest disappointments and losses to cope with. Now there is a more or less permanent loss of a man's sense of immortality, held onto through youth and maybe even middle adulthood. There's no denying that there's a good chance you will die of prostate cancer if nothing else kills you sooner. Most men find relief when a doctor says, "though you have prostate cancer, you will die of something else." Others say that if only they could know how long they still have to live they would cope better. That is an echo of the desire to be in more control and "have it my way," discussed earlier. Few men would really be satisfied if the predicted date of death were in the near future. After a recurrence, coping depends on what treatment you decide on, how well that treatment is tolerated, and how well it ultimately works to reduce or stabilize the PSA and keep the cancer under control. Older men, more often than younger men, must consider other illnesses they have that could compromise or complicate prostate cancer treatment, as well as their overall health. Frequent thoughts about death or dying occur with recall of others known who have died. The older men get, the more likely they are to see other family members and friends die. These ruminations are frightening, demoralizing, and unwelcome. However, with proper support, perspective, and DRAFTing with Emotional Judo, you can manage this next phase of coping with your cancer with calmer anticipation, or less apprehension, and more success living the best you can.

"My Doctor Wants Me to Take Female Hormones . . . Is He Nuts?"

Hormonal therapy, also called *androgen ablation* or *androgen deprivation therapy* (ADT), is a common treatment for prostate cancer. It was discussed briefly in Chapter 6 regarding its impact on men's sexual functioning, intimacy, and close relationships. In early-stage prostate cancer, hormones are used as an adjuvant treatment for primary radiation therapy. It is the common treatment for men whose prostate cancers continue to biochemically progress, as noted by increased PSA levels after definitive treatment, and is used when the disease has already spread outside the area of the prostate or has metastasized to other parts of the body. ADT is also used for salvage radiation therapy if an initial prostatectomy did not cure the cancer. Targeted radiation therapy to treat troublesome metastatic lesions is used to palliate, that is, to relieve or prevent symptoms, often in combination with hormonal therapy.

Androgen ablation agents are synthetically produced to have antihormonal or anti-testosterone effects. Their purpose is to decrease the impact of testosterone that fuels the growth or spread of prostate cancer, essentially starving the tumor. However, these medications have understandable negative effects on natural hormonal secondary sexual characteristics of men. They also cause problematic physical and emotional side effects. Before synthetic androgen blockade medications were available, men would undergo surgical castration with similar clinical benefits and complications. Surgical castration, or orchiectomy, however, has become unpopular, even though testicular prostheses have the look and feel of testicles to decrease the disfigurement and distress of the surgery. You could make a good argument that a one-time surgical orchiectomy is a less expensive therapy over time than periodic injections of a medication; however, surgical castration may be more emotionally and physically scarring than taking hormonal treatments, as ADT allows for intermittent treatment (time off of hormones and away from the side effects).

Testosterone is produced in the testicles, but its hormonal control center is in the brain—specifically in the pituitary gland. The pituitary gland manufactures a protein called gonadotropin-releasing hormone (GNRH) that attaches to a matched receptor that enables the release of luteinizing hormone (LH) and follicular-stimulating hormone (FSH) from the pituitary gland. LH travels to the testes where it stimulates production of testosterone, the hormone men need for a myriad of functions and purposes, including sexual characteristics, erectile functioning, energy, stable moods, body hair growth, the ability to carry out many attention and concentration functions, muscle strength, and bone density. But testosterone can also be the propellant that feeds an existing prostate cancer. These synthetic cancer-fighting hormonal treatments for prostate cancer have traditionally come in two general types. GNRH agonists such as Zoladex (goserelin) or Lupron (leuprolide), or antagonists like Firmagon (degarelix), produced to look like GNRH, ultimately block that connection between the releasing hormone and the hormone receptor. This decreases or downgrades the number of available receptors and blocks release of LH from the pituitary by interrupting the testosterone-producing feedback loop to the brain. This process cuts off the "produce more testosterone" signal from the testicles and significantly diminishes testosterone activity.

The GNRH agonists and antagonists are given in a depot fashion, which means that the medication is injected and then slowly released into the blood according to a predetermined schedule, depending on the particular medicine—over the course of either a month, 3 months, 4 months, or, in some cases, a year. The centrally acting GNRH agonists or antagonists are often taken in conjunction with peripherally acting antiandrogens or androgen antagonists such as Eulexin (flutamide), Casodex (bicalutamide), and Nilandron (nilutamide). These synthetically produced antiandrogens block the targeted receptors at the surface of the testis and decrease local testosterone production. Combined use of the centrally acting GNRH medications and the locally acting antiandrogens is called *complete androgen blockade* or *androgen deprivation therapy*, which reduces testosterone activity as completely as possible. Some of the older hormonal therapies, in particular the estrogen components such as diethylstilbestrol (DES), have fallen out of favor because of the possibility of cardiovascular problems and clot formation.

Over the last few years, new hormonally related medications, abiraterone (Zytiga) and enzalutamide (Xtandi), are improving men's quality of life and adding to longevity. Abiraterone inhibits enzymes in the testes, adrenal glands, and prostate tumor tissue, decreasing circulating levels of testosterone. Abiraterone is given with the steroid medication prednisone in order to maintain physiological actions of the adrenal glands that abiraterone may interfere with. Enzalutamide is an androgen receptor inhibitor. Many men tolerate these newer medications better than the more traditional hormonal treatment.

Many prostate cancer oncologists are cautious about the use of hormonally active agents for non-prostate cancer fighting purposes (i.e., megestrol used as an appetite stimulant or to decrease uncomfortable hot flashes) when trying to achieve androgen blockade. They want to avoid the possibility that the prostate tumor cells will become "immune" and thus desensitized to these medication types by undergoing chemical or genetic mutation; otherwise, the tumor may become resistant to the anti–prostate cancer effects of the androgen blockade. This concern was borne out of the discovery that stopping or withdrawing an anti-androgen treatment like flutamide or bicalutamide after a PSA level has begun to climb can lead to a decrease in the PSA level.

The frustrating list of quality-of-life side effects of hormonal medicines includes sexuality, with decreased libido and erectile dysfunction; body image changes, including decreased testes size and growth of breast tissue; fatigue; hot flashes; attention and concentration problems; cardiovascular difficulties; changes in glucose metabolism and possible diabetic concerns; and emotional symptoms of anxiety, irritability, and depression. These side effects do not affect all men, and the severity of the symptoms varies greatly when they do occur. Even those men who are only getting adjuvant hormonal treatment for a discrete period of time as an addition to a primary treatment of radiation therapy worry about whether the hormones will have permanent effects. Intermittent ADT treatment, described earlier, can give periodic relief from the harsher side effects.

These side effects are sufficient for many men to feel as if they are going through an identity crisis; their bodies feel alien to them. The hormones also increase a man's vulnerability to develop emotional symptoms such as anxiety, sadness, depression, irritability, and tearfulness, often with minimal stressors. The change in testosterone function essentially resets men's emotional thermostat regulation in the brain. Emotional reactions on hormones get triggered with less provocation or prompting, and often with more intensity, than they do without hormones on board. The same reactions can occur with steroid medications. All of these changes have led many men to tell me, "I don't feel like a man anymore." A television commercial or a grandchild's photo may easily bring tears now. A study by William Pirl, a psychiatrist at Massachusetts General Hospital in Boston found that men more likely to get significantly depressed on ADT were those who had significant histories of depression before their prostate cancer diagnosis.

Possible Side Effects of Hormonal Treatment and Decreased Testosterone

Erectile dysfunction and decreased libido

Fatigue and muscular weakness

Gynecomastia (increased breast tissue)

Decreased testicular size

Decreased body hair

Hot flashes

Cardiovascular risk

Diminished attention, concentration and multitasking ability

Diabetes risk or insulin resistance

Loss of bone density

Weight gain

Emotional changes, including anxiety, mood lability, depression, and irritability. These can be direct effects of hormones or reactions to above complications.

Many men become tearful more easily than in the past. There may not be an obvious cause—baby diaper commercials; leaving your son's house after spending a day with your grandkids; not feeling like going out to dinner with friends; or a urinary accident—have all brought tears to many of the men I have treated. **D**etecting and **R**ecognizing the emotional reactions of tears or irritable or depressed moods, as well as **A**cknowledging the rational and not so rational triggers to the situation, either with the mood/activity chart or the DRAFT with EJ techniques described earlier, can help you sense emotional changes more quickly, and then **F**lip them and **T**ransform back to the present using one of your prearranged alternative distracting activities from your quick list. Sometimes these physiological reactions are too quick and intense to manage with EJ and medications are needed to prevent or diminish these upsetting symptoms, as described in Chapter 5.

How Can You (and Others) Find Relief from Your Rage and Moodiness?

Knowledge

Very often, finding out that the hormones may be the cause of snappy changes in your mood or difficulty remembering or multitasking is enough to bring psychological relief and, interestingly, more stability to your mood. Awareness of why you are feeling or responding in a certain way gives you a heads-up to consciously slow down in order to improve your concentration or let a mood pass without questioning your sanity. Knowledge is power. It leads to a greater sense of control and therefore more calm. Distress and frustration grow and intensify when symptoms are experienced "in the dark" as random and unpredictable changes in your body and emotions. But identifying patterns of triggers, including the intensity, duration, and frequency of mood changes, which you can record in your mood/activity chart, can lessen the angst about "out of the blue" chaotic fluctuations. You can clarify what's going on, so you can get a better handle on your reactivity.

Non-Medication Aid

The DRAFT with EJ techniques from Chapter 4 will come in handy again now. Even though your emotional sensitivity may be fueled by ADT now rather than by a reaction to a stressful situation, these techniques can help you identify what is happening, by **D**etecting and **R**ecognizing the emotional reactions you are having now, whether they seem appropriate or not. **A**cknowledge that the reason these reactions are present (at least in part), whether rational or not, is that you are taking a medication to save your life. And if you have already decided to save your life, it makes sense to have the best life possible, with less arguing and less isolation. This is a vulnerability that can be lived with and overcome. At this point, you can again rely on **F**lipping and **T**ransforming, by breathing or meditating, by recognizing what is going well for you, and by finding an alternative activity or task until the emotion runs its course.

Severe and uncomfortable hot flashes, fatigue, and moods can also improve with a variety of medications as well as with other common-sense interventions. Oncologists are able to use intermittent therapy (the on–off schedule of ADT described earlier, depending on PSA levels) for those men who cannot easily tolerate ongoing hormone therapy. Intermittent therapy may help partners and spouses get respite from the wide-ranging consequences of hormonal therapy that a partner and husband go through. Mild exercise and other lifestyle changes can counter many uncomfortable side effects of hormonal therapy, including hot flashes, low energy, and concentration problems.

Sex: If I Don't Feel It, Why Would I Want to Do It?

Many men say that the erectile problems from hormonal therapy are not so troubling to them because the hormones also eradicate their sexual interest or libido: "It used to upset me that I couldn't get hard when I still had an eye or thrill for sex. Now, I don't even think about it." This is difficult for spouses or partners to accept as well. The disappearance of physical intimacy in the relationship can leave a couple with a platonic connection: "We're more like roommates or housemates than a married couple." Sex therapy with a trained therapist can help you express the feelings brought on by sexual dysfunction related to hormonal therapy. Sensate focus techniques described in Chapter 6 can also help a couple learn alternative ways of sharing sexual and physical intimacy and finding pleasure.

Pharmacological and Mechanical Help

As noted in Chapter Sex (6), consultation with a urologist who specializes in male sexual problems due to prostate cancer can also provide information and support to optimize sexual options and satisfaction. The PDE-5 medications that aid erections (sildenafil, tadalafil, and vardenafil) may be less effective when hormonal therapy is on board. Yet men are quite resistant to trying penile injections with vasodilating agents, which have an excellent record of helping men achieve erections in these situations. Many men are unwilling to trying other options such as vacuum erectile devices, penile suppositories, and penile implants to obtain erections because they take time and effort and sometimes a surgical procedure, which can dampen the natural or spontaneous romantic moment. These don't always substitute satisfactorily for "the real thing." Unfortunately, none of these alternatives can replace testosterone's role in stimulating sexual interest. Taking sildenafil, tadalafil, or vardenafil alone with successful results will not get a man in the mood for sex. However, "priming the pump" with a romantic dinner, music, even a sexy movie and physical stimulation can pique sexual interest. Those men who feel emasculated by the hormones also feel a lowered sense of self-esteem. They may think, "Why should I get into a situation where I might feel like a failure?" Though lack of libido takes some pressure off of a man to want to improve erectile dysfunction, it can increase the frustration of a partner who craves physical closeness and intimacy.

Who Am I?

Changes in body appearance by hormones can include growth of breast tissue (gynecomastia), shrinkage of testicles, weight gain, or loss of body hair, which leads many guys to exclaim, "I am not a man anymore. I don't feel like a man and I don't look like a man anymore. Who am I?" Some men avoid previously pleasurable venues such as the gym or the beach because they are embarrassed to get changed in a locker room or take off their shirts, in addition to feeling less energy to do these activities. Some view their body image changes as a barometer as to whether the hormones are still working and get worried when they start to see some of their former bodies making a reappearance, as this means to them that the hormones are no longer working to fight the cancer.

Men have been told that the primary hormonal treatment can keep an advanced prostate cancer in check on average for about 18 months. As we've seen with PSA anxiety, anticipation of recurrence can be experienced from PSA test to PSA test, intensifying as a man nears 18 months of treatment, 2 years, and for a number of PSA tests afterward. One patient I took care of was still watching regularly for hair to return to his forearms and chest 4 years after starting hormonal therapy. It would be a sign, in his mind, that the hormones were no longer working and that he could anticipate his PSA would begin to rise and his cancer progress. Watching for return of hair may have been a good anxiety reliever for this man, but only as long as there were no signs of hair growth. It was a daily at-home proxy for his PSA tests. However, just as with the PSA test itself, other signs that the hormone treatment may have stopped working weren't adopted as an early warning system to find a problem that could be addressed before the cancer got out of control. It was only seen as an on–off signal for the cancer and impending death. When this man thought hair did start to return, his anxiety, and death anxiety in particular, leap-frogged.

"I'm Tired of Being Tired"

Hormonal agents cause muscle weakness, fatigue, and lack of motivation for many men within months of commencing therapy. These symptoms are particularly upsetting to men who led active, productive, and independent lives. Men cut back activities, have less enthusiasm, or stop doing some things altogether. This may result in increased dependence on family or friends, which is a further reminder of how different these men were before the cancer. Family members begin to think the patient is depressed and that an antidepressant is needed. In this instance it may be helpful to review the sections on fatigue in Chapter 7.

Fatigue and lack of motivation are also affected by illness, by muscle weakness independently caused by the hormones, and by other medications, such as opioids for pain, steroids, and chemotherapy. Unless an antidepressant has an activating effect that improves the man's energy, his engagement, interest, and mood would likely remain the same, since this is not an ordinary depression. He may feel depressed because he cannot do more. If asked what he would like to do if I could improve his energy, he would give me a list of interests he would love to participate in. If able, he would gladly do more. On the other hand, the man who has a significant clinical depression would say, "It doesn't matter. I don't care." His depression causes him to feel as if he couldn't care less.

As noted in Chapter 4, reorganizing your schedule and setting realistic daily goals will result in less distress about tiredness and feeling like you cannot get things done. Review your medications with your physician to see if any can be taken at a different time of day or night, substituted with one that does not increase fatigue as much, or may be eliminated altogether—but don't try experimenting on your own.

An activating medication like a psychostimulant or the antidepressant bupropion may also alleviate some or most of your fatigue. I recently treated a man with the psychostimulant methylphenidate who had been demoralized that he had to give up his golf game because of fatigue. He was very grateful that he was able to get back to the game he loved so much. Alternatively try getting in E-Motion (Chapter 7).

"I Sweat Worse Than My Wife Did When She Went Through Menopause"

Hot flashes are caused in men by many of the hormonal treatments for prostate cancer, including orchiectomy. Symptoms include sweating and feelings of intense heat and chills. Women experience similar discomfort during menopause. Rarely, men elect to stop their hormonal therapy because of drenching sweats and chills caused by hot flashes, especially if sleep is disturbed by the sweats with multiple nighttime awakenings that may be further exacerbated by needing to urinate frequently.

You can ask your doctor if you are a good candidate for intermittent hormonal therapy if your hot flashes are very debilitating. It's like having a "drug holiday" until there is sign of the PSA rising again or of the disease progressing in some other fashion.

Short of stopping the hormones intermittently, some lifestyle adjustments can improve management of hot flashes. Alcohol, caffeine, and hot beverages make hot flash episodes more frequent and more intense for many. Therefore, cutting back or cutting out these beverages can bring relief. Cooler clothing in warmer weather or layered clothing in winter may ease hot flashes or help you control your response. Keep rooms, especially bedrooms, cooler all year long. Try to compromise on a moderate temperature with your partner so that she or he does not freeze as you cool down. Small handheld fans can also be refreshing while you are out of your house on a hot day. Some studies report that acupuncture and mindfulness meditation can reduce hot flashes or at least lessen the distress from them.

Antidepressants, particularly the serotonin reuptake inhibitors (SSRIs), such as sertraline (Zoloft), and paroxetine (Paxil), and serotonin-norepinephrine reuptake inhibitors, such as venlafaxine (Effexor) and duloxetine (Cymbalta), have been found to reduce the frequency and intensity of hot flashes. It is not clear whether they relieve the distress of having the hot flash symptoms or alleviate the flashes directly. This is an interesting finding, given that these same antidepressants can also cause flushing and sweating (which sounds like a hot flash to me). Neurontin (gabapentin), an antiseizure medication that is also used for pain control, has also been found to relieve hot flashes, as have some of the older antihypertension medications.

Chemotherapy and Quality of Life

People fear chemotherapy. It is felt by many to be the "old-fashioned, last-ditch effort" or last treatment option available for prostate cancer. Men feel terrorized about what will happen if it doesn't work: "Will it be worth it?" Many are old enough to have seen the harsh effects of chemotherapy from years ago. Debilitating, frightening nausea, vomiting, or diarrhea often made a patient feel much worse before getting better, and many times they did not get much better at all. There have been significant improvements in chemotherapies and in medications that ease the side effects of chemotherapy in the last decade. There is a better understanding of how to use these treatments for improved outcomes. More aggressive treatments are used yet are more easily tolerated than the chemotherapy regimens of the past. But these improvements are not sufficient for some men who decide that the potential *quality of life* deficits are not worth the potential *life-extending* benefits of chemotherapy. Again, without a crystal ball, it is tough to get a glimpse into the future and what either option will actually bring.

Fatigue from chemotherapy is treated the same way as with hormonal therapy. Your oncologist would make sure there isn't a reversible physiological cause of fatigue such as anemia, a thyroid problem, other electrolyte abnormalities, or vitamin deficiencies. Men can track daily fluctuations of their fatigue in a mood/activity chart and see when it is at its worst. Then they can avoid more physically intense activities during those periods. Hydrating and eating as well as you can are important. You might also consider the light exercise activities (walking, stretching, and easy resistance/strength-training exercises) of E-Motion discussed previously. Over the course of a number of weeks, these exercises have been found to either improve energy or at least prevent it from sagging as much as it would without the exercise. Again, an activating antidepressant (i.e., bupropion) or a psychostimulant can be used if there are no medical prohibitions.

You Think You're Not Thinking as Clearly as You Think You Can

"My Concentration Isn't What It Used to Be before the Hormones or Chemotherapy"

Patients treated with chemotherapy have long complained about a "brain fog," more commonly known today as "chemo-brain": problems with attention and concentration while getting, or after receiving, chemotherapy. Many studies have documented deficits in decision-making cognitive functions that include memory, attention, and the ability to multitask, to organize and plan ahead, and to problem solve. These subtle glitches in concentration make it more challenging to carry on routine activities of living. The impact of chemotherapy on concentration is not highly predictable from patient to patient or with all chemotherapy agents. Taking care of bills, other office work, strategic planning, or even handling a phone call when someone rings the doorbell can become daunting and overwhelming. It may be a good idea to ask for basic concentration screening prior to starting your chemotherapy or hormonal therapy, although this is not yet a standard recommendation.

Cognitive dulling has been noted in men with prostate cancer treated with hormones as well. It has been noteworthy to observe men getting hormonal treatment who complain about concentration problems, and then see them after they opt for intermittent treatment. Their reasoning and intellectual fitness subjectively seem much improved after being off the hormones for a few months. Improvement in cognitive sharpness after hormonal therapy has been noted with cognitive behavioral therapy, mindfulness medication, aerobic and resistance exercise, as well as with wakefulness agents or stimulant medications.

Thinking about Dying and Death Does Not Mean Throwing in the Towel

> Sure I worry about dying and suffering; I think most people do at some point after a cancer diagnosis. After all, I've already lived 72 years. But I do not have pain now, I am not suffering physically and I am not in fact dying now. I worry about the events I might miss after I die, like seeing my granddaughter graduate from college. However, I have been fortunate to witness her birth and to spend very happy moments with her and with my entire family. I am writing my memoirs so she will know who her grandpa was. I am laying the foundation for an important legacy.

End-of-life worries shadow men with prostate cancer from the early stages of diagnosis through advanced and progressive, metastatic illness. The focus is sharpened after recurrence of disease. Younger men with prostate cancer tend to be angrier. They mourn and fear different losses than those of older men. They know that cancer can mean death regardless of a hopeful prognosis.

At this stage you have the opportunity to re-evaluate your life, whether older or younger—where you've come from and where you'd like to go—and figure out if there are things that could use some fixing or tweaking given a potentially shortened life span—even though this may not have been in your sights before. Refocusing on future scenarios that include relationships, career, and retirement plans, or giving priority to the smaller joys in life can be powerful value-added life management tools. Hobbies, writing, taking classes, going for walks, or doing exercise or any number of fun undertakings alone or with loved ones help paint a new life image.

Many men tell me they are not afraid of death, as they know that we all die. But very few look forward to "the dying part." They fear the suffering they believe will come along with decreased self-sufficiency, a decreased sense of wholeness, and increased dependence on others. Whether spiritually or with some larger-than-oneself life worldview, these men can accept the finiteness and finality of their physical lives in the natural cycle of life. These viewpoints can change over time. If you have mental images of suffering or of being in pain with advanced disease sometime in the future, even early in your illness while still feeling well, it may not be easy for you to see how you could adjust or cope when that reality hits. Our brains imagine worst-case scenarios in fast-forward speed, which does not allow for time-dependent, real-life adaptation, adjustment, or change along the way. The man who fears a painful dying process and debilitation while his only sign of illness is a rising PSA after surgery or radiation treatment indicating that cure is not likely possible any longer may be jumping the gun when he states, "I'm not going to live with pain or like a vegetable when that happens . . . I will take my life first." He may not say this often or share it with family, and he may not really mean it, but it can negatively impact his interactions with significant others. The reality is that he, like so many other men, will get used to the slow progression and sometimes long remissions of disease progression. If the disease does progress, assuming it does not come too fast or drastically, he, too, will adjust and adapt to the weakening and debilitation of his body as he gets to new baselines, often over the course of months or years. New standards are developed to accommodate for changes and compromises in physical or cognitive functioning.

Other men spend parts of many days contemplating "what it will be like not to be alive anymore." Although they can accept, with some dismay, that death is a natural process, it is hard to fathom that life, and loved ones, will go on without them.

Aging before Dying

In an afternoon therapy session, Jim told me that he had no fear of dying or of death. We spent many sessions discussing the tension between wanting to live on the one hand, but not welcoming the ravages and disappointments of getting older and weaker. Aging and debilitation were more concerning for him than dying. He felt a conflict arise as he thought of his roles as an aging husband, father, and grandfather, while his wife, children, and grandchildren had to deal with their own health, family, relationship, and career problems. He wanted to help and support them and to fix their problems. Yet he described the psychological pain of living long enough to see difficult and tragic circumstances that his grown children and grandchildren had to endure. He felt impotent, not being able to easily repair or prevent these problems as he was able to do when he was younger and more vital.

Earlier in his life he would have had more clout or power to help. He felt he *should* still have it, and felt guilty that he did not. He discussed the frustration of glimpsing his image in the mirror, an image of an aging man who used to be so vital and virile. He said he could see that same reflection in the faces of strangers who offered him seats on the bus or subway; he recalled how when he was younger, he used to be the one to offer seats to the elderly or infirm.

Use of EJ helped Jim eventually transform the images in his mind and his behaviors. He was able to see the changes and losses in his life from a different, more objective vantage point by talking about them. He was able to grieve and not get stuck in a wallowing depression about aging.

He was able to make the best of these situations by taking responsibility for fulfilling and achieving what he could still do that was important to him and his family. He eventually reframed one aspect of his aging doldrums by helping those strangers he met on the bus or subway whom he imagined felt more vital and virile when he accepted their offer of a seat to an elderly man.

Chapter 10

Grieving for Loss of Trust, Physical Wholeness, and Sense of Immortality

Reinvesting in Your Future as a Wise Role Model

Great players who hang up their cleats can become great coaches, great teachers, inspirations and role models; this can be as vital to their legacy as their active playing days.

It's not easy to give up the life you've been familiar with after it has been diverted by prostate cancer. The uncertainty of the future that prostate cancer brings makes men realize how much of their existence they have taken for granted. Throughout this book I have discussed many transient and more permanent losses men and their families experience from the first abnormal PSA test through the positive biopsy, the diagnosis, treatment(s), side effects, and, ultimately, until death, whether from prostate cancer or, for those treated successfully, from any cause.

In this final chapter I review the importance of managing these losses rather than just taking them for granted. This process will help you find light before the end of the tunnel of life. Grieving for these genuine and perceived losses is as important a milestone for spouses and partners as for patients themselves. You can transcend these losses and flourish by identifying, acknowledging, and grappling with them, rather than getting stuck feeling like you are decaying emotionally or spiritually just because your body is declining. This is not unlike a gardener who prunes plants back in order to generate new life and growth.

T-easing into Retirement

Prostate cancer occurs much more frequently in men over the age of 65. Many men I consult with have been retired for a number of years, but not all have been happy and satisfied. Those most frustrated with retirement had dreams and fantasies of a relaxed and restful (R&R) retirement, envisioning themselves not answering to bosses, clients, or time clocks, "doing what they wanted, when they wanted." But many are disenchanted and bored by their "freedom." There is little to show for their golden years. The unstructured contrast to a working life—getting up and out of bed by a certain time; showering; dressing; getting to work by a certain time; being responsible for accomplishing something no matter how menial, important, taxing, or exasperating; concrete or service-minded labor; getting paid for effort; and leaving at the end of the day to go home—leaves many lives wanting and men feeling inadequate. Life feels dull and dreary without that work-oriented structure. Even welcome retirement means adjusting to change and the loss of lifetime habits and daily rituals. Self-identity itself undergoes reconstruction. Retirement may mean escape or relief to those men who were not happy in their jobs. My father couldn't wait to retire early at age 62. He spent his adulthood toiling in oppressive factory work. When he turned 60 and retirement was in sight, he looked forward to having leisure time and not being pressed to answer to anyone but himself. He didn't realize how the absence of structure and a time clock to answer to could be destructive. And some years later he got his lung cancer.

Prostate cancer can aggravate hopeful fantasies of R&R, especially when it shows up right before or early into a planned retirement. Those men with the "all or none" perspective discussed earlier give up hopes of having a more fulfilling retirement as they take on the battle of cancer.

Art was 69 years old. He practiced as a podiatrist for over 35 years. His prostate cancer was diagnosed and treated a few years before I met him. He was planning to retire in about a year, at age 70. He looked forward to traveling around the world with his wife. He had put off retirement since age 65 because he had been so happy with his career and felt so good physically. He had no reason not to assume his health would be as good at 70 as it was at 65, since he was cured of prostate cancer. However, he recently found out that his cancer had returned in an advanced stage. He decided to retire in a few months, a year before his original plan. He had not planned for this curveball. He now faced the premature loss of his profession as well as the loss of his plan. There is a Yiddish proverb that goes "Man plans and God laughs." Art encountered premature and intense grief for his now accelerated retirement plan, yet gratitude for a great career. He made sure to see or speak with all of his patients before selling his practice. He wanted to say goodbye and thank you.

Our therapy focused on the loss of his career, filled with highlights and many rewarding moments when patients thanked him for his excellent care. He talked about the loss of his retirement "plan" and the sadness of what he might *not* get to accomplish in his life. Before cancer he had talked a lot about what he was going to do in the future. He explored the anger about feeling as if life had just pulled the rug out from under him with his fast-forward plans. Instead, he now thought about dying and death and making sure his affairs were in order. He worried about how he would fill up his time without his practice and without his *plan*. What would he do if he didn't have the health and energy to be very active?

Retirement usually goes hand in hand with aging. Careers and work are for the young and middle-aged. Retirement, whether at the age of 60, 65, 70, or 75, implies getting older, weaker, less productive, and perhaps requiring more rest than previously. Neither retirement nor aging signals the imminent loss of life, though each may symbolically highlight limitations, weaknesses, and ultimate decline.

Aging and Mortality

Patient: I hate getting older.
Therapist: Is the alternative really better?

Aging, infirmity, debilitation, and the depletion of energy that worsen with advanced prostate cancer can be difficult to cope with. At the same time, improvements in being able to treat prostate cancer with greater success may set you up to deal with the benefits and drawbacks of otherwise "normal" aging. Gait disturbances, weakness, poorer eyesight or hearing, all common features of aging, can make men feel as if they are fighting a losing battle while wanting to enjoy the fruits of growing children, grandchildren, and hobbies they never had enough time for when they were younger. In a *New York Times* article, "Healthy in a Falling Apart Kind of Way," Jane Brody notes that as we get older we will likely develop various health problems of aging, yet we can still remain independent and feel "healthy." Mindy Greenstein and Jimmie Holland, in *Lighter As We Go*, note that sense of well-being can actually increase as people age.

It is worth taking on the challenge to make time to participate in life-enhancing wonders with your family so they are experienced as victories and joys for all of you to hang on to. The DRAFT with Emotional Judo (EJ) method cues you to **D**etect, **R**ecognize, and **A**cknowledge the understandable, rational, and irrational thoughts, emotions, and behaviors that arise around the physical and emotional challenges of aging and cancer, and ultimately **F**lip and **T**ransform the unhelpful, uncomfortable, and unproductive aspects into calmer, more valuable, and enjoyable ones. DRAFT with EJ can help you make adjustments to cope better with these changes. It will facilitate more contentment with the benefits of aging and less demoralization with the losses of aging.

I got an early taste of the incapacitating essence of aging when my hearing was sacrificed by the surgical removal of my acoustic neuroma brain tumor 9 years ago. I cannot hear from my right ear and there is no hearing aid that can properly help with this. I also cannot localize sound. Don't ask me which smoke alarm in the house is pinging to signal that its battery is dying. I often don't hear when people call me, especially when they are behind me on my right side or I am walking in the opposite direction. In a crowd of people I can do a 360 trying to figure out who is speaking to me if I can't see lips move or recognize the voice. Sometimes I think people are calling me when they're not, when I hear other noises in the background (even a psychiatrist can wonder if he is hallucinating, though I know I am not). I still have daily static-like ringing (tinnitus) in my right ear that I can now disregard most of the time. I have trouble hearing what people say on conference calls—I cannot easily figure out who is talking and often miss the beginning or tail end of sentences (I have often heard a punch line and people laughing, but missed the setup of a joke—quite annoying). It's really bad when more than one person is speaking at a time. Now at age 58, I have had years to get used to this. I felt very old, very quickly, after my surgery. As I adapted, I felt better. I joke about having a great excuse when my wife asks me to do things I don't want to: "Sorry dear, I didn't hear you." Friends and family are pretty tired of my "Sorry, were you talking to me?" jokes, although the humor was a nice bridge for all of us adapting better to my disability. When I cannot accurately hear what someone says, my brain sometimes comes up with odd, yet amusing alternatives. This makes for some very funny puns.

I fear what it will be like when real aging starts to impair my good ear. I could have become incapacitated by the angry, sad, and anxious emotions that stunned me, and I could have avoided many social situations. Instead, I used DRAFT with EJ to adjust. I grieved for this tangible loss as well as the many downstream changes that hearing loss caused for me. I truly believe my "hearing" while listening to patients has improved because I've had to focus more intensely, yet this also has a downstream effect on me by causing me to fatigue more quickly.

Most people experience understandable grief after a loved one dies. Grief is more complicated when losses are less obvious, less instinctual, less tangible, more hidden, and less appropriate for public discussion, such as the loss of a bodily function, a sensory function, a career, the "assurance" of taking an exotic vacation, or the loss of a sense of your own immortality that comes with a cancer diagnosis. The need to grieve for "the future that I used to count on and was still planning and hoping for" still exists.

The losses that pile up on men with prostate cancer include the loss of a future as they've imagined or planned it, however cloudy or clear that image may have been before cancer, and the loss of a sense of security that "all is right with my world and with me." With aging or diminished strength and energy that comes from a serious illness, you may feel more helpless. You may feel like you have little to live for. Losing any independence or autonomy can set in motion a snowballing fear of further losses. You may feel as if you have lost your sense of identity as an individual and as a man. You may grieve the loss of the future as you imagined it. You may have been hoping to be alive for some special event, or to make it to some particular age that you've had in mind for years where you see your grandchildren grow up beside you as you age. These imagined scenarios of the future are not concrete substances that you can literally see and touch right now. However, they can be quite real in your mind. You have worked very hard to make anticipations become real. And you can still make some of them happen.

Professional athletes are coached to visualize over and over again the successful catch, to imagine the perfect home run swing, to see the golf ball going into the hole, the basketball going through the hoop, or the kick of their legs when finishing a race. Why do we make wishes at birthday celebrations? Is that just child's play? Or do we have a better chance of making some wishes come true if we can perceive them more clearly? If we pray, why do we ask for certain things to happen? What's the point of being grateful for what we already have, even if it is not perfect or especially if we want more? We count on life events evolving more or less the way we want, allowing for some wiggle room, as long as the outcomes are relatively close to our goals and desires, whether appropriate, realistic, rational, or not. Looking forward to particular images of retirement, graduations or weddings of children or grandchildren, physical health, or the absence of disability energizes most people. But your hopes and dreams and your desired immortality are now threatened by advanced prostate cancer (or any major illness or life trauma), even if you will still get to participate in many future life-affirming events. Just the fear of their loss can blur the future or distract or derail you from the best present you can have. However, if you navigate your grief well, you can see through the current murkiness that has replaced what used to seem so crystal clear in the nonexistent crystal ball, and live more peacefully and contentedly with a revised and genuine mental picture of what is still attainable.

Grief therapy helps someone cope after the death of a loved one by providing the tools and safety net to deal with the pain and anguish of the loss and adjust to a revised life without a loved one. Whether erections are not rigid, urine leaks, or hearing is lost, when you first hear about your diagnosis or about progression of disease, no one has died. But it may feel as if your dreams, or your plan or guide, or your reason for living died. You can be thrown way off course. The diagnosis of cancer itself along with each treatment decision, treatment, complication, disappointing setback, or regret about options not taken earlier create losses that require acknowledgment, adaptation, or recalculation to move on. DRAFT with EJ can be applied to all of these issues.

When I mention losses and grief to patients and spouses, many recall the five stages of grief described by Elisabeth Kübler-Ross (denial, anger, bargaining, depression, and acceptance) in her groundbreaking book, *On Death and Dying*, and wonder where they are in those stages. These were groundbreaking concepts when developed in the 1960s and are still popular today. However, these stages are not applicable to all people, to all losses, or to all situations. These five aspects of grief may be present at different times or arise together or in different sequences. In fact, some may be completely absent when coping normally with loss.

Thoughts about death and depressed moods may be more intense and frequent if your disease has metastasized and is no longer curable, yet is not necessarily related to a major depression. One man recently told me, "It would be much easier if someone could tell me whether I have 6 months left, 6 years, or longer. Then I can plan better." The logic of this statement is evident. However, its helpfulness in the face of the uncertainty that shrouds death is less so. Physicians have been found to be notoriously bad at predicting time until death, unless someone is within weeks or a couple of months of death. I fear that even an accurate prediction of death more than 2 months into the future would not enhance most people's lives in our goal-oriented society. On the contrary, it could act as a barrier to full engagement and enjoyment of life that is yet to be lived. It's tough, but very possible, to not become preoccupied with the seconds ticking away. It is possible to live more fully in the seconds and days and months. Another man said to me: "I think about dying a little bit every day, and it saddens me. But then I snap out of it and go on with my day, appreciating whatever I can."

Hormonal therapies for advanced prostate cancer, including those that were not available until just a few years ago, can work for many years, even though advanced disease implies "no cure." Many men become fixated and psychologically paralyzed by the idea of no cure. Yet the certainty of death that we all face is tempered by the uncertainty of how, what, when, and where we will die. Others, rather than fixating on death, use the time before dying to mold the best life possible—they see uncertainty as opportunity even in this arena.

If your disease progresses through hormonal treatments, you will likely get one or more chemotherapy agents next. Though these will probably be among the last active treatments available to control your cancer, you can hope for the best possible response with the least severe side effects. Many men hope to stay alive long enough for the next wonder drug to come along. I've now seen many men benefit from that "next miracle medication." Unfortunately, others become crippled by a sense of this being the beginning of the end. They lose sight of the here and now, and the future they have left.

The goals of psychotherapy used with men who have advanced prostate cancer are to help them confront and manage the challenges and losses that encompass end-of-life issues. Psychotherapy can prepare a man to talk with his family and friends about his and their concerns regarding his mortality. These therapy sessions allow men, and family members who participate, to **D**etect and explore worrisome thoughts, sadness, and anger, and to **R**ecognize connections to other challenging, exciting, or frustrating experiences in their lives. They can **A**cknowledge how this situation, and the emotions and thoughts that arise from it, are distinct from others in the past. Then they can **F**lip and **T**ransform their painful though understandable current reactions to the present, and not miss life while they are alive, while preparing themselves and their loved ones for approaching death. This emotional tune-up clears much of the mortality fog and improves subsequent communication and relatedness. Men and their families are less consumed by the idea and fear of death and can live more fulfilled lives until death comes.

I am not naïve to not recognize the finality and sadness of death and the end of long-term relationships. However, focusing only on the "all or none" aspects of living or dying risks losing the potential for living a more fulfilling life. When men grasp this, they understand how to serve as important role models to guide close family and friends during these trying times. Too often, men are ashamed of their perceived or actual diminished strength. They inappropriately think they have little to offer others, and they feel like a burden to those who try to care for them.

> Look at me. I look thinner. I feel weak. What good am I? I don't have anything to offer anyone. I can't easily walk up the stairs to water the plants up there, so I don't water any.

Men and their spouses or partners can learn how to cope with the stressful, anxiety-provoking end-of-life challenges confronting them. There is a large middle ground in between being a super-coper and a failure. They can learn to see themselves as part of the genuine human condition and not isolated and unlucky to have to deal with these life-threatening odysseys.

Your planned-for future may still happen. But once you lose the familiarity of waking up every day assuming that today will be more or less like yesterday, and that tomorrow will have the same opportunities as today, you will move ahead with your life more successfully if you can grieve for that loss. Otherwise, you may spend your life wait-ing for "the train that has already passed" rather than moving on and living an adapted, gratifying life right now. Losses are marked by dif-ferent emotional reactions—tears, anger, sadness, resentment, and anxiety—and behaviors—isolation or impulsivity. But many men expe-rience tearfulness and other emotional reactions as alien and strange. Sometimes it is hard to distinguish between crying that is a biological reaction to a hormone or steroid medication and tears that are a reac-tion to sadness, depression, or sentimentality. Like a stuffed drain, the sludge-like residue can continue to accumulate and prohibit better liv-ing if not adequately understood and handled. Successful grieving fre-quently entails identifying and dealing with uncomfortable emotions that can spew from disappointment, disbelief, and a loss of trust when a cancer comes back or is not easily checked by hard-hitting treatments. These emotions intensify with worsening physical annoyances like fatigue and difficulty sleeping.

When first engaging in psychotherapy for these issues, men have said to me, "So, what I'm hearing from you, Doc, sounds like 'It's not whether you win or lose—it's how you play the game.' Bullshit, Doc! If I die, I lose; end of game. Period!"

The same exercises used in the DRAFT with EJ Playbook (**D**etect, **R**ecognize, **A**cknowledge, **F**lip, and **T**ransform) will help you deal with uncomfortable and intrusive grief and anticipatory grief emotions and place them in proper perspective. Then you can transition them and you to a less burdened state and a more solid psychological footing. You can alleviate inner pain and gain faster resolution of your distress. Though some patients feel they have "no choice" but to accept their cancer state, their passivity or withdrawal from a more active life and loved ones is essentially making a dismissive, non-accepting decision. If loss and sub-sequent grief are not dealt with appropriately, self-defeating thoughts and behaviors can inadvertently derail having a better life. Remember the men I discussed in Chapter 3 who decided to give up golf altogether because they no longer had the stamina to play 18 holes in one morning or afternoon? Those men who cannot stand that their game is just not as good as it used to be because of discomfort when they swing are also giving up fun, relaxing, and cherished time with friends in beautiful settings that tremendously enhanced quality of life for many years. Sure, the competition made games spicier or more interesting and challenging. But an "all in, or all out" strategy may cheat you out of more pleasure in life while you are still here. A psychostimulant, if you can tolerate it, may give you enough energy for a few more holes of golf. Nine holes are better than none. Going to the driving range or a putting green or meeting up with a buddy on the nineteenth hole on a sunny spring day will bring more joy than staying on your couch.

Patients who modify their games or other leisure activities thrive better. They manage the end game better. They turn singles tennis into doubles matches. If that becomes too demanding, they might volley easily with a coach or pro, because the swing and the sound of the ball on the racket on a beautiful day, or the ability to hit an easy backhand is not just good exercise for the body—it is a great workout for the mind and soul as well. I've seen men switch from playing baseball to softball to eventually just having a catch; or giving up the fast-paced sprinting and jumping of five-on-five full-court basketball to half-court games, to shooting free throws in the local schoolyard (with someone who can chase the ball when it gets kicked away). Running morphs into jogging, which transforms into walking. There may come a time when you will "hang up your cleats" for these sports and give them up altogether; at that point, experiment with less strenuous activities.

"All or none" thinking also impacts how you deal with many predicaments that emerge with advanced prostate cancer, just as was true for those who had complications from early-stage disease treatment. If you are concerned about urine leakage you may not go out socially with friends or family, especially if it coincides with decreased energy. You then risk boredom and depression and feeling cheated of camaraderie, which may loop back to worsen fatigue and interest in being more active. It's the same if you have difficulty getting erections. You might shun physical intimacy with your wife or partner and find that you have grown apart. You and your partner may feel lonelier, have self-pity or blue moods, and even become enraged by the unfairness of the circumstances life has brought you. If you are single, you may give up dating altogether because you cannot have intercourse anymore, shunning much of the socializing of pre-cancer days. The belief that "I am a dead man" can become a self-fulfilling, accelerated reality, figuratively as well as physiologically. "I am a dying man" might be more accurate, but that is clearly a "glass half-empty" assessment. If you give up so many of the things that made your life more worthwhile, and you resist finding new or different energy-appropriate alternatives, even toward the end of your life, you may eventually feel that that life is not worth living.

I want to clarify that a "glass half-full" approach to dealing with stressful situations is different from "you have to be positive and think positively all the time." In the world of advanced cancer, that statement is often followed by "or else your cancer will get out of control and you will die." This is another "all or none" statement, leaving few alternatives besides positive or negative thinking and eventual guilt for a cancer which progresses "because you were not positive enough"; this essentially implies that "you gave up." These beliefs are based on the view that stress and even negative or pessimistic thoughts depress immune system function, leading to a body not being able to defend itself sufficiently, which causes the initiation or acceleration of cancer growth. There have been no definitive studies to substantiate these claims over the longer term, though transient weakening effects of stress on immune systems by stress has been shown.

Can negative thoughts lead to poor lifestyle behaviors, such as smoking, drinking, not eating well, or not exercising sufficiently, which could ultimately worsen health in general? Absolutely! Patients have sought consultation with me after hearing the need to adopt these "positive mindset dictates." Men and their family members have asked me to make them think positively. One patient came to see me complaining, "My wife is trying to kill me . . . every time she picks an argument with me, I get upset, and I know my tumor starts growing more." Surely I believe it is better for anyone to be more positive than negative. I also believe it is possible, as our attitudes lie on a spectrum rather than in an on–off split. But not by giving what comes across as an ultimatum: Think positively or you will die. It is difficult to avoid stress and fear and anger. Essentially equating a negative attitude with self-destructive behavior is not useful, unless a major depression leads to suicidal behavior. It does not help to tell a man that if he is not positive enough his tumor will grow and get out of control. That causes more stress for most people. That gives a patient undeserved Almighty responsibility for the outcome of an internal biological process because of how he thinks or feels. Mind over body does not apply here. I once had a patient who felt he let himself and his family down because he could not be strong enough to control his thinking by being more positive as his tumor continued to grow. So he was saddled with a double whammy of progressive cancer and guilt for not being positive enough. Improving behaviors may be more tangible and realistic than initially trying to change emotions and thoughts, and may eventually lead to more positive thinking and emotions because of more engagement in life.

There are men who have always been able to see the bright side during setbacks and remain positive and optimistic regardless of the circumstances. I believe it is their nature. The gentleman I described in the Introduction, Mr. Jonah, who inspired the writing of this book by asking me, "Can you please tell me what I can expect to face emotionally in coping with my prostate cancer, so I can prepare for the crises before they erupt, and therefore handle them better?" was one of those positive thinkers.

It is atypical, however, to maintain a positive attitude when you're fatigued, feeling pain, just saw your PSA go up, feel some moisture in your underwear, or just changed another diaper pad. Most men might feel demoralized because of the stark contrast or disconnect between what they are understandably feeling (angry, worried, despairing) and what they are expected to feel (positive, happy) or want to feel. You might blame yourself for not being positive enough and wonder if your "negative" attitude is self-destructive. From my point of view, that is inappropriate and unhelpful. That is double jeopardy. That your disease progressed is bad enough. That you feel inappropriately responsible for it is even worse. This makes assuming a positive attitude even more difficult, which is a burden you do not deserve or need.

If, on the other hand, you throw caution to the wind when there are setbacks or frustrations and start drinking more alcohol, smoking more, stop exercising, become a non-socializing couch potato, don't take your medications appropriately, and don't eat or hydrate sufficiently, you may find yourself in the middle of the self-fulfilling prophesy that stems from potentially harmful behaviors—you're likely to feel worse physically and psychologically and not optimize your body's potential for healing and better health. The potential for a more hopeful attitude and improved vigor will sail away, beyond the horizon. Lethargy begets lethargy. Unchecked pessimism leads to less healthy behaviors. The unrealistic statements "don't worry" or "everything will be fine" are not believable or helpful for most men who are not accustomed to the positive mindset dictate. But you can be coaxed or coached along the "doing something good is better than doing nothing" spectrum, or the "glass half-full" method of managing stress, and DRAFT your way with EJ and ultimately feel better and more fulfilled.

Family members are understandably concerned when they see their loved ones suffering and in pain. They too are angered or depressed, as they feel powerless to change their loved one's illness. They may feel guilty and frustrated that they could not do enough to prevent or change the course of events. As noted earlier, counseling and support groups can improve the ability of spouses, partners, and adult children and you to cope better with the cancer, even when the cancer is progressing, and even when you may be nearing the end of your life. There is much good care and support available that can help and enrich all of your lives, even when your health is worsening.

A family's good intentions may unfortunately miss the mark when a man has advanced prostate cancer. There are four classic areas of good intentions gone awry that I want to address: information sharing to patient, family, and outsiders; fights over food; activity level; and socializing.

> ### *The Tension of Good Intentions: Four Common Traps of Loving Families*
>
> Information sharing vs. secrets: To tell or not to tell
> Food fights—food for thought: eating vs. grazing
> Staying active vs. idling
> Socializing vs. isolation

To Tell or Not to Tell?

Many families want to protect patients from bad news and emotional demoralization and pain. Patients often want to do the same for family members. One patient I treated became more depressed as his cancer continued to progress. His caring partner wanted to keep bad news from him for fear that it would demoralize or depress him even more. At different oncology office visits she asked the oncology team, "Please don't tell him how high the PSA is. Please don't tell him the cancer has spread. Please don't tell him it's now in his liver." Medical caregivers see that patients understand that things are indeed getting worse by how badly they feel physically and the complaints they make. Staff are aware of patients' frustration of doing less and less. Doctors and nurses ethically feel compelled to keep patients in the loop as long as they have the mental capacity to understand the medical situation and participate in decision-making with informed consent. *Informed consent* means that a patient can understand, and needs to have, appropriate information in order to make treatment decisions, and has the ability to make choices. The family of the patient just described wanted to keep the illusion of good health alive. This is reminiscent of cancer care many years ago, when some family members would ask that a patient not be told that he has cancer. Families encourage patients to continue doing things they have always enjoyed, like traveling; unfortunately, even favorite pastimes can become too physically and emotionally taxing. When they refuse to go along with travel plans, families assume the patient is depressed. Sometimes patients are afraid of not being close to home and not feeling well. Patients can be both anxious and depressed and may or may not benefit from an antidepressant and antianxiety medication and supportive therapy.

Regardless of psychiatric diagnosis, it is difficult to keep medical secrets in large clinics, hospitals, or families. Even with the consent of a patient who clearly understands what is going on and states he does not want certain information given to him about his prognosis or other medical details, it is very difficult to count on all practitioners to know about and abide by a strict "don't ask, don't tell" policy. First of all, the patient has to be aware of this plan, and be able to understand the issues being discussed. It is important for him to let the oncology team know what medical information he wants to know, and to let all of his doctors and nurses know what kinds of information he does not want to know about. Someone may inadvertently "spill the beans." If a patient has the ability to understand the information, he has the responsibility to say he doesn't want to have it and assign a healthcare proxy to make decisions for him. If he is going for tests and procedures, he will have to give consent for these tests, or at least concur that he is agreeable. Partners and patients should have this discussion with doctors and nurses and important others so that all can try to stay on the same page about information sharing. The patient should be as clear as possible about what information he wants to know and what he doesn't want to know.

> I don't want to hear my PSA level, just whether it's going up or down…I don't want to know where the tumor is spreading to…I don't want to hear about time-oriented prognoses.
>
> Let me know what I can do to feel better or stronger.
>
> Don't give me time lines of how much longer 'til I die, but let me know when I need to get my affairs in order.

Men often know what is going on medically even without explicit details from their doctors. They may not want numbers or predictions to obsess about. Families who lovingly try to protect their husbands or partners with news blackouts may find out that the men already know.

Sometimes men play along with the "tension of good intentions," fearing that talking about even their realistic doubts and concerns will sadden their family even more. More often than not, families really do have good intentions, trying to protect loved ones from harsh news and pain. But sometimes having accurate information even about bad news and forecasts can paradoxically be comforting. "I knew I wasn't going crazy" and "Now I can plan for a shortened life and not worry that I won't have time to do what I want to complete and get my affairs in order" are common thoughts of relief. Passively watching the unexplained *random* breakdown of your body may be even more frightening than knowing the details about how cancer is to blame.

Food Fights—Food for Thought: "I Want to Eat; I Just Cannot Eat"

Battles around eating are common when prostate cancer becomes more advanced. Some spouses equate a husband not embracing the highly touted anti-prostate cancer diet of low fat, no red meat, high soy, and green tea with self-destructive, almost suicidal behavior.

John and Jill had horrible arguments about food and eating for the 2 months before our initial visit. More accurately, their quarrels centered on John's not eating. Their verbal battles prompted Jill to ask John's oncologist for a psychiatric referral: "John has a problem—he won't eat. He must be depressed." She was convinced there was something wrong with John psychologically. She hoped I would be able to fix his irritability and unstable moods and get him to see reason, by eating more nutritious and calorie-filled meals.

Jill grew up with the understanding that without nourishment, you cannot thrive. She was devastated by John's slowly deteriorating physical status. He used to lift weights and had always been quite proud of his physique. She knew he couldn't lift the weights anymore; that would be an absurd expectation. But how could he not eat food? She had difficulty accepting his new-found distaste for the foods he used to love. She could not grasp his substantially decreased food intake in the same way that she understood his inability to lift weights. She could not acknowledge that it might be just as absurd to expect John to be able to lift his fork with zest and eat a hearty meal as it would be to lift those weights.

It is not uncommon for some men with advanced prostate cancer to lose their appetite. This can occur for many reasons, including pain, fatigue, medications like chemotherapy, or the cancer itself, which can steal taste or the ability to take in food. Regardless of cultural or ethnic backgrounds, most people believe that if you don't eat well, you don't stay healthy. This is a frustrating dilemma for patients with advanced cancer. I have observed many spouses and adult children arguing with patients over food, out of loving frustration, concern, and worry. Maybe these families always argued about food. But now there is a direct conflict based on clashing perceptions. From the patient's point of view, when you have no appetite, you cannot eat. These men say, "I just I can't eat. I can't force it down. I'll feel sick and throw it up." Their appetite signal has been turned off, and no amount of tender, loving care served with the food will make it go down any easier, faster, or more completely.

I did not think John had a significant depression or even a major psychological disorder when I evaluated him. He wanted to eat; he just couldn't. He wanted to go out with friends; he felt he couldn't because his energy was too low. He wanted to live long enough to see his granddaughter get married, but he knew that he wouldn't. He was sad about all of these shortfalls. Initially, when Jill offered more food to John and begged him to eat, she felt less helpless in the face of encroaching death. She thought they could control this downward spiral with better nutrition and cancer treatment. But since he couldn't follow the sage advice of his wife, he felt helpless, and she did too. They both felt worse.

Remarkably, the painful acceptance of reality through emotional insight gained through acquiring and using appropriate information along with lots of trial and error, or just faith, hope, and good luck, can transform your situation and your reactions and can free you so your life can become better. Experiment with different foods that may be more palatable as your taste buds change because of cancer-fighting agents. Nutritionists and dieticians have excellent suggestions for different food and beverage varieties and preparations to increase caloric and nutritional intake. Serving smaller portions more frequently during the day helps "prime the pump" so that a man does not feel as guilty or angry when he cannot attack a whole plate of food like he used to.

The therapy for "John's problem" turned into brief couples counseling and a referral to a nutritionist and to our integrative medicine service. Both John and Jill worked on understanding the situation from a different angle and from the other's perspective. They made the best of the current reality, rather than losing precious time, energy, and emotion arguing about what "should be" or feeling guilty about "what wasn't." Even though I did not think John had a major depression, I supported Jill's plan to seek help. It was important to see if John was depressed and to get that treated if needed. But it was also important to learn how to communicate about, live with, and improve their circumstances.

Appetite stimulants, or psychostimulants in low doses, can improve the desire to eat. But sometimes these medicines don't work. And these medicines can sometimes make things worse with unwanted side effects. For instance, a steroid medication called megestrol (Megace), used to arouse appetite in people with cancer, is not used for men with prostate cancer who are using hormonal therapy. There is concern that this medicine will speed up the time it takes for the tumor to turn off its response to cancer-fighting hormonal therapy. Remember the benefit–risk balance? If your fatigue is debilitating, it may be worth trying a psychostimulant. If side effects worsen your quality of life, or counter the benefits of the medicine you are taking to fight your cancer, it is not a good trade-off. An antidepressant called mirtazapine causes appetite stimulation as a side effect, in addition to offering relief of anxiety, insomnia, and depression, if present. Unfortunately, it can also cause daytime grogginess, which is not welcome if your energy is already low. You may have to decide which is more debilitating in your benefit–risk balance—appetite or energy, in order to choose to go on the medication. It is also possible that you might get only the benefit and none of the problematic effects. But you won't know that until you try the medication. The "correct" choice may be different for different men in different circumstances at different times.

> John was willing to try a psychostimulant that he tolerated well. It increased his appetite moderately but gave him a boost of energy that was also welcome. John and Jill saw their conflict from a new, common perspective, which led to less arguing and a more loving spirit in their household. This "new normal" was what both John and Jill were looking for and needed. Jill had a chance to deal with some of her fears and sadness about John's worsening health and ultimate death. Her guilt feelings that tried to push him to do what he couldn't, or that made her feel she wasn't doing enough to save him, ultimately transformed into improved understanding and compassionate caregiving.

Staying Active vs. Idling

> Larry enjoyed going to concerts and dinner with his partner Jim for many years. Those evenings out were fun. They enjoyed discussing the performances for days afterward. When Larry's cancer became more advanced, he couldn't easily sit through a concert, and dinner became especially frustrating because he didn't feel like eating much since starting chemotherapy. Going to half a concert was pleasant for a few months, but eventually even that was difficult for Larry. So he and Jim stayed home more, and Jim became concerned that Larry was depressed. In fact, Jim was feeling more depressed about Larry's worsening health. They came into my office together.
>
> Jim noted that Larry had always had a great passion for reading, but he had given this up over the last few months because of decreasing energy and stamina for reading. Jim heard about a book club and decided to join, hoping it would ignite Larry's interest. When Larry found that he was too tired to read, Jim guided the book club to books that could be listened to on CD, so that Larry could stay engaged. When Larry felt too tired to read or listen to the CD, Jim would read to him. Both Larry's and Jim's moods improved despite Larry's declining condition.

Reading is one of the many fuel-efficient passions that can be reawakened if your energy for more taxing activities feels too drained. My colleague Jimmie Holland has started a Vintage Book Club for older people with cancer. The group chooses one of the Harvard classics to read each month. Printing the articles in a large font makes reading more palatable when stamina is low. Then they discuss the readings as a group. Those who cannot make it into the group session join by phone. It is a real fan-favorite.

Energy-efficiency suggestions, as well as medications to enhance your vigor that were discussed in the fatigue section of Chapter 7, apply here as well. Accepting and then accommodating for current energy levels, regardless of how advanced your cancer may be, is beneficial. Doing something is better than doing nothing in terms of pleasure, mental alertness, better physical functioning, and family esprit.

When Sam needed to give up his weekly basketball game after his androgen ablation treatment zapped his energy, he became demoralized. He had always been a good multi-tasker, intermingling high- and low-energy projects. Since he was a kid, he loved playing all sports. Now at age 58 he had to figure out what less physically demanding projects he could do, and how to make them exciting. He started to write short stories and tried painting with watercolors. The painting didn't stick but the writing did. His writing told many of the stories of his life that he wanted his children to have as memories of him, and he hoped that the grandchildren he might never meet would be able to use them to get to know him. He eventually gave up jogging when he noticed his speed was almost a fast walk. In the winter he began to walk regularly, either on a treadmill, through his apartment building hallways, or in a large department store. In the summer, he walked outside, either alone, with a friend he used to play basketball with, or with his wife. His mood improved along with his engagement in activity.

Charles had recently stopped working when he restarted chemotherapy. He quickly became bored when he couldn't go to his fast-paced job as a banker. He dusted off his camera that he rarely had had time to use while working. He started taking it with him whenever he left the house—to doctor visits, to friends' houses, and to family gatherings; he took it on walks to the park or just around the block. He sent prints or digital copies to family and friends of exquisite nature and neighborhood scenes as well as family portraits. He eventually bought a new camera that was lighter and easier to carry around. Charles had a great time documenting life through his photo lens.

A retired teacher getting androgen ablation treatment had been putting on weight and feeling more fatigued. He noticed he wasn't really watching TV while he sat in front of it at home. "There's nothing good on; sometimes I just sit and stare, not following a program at all." He felt too tired to read, which he used to love to do when he was younger. He was happier than expected when he finally accepted a longstanding invitation from his former principal to meet informally with younger teachers at the school to mentor them with advice and encouragement. Initially he thought he should get paid for these discussions to make him feel more worthwhile. However, he quickly noted the great satisfaction he felt just being useful again. He was thrilled when junior teachers appreciatively gave him positive feedback about how helpful his suggestions were with complicated students.

There are many volunteer positions and opportunities men can participate in to match their energy levels and interests. Unfortunately, there is a large gap between what's available and getting that information communicated to patients in an effective way, even with Internet-savvy patients. There is also still a large gap in interest of men to take on these activities. If you are interested in being less bored, check your local library, schools, business associations, and charity organizations, which can lead you to promising work and give you a purpose again in helping others when you think there is little you can still offer.

Socializing vs. Isolation

It is easy to become isolated when you are not feeling well and your ambulating ability has declined. Men who overcome "detaching" behaviors by going out in public with family, friends, or health aides, with canes or walkers, have jumped over a major hurdle to socializing. Even though getting out of the house is an excellent antidote to sadness and demoralization, it takes courage and often a strong push against rising inertia and fatigue to find the "get up and go." It takes a leap of faith for men to transcend the stigmatizing implication of using a wheelchair to make a brief trip to a museum or to a park. Man after man has told me how much more alive he feels by having created a different present than he previously saw projected on his screen of the future. You can spend time with family or friends. You can continue to satisfy some of your culture-appetite. Lastly, you can prevent discouragement and depression, and perhaps slow down overall deterioration from cancer and aging, as you use Emotional Judo to **F**lip and **T**ransform the premature power of death so it does not take your life before you die. I believe this can be a win-win for you and your family.

Can I Say Goodbye Without Really Saying Goodbye? Role Modeling Wisdom and Bravery

Paul was a 70-year-old retired police officer with metastatic prostate cancer. He had difficulty tolerating his last round of chemotherapy and wondered what the future held for him. Paul had lived alone since his wife died years before. He spent hours searching the Internet for clinical trials that might extend his life. He found an experimental protocol that was appropriate for his condition, but noticed that the prognosis was generally unfavorable; if he did this protocol it really would be an altruistic venture that would hopefully benefit others, but not him. He understood that he could die of his illness soon.

His oncologist confirmed the grim outlook. Paul's grandchildren would be visiting from out of town in a few weeks, and he felt that it was time to say goodbye. He cried uncontrollably every time he thought about what he would say to them—he did not really want to say goodbye.

Paul came to see me at the urging of his oncologist. In our first session, he summarized the recent discussion with his oncologist about the likelihood that he would die over the next 3 to 6 months. We discussed what he wanted to say to his family. It became clear that Paul wasn't just having trouble saying a literal goodbye to his grandchildren. He was struggling with how to tell his grandchildren what they meant to him. He struggled with trying to figure out if he had done enough for them—he wanted to know that he was leaving a legacy that had nothing to do with monetary or tangible items. He wanted to know that he really meant something to them. Given his advanced illness, he wanted to make sure that his family understood how important they were to him and the wishes he had for them to have good, worthwhile lives after he died. Every time he thought of what he would say about their relationships and the future without him, he started to cry. He wanted to portray a picture of bravery, the way a cop should. So he did not want to cry in front of his grandchildren. He also thought his tears would upset them. I asked him to describe bravery to me. He began by describing courage and fearlessness, as a police office and former soldier might know it.

If you have pain, don't complain. If something bad happens, and you feel sad, don't cry. Remain the strong one—it's okay for others to "fall apart" but not you; you have to take care of them. If there is uncertainty, trust your gut. You've got good instincts. Plow ahead. Don't acknowledge fear or anxiety during a crisis—and man, this is a crisis. But never give up.

He conveyed all these criteria for bravery with tears rolling down his reddened cheeks. He felt between a rock and a hard place—how could he be brave and cry at the same time?

Paul's perspective of bravery was likely instinctual, yet also refined by years of training, coaching, and reinforcement. It is probably mandatory for anyone in the line of danger, such as police officers confronting criminals, or soldiers fighting an enemy in combat, or rescue workers heading into peril and uncertainty. To some degree, it is also important for a businessman heading into a crucial negotiating session, a young lawyer heading into his or her first battle in a courtroom, or a runner losing stamina during a race in memory of a loved one.

But bravery does not have to have blinders on. It may be defined differently for different situations. People learn to manage the crises of everyday life. They develop the techniques and skills of their trade with years of experience, successes, and mistakes, and then refine them as needed. But there are few training manuals for being ill or dying, apart from religious or biographical accounts.

The bravery principles Paul brought to the table for coping with and living out the end of his life with advanced prostate cancer were counterproductive. Stoicism or a "stiff upper lip" is called for at times in life. It can calm rocky waters for you or for others. But tough approaches do not have to be mutually exclusive of acknowledging and allowing normal emotions to develop, surface, and guide you. *It is especially important to allow some of the hormonal-driven emotions that may be at play to be expressed as you deal with more sensitive issues.* DRAFTing your emotions, thoughts, and behaviors with EJ can help you alter tactics that are not optimal for this part of your life and have more confidence that you can manage these situations well enough. You can take action to transform pessimism and demoralization into a more enriching life for you and your family. You can redefine bravery.

Your voice and actions may be the best model to help those around you experience, acknowledge, and express appropriate loving human emotions better. In fact, you may be the ideal role model to help others deal better with your ill health and end-of life concerns, as well as any relationship, career, or health dilemmas or frustrations that will come along in their lives after you are gone. You can be strong and cry too!

After my mother died of lung cancer, a friend came up to me and said, "Your mother died with dignity. She was so strong. She did not cry at all.

She told me that she was satisfied with her life, and was most proud of seeing her children succeed in life. She was ready to die. I hope I can be that brave when I am dying." I was a little taken aback. I recognized my mother's dignity, strength, and pride, and knew she had a strong back-bone. Yet she shed tears of remorse with me for what she would not be a part of in the future. Though she also expressed anger and sadness about regrets in her life, she felt she had come to terms with them. I observed the mixture of all of these. Either way, I knew she was ready to die and that she had been glad to live. Indeed, there are different strokes for dif-ferent folks at different times and different situations in different fami-lies and different cultures. It is useful to know who is in your presence. You can adjust for their needs and still be true to yourself if you are will-ing to take the responsibility of being a role model, teacher, and guide until you die. I thank my mother for modeling that for me.

> Paul and I spoke of the benefits of saying goodbye to his grandchil-dren in a way that would flesh out a commemoration of his past and a gift, or legacy, for the future, even if, and maybe especially if, he were to shed tears. "Come on, doc, could that really be good for them?" he asked initially. "Isn't it unnatural for children to see a par-ent or grandparent cry? Isn't it better to have a mental picture of "Gramps" as the brave police officer? It's hard to believe you are right on this one."

Our society glorifies the "stiff upper lip." That is the portrait of heroes in the media, in politics, and in sports. It is what my friend saw in my mother. From early on in life, most of us are taught to bury emo-tion and the benefits of a "win at all costs" devotion to a cause. This philosophy can belittle emotional reactions as fitting only for losers. I strongly believed that Paul's grandchildren would benefit from seeing another side of their Gramps' bravery, whether or not it was marked by his tears—that of someone who can talk about how precious life is, and who does not feel shame as he passes on a larger truth about life with heartfelt emotions. They will know how much he loves them and how much he will miss them when he dies. They won't have to guess, even if a formal goodbye was never uttered. He and they will know that it is okay to discuss and share what he wants most for his loved ones, not only by his words or how they are uttered. But if he cries, his tears might teach them an important life lesson: that there are times when keeping a stiff upper lip is not necessarily helpful (especially if they are ignited by medications); in fact, it can potentially backfire as a sign of weakness or shortsightedness if it impedes true, multilevel, multisensory communication and connection. You can send a number of messages at the same time that transmit strength and anxiety, sadness, caring, and bravery. All of these are fundamental symbols of a successful survivor!

We addressed another fear Paul had before he left my office: the Pandora's Box fear. If he cried when talking about his hopes and concerns with his grandchildren, would he start crying about everything else as well, until he died? The answer was simply and truthfully, "No." I felt that if he wasn't crying about everything beforehand, whether as the result of a medication side effect, a major depression, or just natural emotional overflow, the floodgates were not going to open up afterward.

> Paul came back a few weeks later feeling proud of himself and humbled. He had spoken with his grandchildren with tears in his eyes but largely maintained his composure. He focused on his message and the meaning he wanted to convey. His ability to talk about his concerns in therapy and express what was behind his sadness and tears allowed him to focus and accept whatever happened when he spoke with his family. A little rehearsal (yes, there is that practice thing again) didn't hurt, either.

Contemplating and planning for dying and death are not easy. Religion provides a comforting guide to many who face death. Religious faith offers people a vision of what they can expect in death and afterwards. The uncertainty factor is diminished if not removed altogether, the stronger their faith. But what about those who do not have a religious affiliation or are not comforted by faith? Are they doomed?

Frank was a 68-year-old man who told me, "I wish I were religious—I think death would be so much easier. Then there would be something afterwards to believe in. Even if it isn't true or accurate, I would believe it. Right now all I know is that I am going to die, be buried, and decay in the ground. Maybe it's too bad I had that religious stuff drummed out of me a long time ago. I envy those who believe in something."

Frank examined his death fears in therapy as well as his own beliefs of what happens after we die. He was comforted in his exploration and understanding that there is a season for everything, and that life is enhanced by the finiteness of death. He realized this was true not just for him but also for all of nature. He spoke about the legacy he was leaving behind for his family and that he was proud of what he had taught his children about these values since they were born. A chance to investigate one's philosophy on life and death and the emotions that come up from that inspection can be insightful and comforting.

Your legacy goes far beyond a last will and testament; you can prepare a real living will that encompasses aspects of yourself, your philosophies, your beliefs and spirituality, as well as your hopes and dreams developed throughout your life that you have likely taught and modeled for your family, friends, and colleagues and now leave to and for others who will continue living. Frank wanted to clarify some of his beliefs and hopes for his daughter, given relationship problems she had, as he neared death. He decided it would be important for both of them if he could write his thoughts down and present it to her as they spoke. Our therapy helped him put his thoughts on paper and then discuss them with his daughter.

Dr. William Breitbart, Chair of the Department of Psychiatry and Behavioral Sciences at Memorial Sloan Kettering Cancer Center (MSKCC), has an interest in synthesizing what great thinkers and philosophers have discussed through the ages about ideas that are important and consequential to people who face their mortality. He has done this with an eye on advanced cancer patients in particular as they near the end of their lives, to enhance their day-by-day reality. He and psychologist Mindy Greenstein, along with many dedicated researchers, adapted and applied the logotherapy philosophy of Dr. Viktor Frankl, a psychiatrist and Holocaust survivor, to the arena of advanced cancer. They developed meaning-centered psychotherapy (MCP).

Dr. Breitbart has honed this therapy with scientific rigor through many NIH-funded research trials and subsequent teaching seminars. A number of men with prostate cancer have participated in these trials and benefited from this psychotherapy in both group and individual formats. MCP has helped countless men and women with advanced cancer discover how to transcend the demoralization and inevitability of their cancer fate and ultimate death, and find a sense of meaning and purpose in their lives before they die. Workshops on MCP for therapists at international conferences are often oversubscribed. Therapists learn a therapeutic path to help their patients deal with desperate situations. I believe the principles of MCP also help these therapists live their own lives more fully.

The Will to Live with Dignity at the End of Life

It is not uncommon to hear families lament, "He just lost the will to live, and died." Family and caregivers assume that losing the will to live is synonymous with depression, and if only that could be treated, the patient would want to live and be able to will himself to longer life. Sometimes this is accurate and treating a depression or improving a debilitating symptom brings back a will to live. However, a major depression is not always the cause of this demoralized state. The belief that a patient can summon the will to live and defy death with the proper outlook or attitude again shifts the responsibility of living or dying onto the ill person and removes it from the hands of fate, the cancer, the healthcare system, or God. Family members then look to mental health practitioners to resuscitate the will to live.

Dr. Harvey Chochinov, a psychiatrist in Canada, continues to research the nuances of the will to live (WTL). He found that the WTL fluctuates dramatically and frequently in the last weeks of life. WTL is dependent on a combination of existential, psychological, and physical factors, including depression, anxiety, and shortness of breath, a sense of well-being, hopelessness, burden to others, and a person's sense of dignity. The WTL fluctuates as these other symptoms fluctuate over time—they are not usually stuck in "low gear" unless a major depression and hopelessness take hold. I believe it is much more appropriate to blame *the illness* for its debilitating aspects and disappearance of will than *the person*, who may be exhausted or demoralized by their symptom burden.

Healthcare providers then have to commit their best to improve the symptoms that impede the WTL. This can be done with many modalities. Medications ease uncomfortable physical symptoms such as shortness of breath, pain, nausea, and fatigue. Psychotherapy, antidepressants, and antianxiety medications treat depression and anxiety. Support for patients and families to relieve hopelessness and isolation and have appropriate realistic goals helps all prepare for the inevitability of and acceptance of death while maintaining an intimate connectedness, instead of seeing death as an evil to prevent at all costs. Dr. Chochinov developed dignity therapy, which helps families deal these end-of-life issues. Dignity therapy facilitates patients reciting the highlights of their life stories while creating a transferrable, tangible legacy to hand over to loved ones—in writing, video, audio, art, or other media.

A Legacy: Role Modeling for the Future while Facing Your Last Frontier

A number of men have essentially told me, "I don't want my kids (or grandkids) to see me or remember me like this. I'm so weak, I feel useless. I can't interact with them like I used to." These men become frustrated by the onset of worsening health or decreased physical ability.

Navigating this life phase successfully may be the most important legacy you can leave: just like Paul the police officer did, you can model with appropriate human emotion, humor, and love how to realistically face difficult situations that may not be reversible or fixed. Most men do not easily adopt my suggestion that "this is a great opportunity to be a meaningful role model for your family regarding the management of life challenges." It doesn't make sense to them theoretically, let alone practically: "That's not for me, doc. Just look at me. I'm no role model anymore."

This is a common initial response. Role-modeling is not a matter of putting on a good face when the family is around, or acting tough as nails when the going gets rough. It is important to acknowledge that aging, ill health, and debilitation happen to all of us to different degrees, if we live long enough. Many years ago, a patient was startled to hear what I thought when he described how unfair it was that he had to deal with a newly diagnosed advanced prostate cancer, that he was not eligible for any of the primary treatments that could provide a cure, and that he now faced one medical insult after another. All I said was, "It's frustrating when stuff happens." It was as if a light bulb went on for him when he heard it from me. "Stuff happens." I thought this elderly, very proper businessman would more easily hear this more polite version of the street phrase "shit happens." I was right. He quoted this to all of his friends when they had setbacks, health or otherwise. He became a role model for accepting situations he did not want or expect, expressing sadness or frustration, anger or worry when circumstances did not go the way he would have preferred, and then doing what he needed to in order to transform the unhelpful, uncomfortable thoughts, emotions, and behaviors to have as good a present and future for as long as he had to live. In some ways, the work we did together helped model what eventually became the DRAFT with EJ techniques described in this book. He did this with great purpose before he died a few years later.

Alan was an elderly gentleman with metastatic prostate cancer who taught me about the importance of accepting current circumstances in the service of others. As he was rolled into my office in a wheelchair, I saw fatigue on his face, but his head was held with a sense of dignity. He was frustrated with his loss of energy and not being able to do the things he enjoyed for any reasonable length of time. When we spoke about leaving a legacy for his family, he said that he had tried to give those lessons when he was younger. He used to spend "quality" time with each of his grandchildren, taking each to dinner and to a favorite activity of theirs afterward (just as he had done with his children when they were growing up). He got to know his grandchildren well, and they knew him. He enjoyed when they came into town (they each lived in different parts of the country) to visit him. He felt blessed that they had picked up his lessons. He told me about teaching his children and grandchildren to play backgammon, a game he had loved since he was a child. When they visited they each played Grandpa a few games. As he got weaker, he did not think it made sense for them to travel such long distances for such short visits. When he suggested fewer visits, his family resisted, lovingly. The more ill he became, the more time he felt he had on his hands, and the more depressed he got. But Alan did not want to be a burden on others. He wondered what purpose he had left. He had always been a go-getter and do-gooder. Until recently, he had kept himself occupied with his job, doing charity work, or spending time with his family.

He felt badly that his wife Alice was "reduced" to caring for him. Though she spent time with her friends and got to read books, they had few passive hobbies in common, since they had always gone out or entertained before Alan got ill. I asked Alan why he and Alice didn't play backgammon together. "She doesn't play." I asked why he had never taught her. "I didn't think she was interested." We brought Alice into the room and I asked her why she didn't play backgammon. Alice said, "I never learned how." I asked why she had never asked Alan to teach her. She said, "It looked complicated, so I never tried. And besides, he was having a great time playing with the children and grandchildren. That was their thing." Alan gladly took on the challenge to teach Alice how to play backgammon. About a month later, Alan came into a session smiling, and stated that his pupil had gotten very good. She had beat him in a game of backgammon that week. More than the quality of their game, they got to spend quality time together, when otherwise, the moments together might have been lost.

Good role-modeling can help you find new sources of worth and meaning. It also helps teach others about how to cope with your illness. Life usually presents financial, career, health, and/or relationship challenges that can be demoralizing and debilitating and can make most of us feel vulnerable or threatened. Your adult children and grandchildren will face these types of crises after your death, and hopefully they will hang on to your real-life example of how you went through one of the toughest crises people know. Hopefully, that will guide them to accept and manage their own predicaments more successfully with helpful emotion, humor, and resolve to love and facilitate better living for themselves and others until the end of *their* lives. Unless someone eventually invents a true crystal ball, there will be no guarantees about outcomes. But your friends and family can have a sense of how to roll with the punches when "stuff happens," just like you have. Show them how to live a better life and contradict the standard misconceptions about coping.

You can do this in person, like Paul did. Or you can record your lessons of living and dying if you want. People do this in letters to be read while they are still alive, and some to be read after their deaths. Some do it in written story form, and others with video or audio recordings. Some convey their messages in different art forms. Pick the style you are comfortable with. In fact, it's not a bad idea to ask a tech-savvy grandchild, niece, or nephew to help you out. But communicate it somehow. You then can epitomize Erik Erikson's last stage of life, in which adults reflect back on their lives, assess what they've attained and given to others, and,

---

Treatment for Managing and Living Better with Prostate Cancer

Rx: Manage and live better with prostate cancer

Sig: Use your cancer experience to become a role model.

Model how to meet the challenges of life with strength, with human vulnerability and emotion, and with the perseverance and humor to overcome, to change, and to have a better life.
DRAFT with Emotional Judo
Prepare your legacy for family, friends, and caregivers.
Use oral or written stories, letters, videos, or pictures.

Refills: Infinite

Dispense: Until you die

hopefully, feel a sense of fulfillment, or ego integrity, with an aura of wisdom, rather than regret, bitterness, or despair.

As men become frailer, they fear the eventual loss of independence, regardless of how old they are: "I'm a burden on my family—I can't do anything for myself." They may be used to taking care of others, but as their responsibilities become tougher to fulfill, their ability to carry out tasks with the same stamina and confidence is lessened, and their freedom feels compromised. They feel saddened by being less autonomous, feeling less whole, and less in control. Many men feel like psychological and physical burdens when they rely on others for physical help. Asking these men, "If the roles were (God forbid) reversed, how much would you view taking care of your wife or partner (or your child) as a burden?" puts the overarching issue into a different perspective, and allows for a different discussion that could not be addressed beforehand. Men are temporarily placed in the role of "the healthier other" and they can observe the situation more objectively. Feeling like a burden on wives or partners is frustrating; it is especially upsetting and guilt-inducing when men think about their grown children as caregivers. "They have their own lives to live; they shouldn't be worrying about me. I don't want to be a distraction to them."

Taking care of an ill person is not easy and requires sacrifices. Yet it is also has the potential for vital moments of connection and completion. When an adult child gets a chance to "give back" and feel like they matter in your life, they feel essential and whole. When a spouse or partner or adult child feels useful even in the midst of a progressing cancer, they can resolve regrets for not being able to control the cancer or not caring sufficiently; in fact they may realize they can handle just about anything that comes up in the future. A loved one who is helpful, supportive, and caring, knowing there will be no payback, may epitomize the bedrock of our humanity. "Don't worry, everything will be all right," may sound nice, but this does not always bring relief to an ill person who does require help. More down-to-earth and realistic is, "This is tough stuff for both of us, but we will figure it out and deal with it together. I'm here to help you, so you don't have to worry so much." A patient can shrug off the former statement upsettingly, even if it was well intentioned, with

"They don't know what they are talking about," and not receive the comfort or reassurance that was hoped for. The latter statement is sensible, validates reality, and gives a sense of a team that can act as a "worry proxy." An adult child knows that when death happens, there is no going back. Being able to share this experience and be part of helpful and supportive attempts to comfort and ease a loved one's suffering or burden is an important way to feel more whole as a human and facilitate grieving later on.

This is what *Managing Prostate Cancer: A Guide for Living Better* has been all about. There is nothing good about a prostate cancer diagnosis, but there can be opportunities for silver linings if you are open to them. A cancer diagnosis does not have to be equated with a life of misery, desperation, or depression. You can develop your playbook to manage your emotions, thoughts and behaviors regarding primary or secondary treatments to live the best life possible. With this book, you have that playbook to help you deal with the very real, yet not always tangible, psychological, emotional, and physical ramifications of this cancer and to be on top of your life game from diagnosis through cure. And if there is recurrence or progression of disease and no chance of cure, you can be on top of your life game for the rest of your life.

As Yogi Berra said, "It ain't over 'til it's over." And when it's over, your legacy continues.

APPENDIX

References

American Cancer Society. *Sexuality and Cancer: For the Man Who Has Cancer and His Partner* (The original material for this booklet was prepared for the American Cancer Society by Leslie R. Schover, PhD, Associate Professor, Behavioral Sciences, University of Texas M.D. Anderson Cancer Center). *This is an easy-to-read booklet that discusses sexual challenges after prostate cancer and interventions for improvement.*

Herbert Benson with Miriam Z. Klipper. *The Relaxation Response.* 2000, New York: Harper Torch. *This book describes brief relaxation and meditative techniques that help reduce the stress and suffering from heart conditions, high blood pressure, chronic pain, and insomnia.*

William S. Breitbart and Shannon R. Poppito. *Meaning-Centered Group Psychotherapy for Patients with Advanced Cancer.* 2014, New York: Oxford University Press. *Meaning-centered psychotherapy, an intervention developed and tested by the Department of Psychiatry and Behavioral Sciences at Memorial Sloan Kettering Cancer Center, is a 7-week program that utilizes a mixture of didactics, discussion, and experiential exercises that focus on particular themes related to meaning and advanced cancer. The program is based on the philosophy of Viktor Frankl and logotherapy.*

Jane Brody. Falling apart in a healthy sort of way. *New York Times*, March 2, 2015. *This article explores the tension of maintaining a healthy outlook even as we age and develop medical illnesses.*

David Burns. *Feeling Good: The New Mood Therapy*. 2008, New York: Harper. *This book provides an excellent background to cognitive behavioral therapy and guides people in enacting methods to improve mood and anxiety.*

Suzanne Chambers. *Facing the Tiger: A Guide for Men with Prostate Cancer and the People Who Love Them*. 2014, Samford Valley: Australian Academic Press. *This book provides practical strategies to help cope with the emotional and psychological stress of living with prostate cancer. The book has a companion iPad app, launched by the Prostate Cancer Foundation of Australia, that is designed to help men cope with the distress of prostate cancer. It contains videos, exercises, and advice to meet the challenges of the condition.*

Harvey Max Chochinov. *Dignity Therapy: Final Words for Final Days*. 2012, New York: Oxford University Press. *Dignity therapy is a well-tested intervention to address the psychological, existential, and spiritual challenges faced by patients and their families as they grapple with the end of life.*

John Gray. *Men Are from Mars and Women Are from Venus: The Classic Guide to Understanding the Opposite Sex*. 2012, New York: Harper Collins. *This book explores the differences in needs, desires, and behaviors between men and women, with suggestions on how to improve understanding and communication.*

Mindy Greenstein and Jimmie Holland. *Lighter as We Go*, 2014, New York: Global OUP. *This book discusses the benefits of growing older with suggestions on how to get there.*

Jon Kabat-Zinn. *Full Catastrophe Living* (revised edition): *Using the Wisdom of Your Body and Mind to Face Stress, Pain and Illness*. 2011, New York: Bantam. *This book describes the background and uses of the mindfulness-based stress reduction program—a mind–body approaches derived from meditation and yoga to counter-act stress. Use of these mindfulness practices can help manage chronic pain, promote optimal healing, reduce anxiety and feelings of panic, and improve overall quality of life.*

A.B. Kornblith, H.W. Herr, U.S. Ofman, H.I. Scher, and J.C. Holland. Quality of life of patients with prostate cancer and their spouses. The value of a data base in clinical care. *Cancer*. 1994 Jun 1;73(11):2791–2802. *This study examined the nature and extent of problems in patients' and spouses' adaptation to prostate cancer and quality of life.*

Elisabeth Kübler-Ross. *On Death and Dying*. 1969, New York: Scribner. *In this classic book, Dr. Kübler-Ross first explored the five stages of death: denial and isolation, anger, bargaining, depression, and acceptance, giving readers a better understanding of how death affects the patient and caregivers.*

Marsha M. Linehan. *Skills Training Manual for Treating Borderline Personality Disorder*. 1993, New York: Guilford Press. *This book is a step-by-step guide to teaching interpersonal effectiveness, emotion regulation, distress tolerance, and mindfulness.*

Peter Mueller, from The Cartoon Bank, Inc. "I want a new prostate." 1995. https://www.cartoonbank.com/

C.J. Nelson, S. Lacey, J. Kenowitz, H. Pessin, E. Shuk, and J.P. Mulhall. Men's experience with penile rehabilitation following radical prostatectomy: a qualitative study with the goal of informing a therapeutic intervention. *Psychooncology.* 2015, Feb 24. *This article discusses the pilot research program using acceptance and commitment therapy to help men better utilize erectile rehabilitation to improve erectile dysfunction after radical prostatectomy.*

Frank Penedo, Michael Antoni, and Neil Schneiderman. *Cognitive-Behavioral Stress Management for Prostate Cancer Recovery (Treatments That Work).* 2008, New York: Oxford University Press. *Cognitive behavioral stress management (CBSM) and relaxation training constitute the two components of this comprehensive program for men with localized prostate cancer who have difficulty readjusting to life after surgery as a result of treatment related side effects. The book provides stress management skills, including cognitive restructuring, coping strategies, and social support. Issues of sexuality and communication are also addressed.*

Gerald Perlman and Jack Drescher. *A Gay Man's Guide to Prostate Cancer.* 2005, Boca Raton, FL: CRC Press. *This book explores the medical and psychological aspects of prostate cancer, focusing on the unique concerns of gay men.*

W.F. Pirl, G.I. Siegel, M.J. Goode, and M.R. Smith. Depression in men receiving androgen deprivation therapy for prostate cancer: a pilot study. *Psychooncology.* 2002 Nov-Dec;11(6):518–523. *This study examined the prevalence rates and risk factors associated with major depression in this population, finding that men most at risk for developing depression while getting androgen deprivation therapy were those who had significant past histories of depression.*

J.O. Prochaska, J.C. Norcross, and C.C. DiClemente. *Changing for Good: A Revolutionary Six Stage Program for Overcoming Bad Habits and Moving Your Life Positively Forward.* 2007, New York: W. Morrow. *This book describes the stages that people employ to undergo difficult behavioral changes.*

A.J. Roth, A.B. Kornblith, L. Batel-Copel, E. Peabody, H.I. Scher, and J.C. Holland. Rapid screening for psychologic distress in men with prostate carcinoma: a pilot study. *Cancer.* 1998 May 15;82(10):1904–1908. *This article discusses the testing of the distress thermometer screening method in a prostate cancer clinical setting.*

A.J. Roth, C. Nelson, B. Rosenfeld, H. Scher, S. Slovin, M. Morris, N. O'Shea, G. Arauz, and W. Breitbart. Methylphenidate for fatigue in ambulatory men with prostate cancer. *Cancer.* 2010 Nov 1;116(21):5102–5110. *This study reports on a randomized, placebo-controlled research project to evaluate the efficacy of meth-ylphenidate to treat fatigue in prostate cancer patients.*

Leslie Schover. *Sexuality and Fertility after Cancer.* 1997, New York: Wiley. *This book is written for cancer survivors, providing information on staying sexually active after cancer treatment. It examines the emotional and physical impact of breast, prostate, and other cancers, plus has sections on dating and sexual orientation.*

Nate Silver. *The Signal and the Noise: Why So Many Predictions Fail—But Some Don't.* 2012, New York: Penguin Press.

George Vaillant. *Aging Well: Surprising Guideposts to a Happier Life from the Landmark Harvard Study of Adult Development.* 2003, Boston: Little, Brown and Company. *This book highlights a series of studies from Harvard University following 824 subjects from their teens to old age that illustrate some interesting factors involved in reaching happy, healthy old age.*

Barbara Rubin Wainrib, Jack Maguire, and Sandra Haber. *Men, Women, and Prostate Cancer: A Medical and Psychological Guide for Women and the Men They Love.* 2000, New York: New Harbinger Publications. *This book provides infor-mation on prostate cancer, including diagnosis, treatment options, and recovery, and provides advice for women on how to deal with the emotional issues surround-ing this disease.*

Additional Reading

Steven Hayes with Spencer Smith. *Get out of Your Mind and into Your Life: The New Acceptance and Commitment Therapy.* 2005, Oakland, CA: New Harbinger Publications. *This book reviews the basics of acceptance and commitment therapy with plentiful exercises to help identify core struggles, break them down into man-ageable pieces, and develop effective ways to improve suffering.*

Jimmie Holland and Sheldon Lewis. *The Human Side of Cancer: Living with Hope, Coping with Uncertainty.* 2001, New York: Harper. *This book, written by the founder of the field of psycho-oncology, Jimmie Holland and coauthor Sheldon Lewis, combines sensitive advice and explanations with quotes and anecdotes of patients with all types of cancer, research summaries, self-help tips, and checklists. The book is for both the cancer survivor and family members. A range of avail-able strategies, both physical (e.g., medications) and psychological (e.g., support groups), to cope with severe depression, fear of surgery, and sleeplessness as well as aiding the terminally ill are discussed.*

John Mulhall. *Saving Your Sex Life—A Guide For Men with Prostate Cancer.* 2008, Munster, IN: Hilton Publishing. *This book explains the role of testosterone, the functions of the prostate, and the common difficulties men encounter with prostate cancer. It focuses in particular on sexual health and erectile dysfunction.*

Arthur M. Nezu, Christine Maguth Nezu, Stephanie H. Friedman, Shirley Faddis, and Peter S. Houts. *Helping Cancer Patients Cope: A Problem Solving Approach.* 1998, Washington, DC: American Psychological Association. *This book reviews good problem-solving skills that help people cope better with major life events such as cancer.*

Peter Scardino and Judith Kelman. *Dr. Peter Scardino's Prostate Book, Revised Edition: The Complete Guide to Overcoming Prostate Cancer, Prostatitis, and BPH.* 2010, New York: Avery Press. *This book is written by an eminent urologist and prostate cancer surgeon, now chairman of the Department of Surgery at Memorial Sloan Kettering Cancer Center in New York. It educates the reader about the normal prostate and its function; presents common prostate problems, including prostatitis and an enlarged prostate; and prostate cancer. Issues related to risk factors, prevention, and detection are also discussed. Available treatment options and their resultant statistics, including side effects that many men are curious about but are afraid to bring up with doctors, are discussed in detail.*

Patrick C. Walsh and Janet Farrar Worthington. *Dr. Patrick Walsh's Guide to Surviving Prostate Cancer.* 2002, New York: Grand Central Life & Style. *This book reviews how the prostate works, prostate cancer prevalence, and the reasons men develop prostate cancer, including age, race, family history, and diet. The book informs readers about getting a proper diagnosis, the results of biopsies, and the disease. Explanations are provided for surgical and other types of treatment, side effects, and postsurgical complications.*

Abbreviated List of Reliable Information Sources

American Cancer Society: http://www.cancer.org/

ASCO, The American Society of Clinical Oncology: http://www.cancer.net/ (doctor approved patient information from ASCO).

Caring Bridge: http://www.caringbridge.org/

Guided Mindfulness Meditation: Practices with Jon Kabat-Zinn: http://www.mindfulnesscds.com/

National Cancer Institute—PDQ: http://www.cancer.gov/cancertopics/pdq

National Comprehensive Cancer Network (NCCN): http://www.nccn.org/

Prostate Cancer Foundation: http://www.pcf.org

The NCCN Clinical Practice Guidelines in Oncology (NCCN Guidelines®) are a statement of evidence and consensus of the authors regarding their views of currently accepted approaches to treatment. Any clinician seeking to apply or consult the NCCN Guidelines® is expected to use independent medical judgment in the context of individual clinical circumstances to determine any patient's care or treatment. The National Comprehensive Cancer Network® (NCCN®) makes no representations or warranties of any kind regarding their content, use, or application, and disclaims any responsibility for their application or use in any way. The NCCN Guidelines are copyrighted by National Comprehensive Cancer Network®. All rights reserved. The NCCN Guidelines and the illustrations herein may not be reproduced in any form without the express written permission of NCCN. ©2013.

Abbreviated List of Support Groups

Cancer Support Community: http://www.cancersupportcommunity.org

Gilda's Club: http://www.gildasclubqc.org/ (local groups have individual websites)

Malecare: www.malecare.org

Man to Man: www.cancer.org/Treatment/SupportProgramsServices/MantoMan/index

Us Too: http://www.ustoo.org/

INDEX

Note: Page numbers followed by the italicized letters *b* and *f* indicate material found in boxes or figures.

abiraterone (Zytiga), 280
acceptance and commitment therapy
    (ACT), 111, 113, 216
Acknowledge (as DR**A**FT technique).
    See also DRAFT technique/
    situations
    in catastrophizing scenario, 150,
        151–152
    with EJ for insomnia, 171
    in *Emotional Judo (EJ)* playbook,
        141–142
    emotions and thoughts, 48, 130,
        134–135
    in generalizing scenario, 153
active muscle relaxation, 122. *See also*
    relaxation
active surveillance
    after biochemical recurrence, 276
    as current treatment option, 34*b*
    vs. "definitive" treatment, 90
    PSA tests in, 57
    as treatment route, 56–57
activities. *See also* exercise
    modification of, 305

quick list of, 86–87, 146*b*
    schedule and pace of, 163*b*
    staying active, 251*b*
    when preparing for treatment,
        87, 88*b*
activity levels, 314–316. *See also*
    end-of-life issues
Adderall, 197*t*
addiction
    benzodiazepines and, 185–186*t*
    as misunderstood, 180
    pseudo-addiction, 181
ADHD (attention deficit-hyperactivity
    disorder), 196
ads, prostate-cancer related, 61
advanced cancer
    appetite loss in, 312
    coping with, 4
    denial in, 67*b*
    fatigue and, 245
    imagined scenarios of, 274
    meaning-centered psychotherapy
        (MCP) and, 322–323
    positive/negative thinking and, 306

advanced directives, 55
African descent, prostate cancer risk
    in men of, 3, 17
aging
    burden of cancer and, 3–4
    retirement and, 297–298
    sense of loss and, 22
Aging Well (Vaillant), 231
akathisia (medication side effect), 195
alcohol
    anxiety and, 44
    use of, 80–81
Alcoholics Anonymous, 81
"all or nothing" thinking, 149, 156,
    207, 222, 297, 303, 305–306
alprazolam (Xanax), 178–179,
    186t, 201
alprostadil, 219
Ambien (zolpidem), 198–199, 200t
American Cancer Society, 63, 100,
    210, 335
amitriptyline, 193
amphetamine, 197t
androgen ablation therapy, 192, 196,
    246b, 278–279, 315, 316. *See
    also* hormonal therapy
androgen antagonists, 280
androgen deprivation therapy (ADT),
    277–279, 281–284. *See also*
    hormonal therapy; intermittent
    therapy (ADT treatment)
anesthesia, concerns about, 39, 40
anger, as common reaction, 21
antiandrogens, 280
antidepressants. *See also* anxiety
    medications; medication
    for anxiety, 183–184, 186t
    carcinogenic concerns, 194
    choice of, 189–190
    by class, 191–193
    with hormonal therapy, 288
    myths vs. reality, 193–194
    scouting report on, 197t

    secondary side effects, 195–196
    suicidal concerns, 194–195
    tricyclic antidepressants
        (TCAs), 193
anti-inflammatory medications, 244
antipsychotics, 184–185, 186t
anxiety. *See also* PSA anxiety
    vs. depression, 98
    fight or flight reactions, 100, 102
    medical causes of, 177–178
    in the medically ill, 95–96, 174
    PSA tests and, 69, 102–105,
        111, 139
    psychiatric medicine benefits for,
        174–175
    signs/symptoms of, 104b, 177
    therapeutic/coping techniques for,
        110–111
    "thought trap" avoidance, 46–50
anxiety medications. *See also*
    medication
    addiction worries, 180–181, 182b
    antidepressants for, 183–184, 186t
    classes of, 178
    common side effects, 179
    physical dependence, 180, 182b
    psychological addiction, 181, 182b
    rebound anxiety, 179
    scouting report on, 185–186t
    tolerance, 180, 182b
    withdrawal symptoms, 180
appetite, loss of, 311–314
appetite stimulants, 313
armodafinil (Nuvigil), 197t, 253
assertive, being, 51
Ativan (lorazepam), 178–179, 186t,
    200, 200t
attention deficit-hyperactivity
    disorder (ADHD), 196

baby boomers, diagnoses among, 3–4
Batel-Copel, Laure, 99
Beck, Aaron, 112

behavior. *See also* cognitive behavioral therapy (CBT); DRAFT technique/situations
  development of new, 9–10
  in preventive health, 21–22
  risky thought processes and, 146–149
  unhelpful, 130–132
behavioral changes, stages of
  action, 227–228
  contemplation, 226–227
  pre-contemplation, 226
  preparation, 227
  reinforcing and maintaining, 228
"belly breathing," 121. *See also* breath
benign prostatic hypertrophy, 25
Benson, Herbert, 117
benzodiazepines, 178, 185–186*t*, 200, 201
biases, among medical practitioners, 56
biochemical addiction, to anxiety medications, 182*b*
biofeedback techniques, 238–239
biopsies
  anxiety and, 24–27
  in Gleason score, 31
  risks/discomforts of, 30
bleeding
  rectal, 41*t*, 243–244
  urinary, 39, 241
blogs, as decision-making tool, 62
bodily functions, discussion of, 54
bowel problems. *See also* urinary and bowel complications
  case study examples, 243–245
  expectation errors, 233
  as quality-of-life issue, 243
  worries about, 74–75
Box Relaxation Technique, 169*f*
brachytherapy, 48
bravery, 317–321

breast tissue growth (gynecomastia), 285
breath
  Box Relaxation Technique, 169*f*
  breathing exercises, 115
  observation of, 120–122
  in relaxation techniques, 116–119, 122–126, 167
Breitbart, William, 322–323
Brody, Jane, 298
bupropion (Wellbutrin), 183, 195, 197*t*, 253
Burns, David, 113
buspirone (Buspar), 184, 186*t*, 197*t*
buyer's remorse
  avoiding, 36*f*
  fear of, 33–42, 48, 92–93

caffeine
  anxiety and, 44
  sleeplessness and, 165
Cancer Support Community, 336
caregivers, spouses/partners as, 97
CaringBridge, 96, 335
The Cartoon Bank (Mueller), 31
Casodex (bicalutamide), 280
castration, surgical, 279
catastrophizing scenarios, 149–152
catheterization (self), 241–242
Celexa (citalopram), 183, 186*t*, 191, 197*t*
Chambers, Suzanne, 102
"chemo-brain," 289
chemotherapy
  antidepressants and, 195–196
  appetite and, 312
  exercise and, 251
  fatigue and, 245, 246*b*, 247, 286, 289
  memory/concentration issues, 289–290
  quality of life of, 288–290
  staying active during, 314–315
  in treatment progression, 302, 317

chlorpromazine (Thorazine), 185
Chochinov, Harvey, 323–324
citalopram (Celexa), 183, 186*t*,
    191, 197*t*
clamps, for urinary dribbling,
    238–239
clarification/explanation
    decreasing distress with, 152
    of medical situations/treatment
        recommendations, 51
    of statistics, 52*b*, 53*b*, 54
    superstitions and, 157
clonazepam (Klonopin), 178–179,
    186*t*, 200, 200*t*
Cognitive-Behavioral Stress
    Management for Prostate Cancer
    Recovery Workbook (Treatments
    That Work) (Penedo), 113
cognitive behavioral therapy (CBT)
    for distress relief, 276
    in DRAFT with EJ strategy,
        111–113, 128, 149
    energy/mood levels and, 251, 253*b*
    family/spouse/partners and, 259
    hormonal therapy and, 290
    irrational thoughts and, 72
cognitive dulling, 290
communication. *See also* questions;
        spouses/partners
    of couples, 57–61, 264–268
    dreaded discussions, 82–85
    guidelines for improved, 269*b*
    between patients and
        physicians, 51
    "red flags" in, 86*b*
    tension of good intentions in,
        257–263
comparisons to others' experiences,
    47, 155–156
concerns
    about anesthesia, 39, 40
    about masturbation, 73, 221
    about radiation therapy, 40*b*
    about surgery, 39

about urinary and bowel
    complications, 73–75, 236–242
compartmentalization of, 66–67
denial of, 65–66
sexual, 73–74
suppression of, 67*b*
talking to experts about, 40*b*
treatment-related, 70*b*, 71*b*
Concerta, 197*t*
coping/coping techniques. *See also*
        DRAFT technique/situations
    for anxiety/depression, 110–111
    gender differences in, 261–262
    in sexual functioning, 209–210
    for sleeplessness, 164–166
    for spouses/partners, 255–256
    using *Emotional Judo* (EJ), 6
"couple's cancer," 208. *See also*
        intimacy and relationships
cryosurgery, 33, 34*b*
cultural backgrounds, prostate cancer
    risk among, 3
Cymbalta (duloxetine), 183, 186*t*,
    191–192, 197*t*, 288
cystitis, 241, 242
cystoscopy, 241

dating challenges, 222–223
death/dying. *See also*
        end-of-life issues
    certainty of, 302
    "death anxiety," 256, 286
    DRAFT technique for,
        303–304
    psychotherapy for, 292–293,
        321–322
    thinking about, 290–292
"definitive" treatment
    vs. active surveillance, 90
    psychological distress and, 6
    return of cancer following, 31,
        273–274, 279
    rising PSAs following, 150, 277
    urinary function after, 237

denial
  characteristics of, 67*b*
  of concerns, 65–66
  of prior illness, 17–18
  second opinions and, 66
depression
  vs. anxiety, 98
  identification of, 107–110
  medical causes of, 177–178
  in the medically ill, 95–96, 174
  professional help for, 109–110*b*
  psychiatric medicine benefits for,
    174–175
  suicide, thoughts of, 188–189
  symptoms of, 177, 187–188
  therapeutic/coping techniques for,
    110–111
  urinary complications and, 237
depression medications, 183–184.
    See also antidepressants;
    anxiety medications;
    medication
desipramine, 193
diagnosis/diagnoses
  ability to function, 177
  difficulty accepting, 17
  in men over 65 years old, 3–4
  preventive health behaviors
    and, 21–22
  questions following, 13–14
  response/reactions to, 1–2, 14*b*,
    20–21, 64–67
  in US annually, 2–3
diarrhea, 41*t*, 103, 140, 178, 186*t*,
    243, 288
diazepam (Valium), 178–179, 186*t*, 200t
diet
  arguments over, 311–314
  behavioral changes and, 226
  benefits of, 79, 81*b*
  bowel complications and, 244
  changes to, 52b, 54, 78
  in development of prostate
    cancer, 16, 31

dietitian, suggestions from, 253, 313
  exercise and, 128
  importance of, 148, 249, 251
diethylstilbestrol (DES), 280
dignity, living with, 323–324. *See also*
    end-of-life issues
dignity therapy, 324. *See also* therapy
    (psychotherapy)
disagreements, among medical
    practitioners, 56
distraction technique. *See also quick
    list* of activities
  in DRAFT with EJ strategy, 48,
    130, 162*b*
  exercise as, 75, 78
  information gathering as, 72
  for sleeplessness, 164, 198
  for urinary incontinence, 240
distress
  vs. depression/anxiety, 98–100
  signs of, 104*b*
  of spouses/partners, 3
  therapeutic/coping techniques for,
    110–111
Distress Thermometer, 99–100
"doctor's office" anxiety, 50
doctor visit
  being assertive during, 51
  preparation for, 43–44
  questions for oncology
    team, 52–53*b*
  "white coat syndrome" during, 50
Do Not Resuscitate order, 55
"don't ask, don't tell" policy, 259. *See
    also* communication
downward spiral, expectation
    of, 95–96
doxepin, 198
DRAFT: Acknowledge
  in catastrophizing scenario, 150,
    151–152
  with EJ for insomnia, 171
  in *Emotional Judo (EJ)* playbook,
    141–142

DRAFT: Acknowledge (*Cont.*)
  emotions and thoughts, 48, 130,
    134–135
  in generalizing scenario, 153
DRAFT: Detect
  in catastrophizing scenario,
    149–150, 151
  detection of uncomfortable/
    unhelpful emotions, thoughts
    and behaviors, 130–132
  with EJ for insomnia, 171
  in *Emotional Judo (EJ)* playbook,
    138–140
  in generalizing scenario, 153
DRAFT: Recognize
  in catastrophizing scenario,
    150, 151
  with EJ for insomnia, 171
  in *Emotional Judo (EJ)*
    playbook, 140
  emotions/thoughts/behaviors,
    132–134
  in generalizing scenario, 153
DRAFT technique/situations
  for aging challenges, 298–299
  all-or-nothing thinking, 156
  for approaching death, 303–304
  for behavioral change, 228–231
  catastrophizing scenarios, 149–152
  changing perspectives, 157–158
  cheat sheet for, 162*b*
  comparisons to others'
    experiences, 155–156
  generalization scenarios, 153–155
  for intimacy and relationships,
    211–213
  mnemonic/acronym, 130
  mood/activity charts, 158–163
  in spouse/partner communication,
    256–257
  strategies in, 48
  superstitions and magical
    thinking, 157
DRAFT: The Flip

in catastrophizing scenario,
    150–151, 152
  described, 135–136
  with EJ for insomnia, 171–172
  in *Emotional Judo (EJ)* playbook,
    142–144
  in generalizing scenario, 153–154
DRAFT: Transformation
  in catastrophizing scenario,
    151, 152
  described, 136–137
  with EJ for insomnia, 172
  in *Emotional Judo (EJ)* playbook,
    144–146
  in generalizing scenario, 154–155
dreaded discussions. *See also*
    communication
  communication needs, 84–85
  "Everything will be fine," 83–84
  "How are you feeling? 82–83
Drescher, Jack, 215
duloxetine (Cymbalta), 183, 186*t*,
    191–192, 197*t*, 288

eating, battles around, 311–314
Effexor (venlafaxine), 183, 186*t*,
    191–192, 197*t*, 288
E-motion, 250–253
Emotional Judo (EJ). *See also* DRAFT
    technique/situations; relaxation
  awareness of thought processes/
    behaviors in, 146–149
  cheat sheet for, 162*b*
  as coping mechanism, 6
  DRAFT technique in, 7, 48
  playbook for, 137–146
  schools of psychotherapy in, 111
  scientific disclaimer, 127–130
  term usage, 127
emotional reactions
  dealing with, 27
  to diagnosis, 14*b*, 18, 64–67
end-of-life issues. *See also* death/
    dying; grief

activity levels, 314–316
fights over food, 311–314
information sharing, 309–311
leaving a legacy, 324–329
living with dignity, 323–324
modifying leisure activities, 305
saying goodbye, 317–323
socializing, 317
end-stage disease, 4, 275. *See also*
advanced cancer
energizing side effects, 183, 187, 192,
195–196, 253*b*
energy-efficiency suggestions, 315
energy/mood levels, depression
and, 98
enzalutamide (Xtandi), 280
erectile assists, 221*b*
erectile dysfunction (ED)
after prostatectomy, 205–207
alternative routes to erection,
218–221
biological complications, 206–207
causes of, 205
discussion of, 54
managing expectations, 203
penile rehabilitation, 204, 216–221
quality-of-life-issues, 235–236
erectile-stimulating medications, 74
erectile suppositories, 221
escitalopram (Lexapro), 183, 186*t*,
191, 197*t*
eszopiclone (Lunesta), 198–199, 200*t*
Eulexin (flutamide), 280
exam room, waiting in, 46*t*
exercise. *See also* activities; behavioral
changes, stages of
author's use of, 78
breathing exercises, 115
chemotherapy and, 251
diet and, 128
as distraction technique, 75, 78
for energy level/mood
improvement, 249–251
fatigue/low energy and, 250–251

for insomnia/sleeplessness,
167–170
Kegel exercises, 71, 234, 237–240
as preparation for
treatment, 75–79
recurrence and, 248
for relaxation, 116–120, 125–126
exercise group (PEX), 78
expectant monitoring, 56. *See also*
active surveillance
experts, speaking about concerns
with, 40*b*
explanation/clarification
decreasing distress with, 152
of medical situations/treatment
recommendations, 51
of statistics, 52*b*, 53*b*, 54
superstitions and, 157
external beam radiation therapy,
33, 34*b*

Facing The Tiger: A Guide for Men with
Prostate Cancer and the People
Who Love Them (Chambers), 102
faith and spirituality, 88–92, 321. *See*
also religion/religious faith
family history
in generalizing, 153
prostate cancer risk and, 17, 22
PSA tests and, 23, 30
family members. *See also* end-of-life
issues; spouses/partners
fights over food, 311–314
information sharing, 309–311
fatigue/low energy. *See also*
psychostimulants
causes of, 245–246
exercise and, 250–251
expectation errors, 233
with hormonal therapy, 286–287
mood/activity chart use, 247–248
post-treatment recuperation and,
246–247
suggestions for, 253*b*

FDA (U. S. Food and Drug Administration), 194
fears, sharing of, 97
Feeling Good: The New Mood Therapy (Burns), 113
feelings, men's hesitancy to describe, 236
fiber, dietary, 244. *See also* diet
fight or flight reactions, 100, 102
Firmagon (degarelix), 280
five stages of grief, 301
The Flip (as DRAFT technique). *See also* DRAFT technique/ situations
   in catastrophizing scenario, 150–151, 152
   described, 135–136
   with EJ for insomnia, 171–172
   in *Emotional Judo (EJ)* playbook, 142–144
   in generalizing scenario, 153–154
fluoxetine (Prozac), 183, 186*t*, 191, 195, 197*t*, 253
Focalin, 197*t*
follicular-stimulating hormone (FSH), 279
food, fights over, 311–314. *See also* end-of-life issues
Food and Drug Administration (FDA), 194
Frankl, Viktor, 322
Freud, Sigmund, 112
Full Catastrophe Living: Using the Wisdom of Your Body and Mind to Face Stress, Pain and Illness (Kabat-Zinn), 113

gabapentin (Neurontin), 288
gamma-aminobutyric acid (GABA), 184
A Gay Man's Guide to Prostate Cancer (Perlman and Drescher), 215
genders, coping differences of, 261–262

generalizations
   anticipatory grief and, 73
   comparisons to others' experiences, 47, 155–156
   in DRAFT model example, 153
   example scenario, 153–155
   second opinions and, 49
Gilda's Club, 336
Giuliani, Rudolph, 47–48
Gleason score, 31, 42, 66, 155–156
God
   anger at, 89
   bargaining with, 24
   faith in, 90–91
gonadotropin-releasing hormone (GNRH), 279–280
goodbye, saying, 317–323. *See also* end-of-life issues
good intentions, tension of, 257–263, 311
"go-to" activities, 87, 88*b*
Gray, John, 225
Greenstein, Mindy, 298, 322
grief
   anticipatory, 73
   as complicated, 300
   DRAFT technique for, 304
   five stages of, 301
   for losses, 26–27
grief therapy, 301
Guided Mindfulness Meditation, 335
gynecomastia (breast tissue growth), 285

haloperidol (Haldol), 185
Hayes, Steven, 113
healthcare proxy, 55, 310
"Healthy in a Falling Apart Kind of Way" (Brody), 298
holding hands, 268. *See also* sensate focus therapy
Holland, Jimmie
   on burden of aging and cancer, 4

Distress Thermometer scale use, 99
Lighter As We Go, 298
prostate cancer program and, 25
recognition of patient distress, 2
Vintage Book Club of, 315
hormonally related medications,
    280–281
hormonal therapy
    androgen ablation agents,
        279–281
    DRAFT technique in, 282–284
    in early-stage prostate cancer,
        278–279
    emotional reactions, 281–282
    fatigue/low energy, 286–287
    hot flashes, 287–288
    identity crisis in, 285–286
    memory/concentration issues,
        289–290
    moodiness, relief from, 283–285
    pharmacological/mechanical help,
        284–285
    side effects, 281–282
hot flashes, 287–288
hyperbaric oxygen (HBO)
    therapy, 241

identity crisis, as hormonal
    side-effect, 281
"if only" thinking, 66, 165
imipramine, 193
implants/prosthetic options, 221
incontinence. *See* urinary and bowel
    complications
information sharing, 96–97,
    309–311. *See also*
    end-of-life issues
informed consent, 309
insight-oriented therapy
    in *Emotional Judo (EJ)*, 111–112,
        115, 126, 128, 149
    as psychotherapy choice, 259
insomnia/sleeplessness. *See also*
    fatigue/low energy

coping with, 164–166
DRAFT with EJ for insomnia,
    171–172
in the medically ill, 95–96
medications for, 198–201
psychiatric medicine benefits for,
    174–175
relaxation exercises, 167–170
suggestions for, 165–167
insurance companies, mental health
    coverage, 262
intermittent therapy (ADT
    treatment), 279, 281, 284,
    287–288, 290
Internet, as decision-making
    tool, 61–62
intimacy and relationships. *See
    also* erectile dysfunction (ED);
    sexual satisfaction; spouses/
    partners
    attitude adjustments, 209–211
    "couple's cancer," 208
    DRAFT technique for, 211–213
    in gay couples, 215
    women's physiological
        changes, 215
    worries about sex, 204*b*
irrational thoughts, 115, 149, 298
isolation, feelings of, 4, 317

Kegel exercises, 71, 234, 237–240
KISS (**K**eep **I**t **S**imple **S**illy) method, 9
Klonopin (clonazepam), 178–179,
    186*t*, 200, 200*t*
Kornblith, Alice, 99, 261
Kübler-Ross, Elizabeth, 301

last will and testament, 55
leakage
    rectal, 244
    urinary, 74, 207, 236, 240, 305
    venous, 217
legacy, leaving a, 324–329. *See also*
    end-of-life issues

leisure activities, modification of, 305
lethargy. *See* fatigue/low energy
Lexapro (escitalopram), 183, 186*t*, 191, 197*t*
LH (luteinizing hormone), 279–280
life expectancy
    active surveillance and, 56
    for treatments, 41*t*
    in younger men, 23
lifestyle behaviors, 21–22
lifestyle choices, 79–81
Lighter as We Go (Greenstein and Holland), 298
living with dignity, 323–324. *See also* end-of-life issues
lorazepam (Ativan), 178–179, 186*t*, 200, 200*t*
losses
    acknowledging/grieving for, 26–27
    of aging, 298
    fear of, 300
    importance of managing, 295–296
Lunesta (eszopiclone), 198–199, 200*t*
Lupron (leuprolide), 280
luteinizing hormone (LH), 279–280

magical thinking, 61–64
magnesium sulfate, 198
Malecare, 336
Managing Prostate Cancer: A Guide for Living Better (Roth), 4, 6, 329
Man to Man, 336
mantras, 122
Masters and Johnson, 210
masturbation, concerns about, 73, 221
MD Anderson Cancer Center, 210
meaning-centered psychotherapy (MCP), 321–323. *See also* therapy (psychotherapy)
medical updates
    for families and friends, 96–97
    information sharing, 309–311

medication. *See also* antidepressants; anxiety medications; *specific medications*
    antiandrogens, 280
    anti-inflammatory, 244
    antipsychotics, 184–185, 186*t*
    appetite stimulants, 313
    choice of, 189–190
    for depression and fatigue, 197*t*
    erection-enhancing, 216–217
    fatigue/low energy symptoms and, 249
    feelings/emotional responses to, 173
    psychostimulants, 196, 197*t*, 252, 253*b*, 313
    reactions to, 95
    side effect fears, 175–176
    for sleep, 198–201
    steroids, 246*b*, 252, 280, 281, 304, 313
meditation, 86–87, 124*b*. *See also* mindfulness meditation; relaxation
megestrol (Megace), 313
melatonin, 198
Memorial Sloan Kettering Cancer Center (MSKCC)
    author's experience at, 15
    on burden of aging and cancer, 4
    Distress Thermometer scale, 99
    on facing mortality, 322
    on penile rehabilitation, 216
    quality of life study, 261
    recognition of patient distress, 2
    on sexual dysfunction, 74
    statistical model development, 31
Men Are from Mars and Women Are From Venus (Gray), 225
mental health coverage, 262
Metadate, 197*t*
methylphenidate (Ritalin), 197*t*, 252
mindfulness-based stress reduction (MBSR), 113, 117
mindfulness meditation

in cognitive sharpening, 290
in *Emotional Judo (EJ)*, 111
for energy/mood levels, 251, 253
focus on breath, 117, 118
for help in sleeping, 166
for hot flash reduction, 288
in prescription for relaxation, 126
for stress/tension reduction, 113–115
mirtazapine (Remeron), 183, 186*t*,
    192, 197*t*, 198, 313
modafinil (Provigil), 197*t*, 252, 253
mood/activity charts, 158–163,
    247–248
mood stabilizers, 184–185
Mueller, Peter, 31
Mulhall, John, 74, 216

National Cancer Institute, 63, 335
National Comprehensive Cancer
    Center Network (NCCN),
    99–100, 335
NCCN Clinical Practice Guidelines in
    Oncology (NCCN Guidelines®),
    335–336
negative thoughts, 306–308
Nelson, Chris, 113, 216
neuroleptics, 184–185, 186*t*
Neurontin (gabapentin), 288
neurovegetative symptoms, 107,
    108, 188
new behaviors, development of, 9–10.
    See also behavioral changes,
    stages of
"new normal," acceptance of, 10
Nilandron (nilutamide), 280
nomograms/predictive nomograms,
    38, 42, 61
non-benzodiazepine hypnotics
    (Z-Drugs), 199, 200*t*
nortriptyline, 193
Nuvigil (armodafinil), 197*t*, 253

office visit, preparation for, 43–44
olanzapine (Zyprexa), 184, 186*t*

oncology team
    biases/disagreements among, 56
    questions for, 52–53*b*
On Death and Dying
    (Kübler-Ross), 301
open radical prostatectomy, 33
orchiectomy (surgical castration), 279
orgasms
    dry, 207
    medications and, 190
    partners,' 268
    penile stimulation and, 223
    le petit mort, 223–224
    questions regarding, 39
    relationship intimacy and, 222
    in sensate focus therapy, 210–215
    without erection, 221
OTC medications (for sleep),
    198–199

panic/panic attacks
    author's experience of, 174
    medications for, 178, 183–184,
        185–186*t*
    signs/symptoms of, 103, 104*b*, 180
papaverine, 219
paroxetine (Paxil), 183, 186*t*, 191,
    197*t*, 288
partners/spouses. *See also* intimacy
    and relationships; sexual
    satisfaction
    as caregivers, 97
    communication needs of, 84–85,
        257–263
    coping strategies for, 255–256
    distress of, 3
    DRAFT technique/situations for,
        256–257
    exercising with, 78–79
    healing of relationships, 256
    questions following diagnosis, 16
    role in treatment decisions, 57–61
Paxil (paroxetine), 183, 186*t*, 191,
    197*t*, 288

PDE-5 inhibitors, 217, 285
Peabody, Elizabeth, 99
Penedo, Frank, 113
penile injections, 217–219
penile pump, 219–220
penile rehabilitation
    erection-enhancing medications,
        216–217
    as urological specialty, 216
penile tumescence, 205
Perlman, Gerald, 215
perspective, changing of, 157–158,
    247–250
PEX (exercise group), 78
Peyronie's disease, 219
phentolamine, 219
phosphodiesterase type 5 (PDE-5)
    inhibitors, 217, 285
physical dependence, on anxiety
    medications, 180, 182b
physical motion. See exercise
physical tolerance, of anxiety
    medications, 180, 182b
Pirl, William, 282
positive attitude, 306–308
prayer, 89, 231. See also faith and
    spirituality; God
predictive nomograms, 38, 42, 61
preparing for treatment
    communication needs, 84–86
    concerns and questions, 70b, 71b
    diet and, 79
    dreaded discussions, 82–83
    exercise in, 75–79
    faith and spirituality, 88–92, 321
    "go-to" activities, 87, 88b
    lifestyle choices, 79–81
    meditation, 86–87
    period of waiting, 69–70
    relaxing, 87
    sexual concerns, 73–74
    speaking with other
        patients, 71–72
    therapeutic writing, 86

urinary incontinence concerns, 73
preventive health behaviors, 21–22
problem-solving therapy, 111
Prochaska, J. O., 226
proctitis, radiation-induced, 243
prognosis, for prostate cancer, 4
prophylactic penile injection therapy,
    217–219
pros and cons lists, 41, 41t
prostate cancer, vs. other types of
    cancer, 16–17
Prostate Cancer Foundation, 335
prostate cancer risk, in different
    groups, 3
prostatectomy, 48
prostate gland, size of, 25
prosthetic options/implants, 221
proton beam therapy, 33, 34b
Provigil (modafinil), 197t, 252, 253
Prozac (fluoxetine), 183, 186t, 191,
    195, 197t
PSA anxiety, 24, 103–107, 286
PSA tests
    in active surveillance, 57
    anxiety and, 69, 102–105, 111, 139
    as cancer management option, 6
    distress over, 4
    in DRAFT model example, 132–133,
        140, 142, 150–152, 154
    emotional reactions to/preparation
        for, 65–66, 101
    family histories and, 21–22, 23
    goals of, 30, 147
    in mood/activity chart, 162t
    questions for oncology team, 52b
    in recurrent prostate cancer,
        274–276, 286
    screening controversy, 30–31
    sleep loss and, 200
    spouse/partner communication,
        258, 260–261, 266
    trends of results, 106
    uncertainty and, 295
    "what if" questions and, 148

pseudo-addiction, 181
psychiatric medication. *See*
    medication
psychological addiction, 181, 182*b*
psychological difficulties/distress
    family histories and, 6
    following diagnosis, 15
    interference of, 5
psychostimulants, 196, 197*t*, 252,
    253*b*, 313
psychotherapy. *See also* cognitive
    behavioral therapy (CBT);
    DRAFT technique/situations;
    sex therapy
    for acceptance of "new normal," 227
    ACT approach, 113
    bowel problem case study, 243–245
    coping with loss, 224, 297
    for couples, 59–60, 263,
        264–266, 313
    for dating issues, 222
    for death and dying, 292–293,
        321–322
    for depressive symptoms, 108
    dignity therapy, 324
    for dreaded discussions, 82–83
    gender differences in, 261–262
    goals, in advanced prostate cancer,
        302–304
    for grief, 301
    individual vs. family focus, 259–260
    insight-oriented, 112, 115, 126
    interactivity of, 5
    meaning-centered (MCP), 321–323
    medications and, 111
    stigma and, 262
    treatment decisions and, 29
    for worry/anxiety, 101–102, 174
pump (penile pump), 219–220

quality-of-life-issues
    active treatment and, 56–57
    after cancer treatments, 235–236
    chemotherapy and, 288–289

questions
    about causes, 17
    following diagnosis, 13–14
    intrusion of, 26
    for oncology team, 52–53*b*, 54
    on orgasm, 39
    on PSA tests, 52*b*, 148
    of spouses/partners, 16
    "Why me?," 13–15, 16, 20
quetiapine (Seroquel), 184, 186*t*
quick list of activities, 86–87, 146*b*

racial backgrounds, prostate cancer
    risk among, 3
radiation-induced bladder cystitis,
    241, 242
radiation oncology, specialist
    questions regarding, 53*b*
radiation proctitis, 243
radiation therapy
    bladder cystitis and, 241, 242
    as current treatment option,
        33, 34*b*
    external beam, 33, 34*b*
    fears/concerns about, 39, 40*b*
    proctitis and, 243
    pros and cons lists, 41*t*
    salvage, 279
    targeted, 279
ramelteon (Rozerem), 198–199, 200*t*
reactions
    dealing with, 27
    to diagnosis, 14*b*, 18, 64–67
rebound anxiety, 179
Recognize (as D**R**AFT technique). *See
    also* DRAFT technique/situations
    in catastrophizing scenario,
        150, 151
    with EJ for insomnia, 171
    in *Emotional Judo (EJ)*
        playbook, 140
    emotions/thoughts/behaviors,
        132–134
    in generalizing scenario, 153

rectal urgency/leakage. *See* bowel
    problems
recuperation time
    after treatment/surgery, 52–53*t*,
        96–97, 112, 205, 233–234,
        236, 246
    emotional, 49, 277
    variables in, 38
recurrence. *See also* hormonal therapy
    anxiety/fear of, 3, 6
    coping with, 4
    disbelief over, 274
    end-of-life worries, 290–291
    exercise and, 248
    fear of dying, 292–293
    issues related to, 7
    PSA tests and, 151
    spouses/partners and, 276
    treatment choice and, 35, 61
regrets, over treatment
        choice, 92–93
relationships and intimacy. *See also*
        erectile dysfunction (ED); sexual
        satisfaction; spouses/partners
    attitude adjustments, 209–211
    "couple's cancer," 208
    DRAFT technique for, 211–213
    in gay couples, 215
    women's physiological
        changes, 215
    worries about sex, 204*b*
relaxation
    active muscle relaxation, 122–124
    breath observation, 120–122
    mindfulness meditation for,
        113–115
    prescription for, 117*b*, 126*b*
    quick guide to, 124*b*
    as skill to learn, 115–116
    techniques/exercises for, 116–120,
        125–126
    word/phrases/mantras, 122
religion/religious faith, 88–92, 321.
        See also God; prayer

Remeron (mirtazapine), 183, 186*t*,
        192, 197*t*, 198, 313
repression, characteristics of, 67*b*
Restoril (temazepam), 200, 200*t*
retirement
    aging and, 297–298
    lack of structure after, 296–297
    prostate cancer occurrence
        after, 296
risk
    of biopsies, 30
    family histories and, 17, 22
    of prostate cancer, 3
    in thought processes/behaviors,
        146–149
Ritalin (methylphenidate), 197*t*, 252
robotic-assisted laparoscopic
        prostatectomy, 33
role-modeling, 325–326
Roth, Andrew J.
    author's diagnosis/odyssey, 18–20
    experience of aging, 299
    information overload of, 64
    "magical thinking" of, 62
    panic attack experience of, 174
    physical exercise use, 78
    recuperation expectations of, 234
    "white coat syndrome" and, 50
    wife as ally of, 60
Rozerem (ramelteon),
        198–199, 200*t*

salvage radiation therapy, 279
satisfaction. *See* sexual satisfaction
saying goodbye, 317–323. *See also*
        end-of-life issues
Scardino, Peter, 31
Scher, Howard, 2, 15, 99
Schover, Leslie, 210
screening, controversy about, 30–31
second opinions
    case study example, 1
    denial and, 66
    generalizations and, 49

importance of, 29
information overload, 64
from multiple practitioners, 56
partners and, 56, 260
as reaction to diagnosis, 14*b*
self-catheterization, 241–242
self-destructive behavior, 307
sensate focus therapy, 210–214. *See also* sex therapy
Serenity Prayer, 231
Seroquel (quetiapine), 184, 186*t*
serotonin, 183, 191–192, 288
serotonin-norepinephrine reuptake inhibitor (SNRI), 181, 183, 191–192, 197*t*, 288
serotonin-specific reuptake inhibitor (SSRI), 181, 183, 191, 197*t*, 288
sertraline (Zoloft), 183, 186*t*, 191, 197*t*, 288
sex
  interest in, 284
  as not just about sex, 268–269
sex therapy, 215, 284. *See also* sensate focus therapy
sexual functioning. *See also* erectile dysfunction (ED)
  ADT's impact on, 278
  after treatment, 190
  coping with changes in, 209–210
  "guarantees" and, 36
  medical issues and, 205
  "new normal," acceptance of, 208
  self-definition and, 26
  treatment decisions and, 58
Sexual Functioning for the Man Who Has Cancer and His Partner (American Cancer Society), 210
Sexuality and Fertility after Cancer (Schover), 210
sexual satisfaction
  in dating challenges, 222–223
  in long-term relationships, 221
  sense of loss, 224–225

stages of behavior changes, 226–228
side effects. *See also* medication
  of anxiety medications, 179, 189
  energizing, 183, 187, 192, 195–196, 253*b*
  sexual, 57–58, 73–74
  spouses/partners and, 189
  of treatments, 26
The Signal and the Noise (Silver), 38
sildenafil, 217, 285
Silver, Nate, 38
single men, supportive networks for, 60–61
sitz baths, 244
sleep apnea, 201
sleep hygiene, rules for, 166
sleeplessness/insomnia. *See also* fatigue/low energy
  coping with, 164–166
  depression and, 98
  DRAFT with EJ for insomnia, 171–172
  in the medically ill, 95–96
  medications for, 174–175, 198–201
  relaxation exercises, 167–170
  suggestions for, 165–167
smoking, 79–80
SNRI (serotonin-norepinephrine reuptake inhibitor), 181, 183, 191–192, 197*t*, 288
socializing/social engagements, 74, 317
Sonata (zaleplon), 198–199, 200*t*
sphincter control, 239–240. *See also* urinary and bowel complications
spouses/partners. *See also* intimacy and relationships; sexual satisfaction
  as caregivers, 97
  communication needs of, 84–85, 257–263

spouses/partners. (*Cont.*)
  coping strategies for, 255–256
  distress of, 3
  DRAFT technique/situations for,
    256–257
  exercising with, 78–79
  healing of relationships, 256
  questions following diagnosis, 16
  role in treatment decisions, 57–61
SSRI (serotonin-specific reuptake
    inhibitor), 181, 183, 191,
    197*t*, 288
stages of grief, 301
statistics
  asking for explanations, 51, 52*b*,
    53*b*, 54
  generalizations and, 49
  in informed decisions, 38–39
  in pros and cons lists, 41
  of surgical outcomes, 42
  usefulness of, 37
steroid medication, 246*b*, 252, 280,
    281, 304, 313
stool softeners, 244
suicide, thoughts of, 109, 188–189,
    194–195
suppositories, 221
suppression
  characteristics of, 67*b*
  of concerns, 65–66
surgeon
  choice of, 53
  statistical outcomes of, 42
surgery
  concerns about, 39, 39*b*
  current treatment
    options, 33–34*b*
  pros and cons lists, 41*t*
surgical castration
    (orchiectomy), 279
survival/survival rates
  lack of guarantees, 5–6
  physical/emotional distress
    despite, 3

symptoms, men's hesitancy to
    describe, 236

tadalafil, 217, 285
targeted radiation therapy, 279
TCAs (tricyclic antidepressants), 193.
    See also antidepressants
telling others about cancer. *See also*
    end-of-life issues
  family members, 309–311
  following diagnosis, 81–82
  sharing of fears, 97
temazepam (Restoril), 200, 200*t*
tension of good intentions,
    257–263, 311
testicular prostheses, 279
testosterone, 204, 205, 248,
    279–282, 285
therapeutic writing, 86–87
therapy (psychotherapy). *See also*
    cognitive behavioral therapy
    (CBT); DRAFT technique/
    situations; sex therapy
  for acceptance of "new
    normal," 227
  ACT approach, 113
  bowel problem case study,
    243–245
  coping with loss, 224, 297
  for couples, 59–60, 263,
    264–266, 313
  for dating issues, 222
  for death and dying, 292–293,
    321–322
  for depressive symptoms, 108
  dignity therapy, 324
  for dreaded discussions, 82–83
  gender differences in, 261–262
  goals, in advanced prostate cancer,
    302–304
  for grief, 301
  individual vs. family focus,
    259–260
  insight-oriented, 112, 115, 126

interactivity of, 5
meaning-centered (MCP),
    321–323
medications and, 111
need for, 101–102
sensate focus, 210–214
stigma and, 262
treatment decisions and, 29
for worry/anxiety, 101–102, 174
The Relaxation Response
    (Benson), 117
Thorazine (chlorpromazine), 185
thoughts. *See also* DRAFT technique/
    situations
irrational, 72, 115, 149, 298
negative, 306–308
processes/behaviors and,
    146–149
of suicide, 109, 188–189,
    194–195
uncomfortable/unhelpful, 131*b*
thought trap, avoidance of,
    46–50, 96
tolerance, of anxiety medications,
    180, 182*b*
Torre, Joe, 147
tranquilizers (major), 184–185
Transformation (as DRAF**T**
    technique). *See also* DRAFT
    technique/situations
in catastrophizing scenario,
    151, 152
described, 136–137
with EJ for insomnia, 172
in *Emotional Judo (EJ)* playbook,
    144–146
in generalizing scenario, 154–155
trazodone, 198
treatment, preparing for
communication needs, 84–86
concerns and questions, 70*b*, 71*b*
diet and, 79
dreaded discussions, 82–83
exercise in, 75–79

faith and spirituality, 88–92, 321
"go-to" activities, 87, 88*b*
lifestyle choices, 79–81
meditation, 86–87
period of waiting, 69–70
relaxing, 87
sexual concerns, 73–74
speaking with other
    patients, 71–72
therapeutic writing, 86
urinary incontinence concerns, 73
treatment decision/choice. *See also*
    active surveillance; "definitive"
    treatment; hormonal therapy;
    questions
active treatment vs. active
    surveillance, 33
current treatment
    options, 33–34*b*
dealing with trials of, 4–5
fear of buyer's remorse, 33–42,
    48, 92–93
as individualized, 47–48
magical thinking in, 61–64
partners' role in, 57–61
pros and cons lists, 41*t*
wishful thinking and, 31–32
tricyclic antidepressants (TCAs), 193.
    See also antidepressants
tumescence, 205

unhelpful behaviors, 130–132. *See
    also* **D**RAFT: Detect; DRAFT
    technique/situations
United States, diagnosis of prostate
    cancer in, 2–3
urinary and bowel complications. *See
    also* bowel problems
concerns about, 73–75
discussion of, 54
expectation errors, 233
quality-of-life-issues, 235–237
spouse/partner and, 58
strategies to decrease, 237–242

urinary and bowel
complications (*Cont.*)
taking control of, 240*b*
in untreated cancer, 26
urology, specialist questions
regarding, 52–53*b*
U. S. Food and Drug Administration
(FDA), 194
Us Too, 336

vacutainer, 219–220
Vaillant, George, 231
Valium (diazepam), 178–179,
186*t*, 200*t*
vardenafil, 217, 285
venlafaxine (Effexor), 183, 186*t*,
191–192, 197*t*, 288
Vintage Book Club, 315
Vyvanse, 197*t*

waiting room, waiting in, 44–46
walking, for fatigue relief, 251. *see
also* exercise
watchful waiting, 56. *See also* active
surveillance
websites, as decision-making tool, 62
Wellbutrin (bupropion), 183,
192–193, 195, 197*t*, 253
"white coat syndrome," 50
will to live (WTL), 323–324
wishful thinking
becoming trapped in, 66
treatment choice and, 31–32
withdrawal symptoms, from anxiety
medications, 180

women
coping/coping techniques of,
261–262
menopausal/postmenopausal,
225
physiological changes in, 215
sexual dysfunction in, 216
worry. *See also* Acknowledge (as
DRAFT technique); anxiety;
anxiety medications; distress;
PSA anxiety
about erections, 207
detection of, 131*t*, 153
distraction to avoid, 164–165
"Don't Worry" statements, 83–87,
308, 328–329
mood activity chart, 248*t*
psychotherapy and, 101
sleeplessness and, 198
"worry proxy," 148, 329
"worry snowball," 121

Xanax (alprazolam), 178–179,
186*t*, 201

zaleplon (Sonata), 198–199, 200*t*
Z-Drugs (non-benzodiazepine
hypnotics), 199, 200*t*
Zinn-Kabat, Jon, 113–114
Zoladex (goserelin), 280
Zoloft (sertraline), 183, 186*t*, 191,
197*t*, 288
zolpidem (Ambien), 198–199, 200*t*
Zyprexa (olanzapine), 184, 186*t*